Down's Syndrome

Down's Syndrome

The psychology of mongolism

DAVID GIBSON

Professor of Psychology
University of Calgary, Alberta, Canada

CAMBRIDGE UNIVERSITY PRESS

Cambridge
London   New York   Melbourne

Published by the Syndics of the Cambridge University Press
The Pitt Building, Trumpington Street, Cambridge CB2 1RP
Bentley House, 200 Euston Road, London NW1 2DB
32 East 57th Street, New York, NY 10022, USA
296 Beaconsfield Parade, Middle Park, Melbourne 3206, Australia

First published 1978

Printed in Great Britain at the
University Press, Cambridge

Library of Congress Cataloguing in Publication Data
Gibson, David, 1926–
Down's syndrome.
Bibliography: p.
Includes index.
1. Down's syndrome.   I. Title.
RC571.G5   616.8'58842   77–87381
ISBN 0 521 21914 0

To
H.F.F.
and
N.F.W.

Contents

Preface

The study of Down's syndrome has become a fractionated business, each discipline pressing exclusive views about mechanisms and management. The result has been a confusing array of books, pamphlets and technical articles about Down's syndrome (close to 1000 published items to date on psychological matters alone) which mostly fail to enlighten. The purpose of this book is to integrate the vast behavioural literature in such a way that the traditional assumptions can be inspected and conclusion drawn in support of a multidisciplinary research and remedial approach. The desired audience is both professional and lay because, despite the unavoidable jargon of the field, the state of our knowledge is not so technically complex that the literate parent or community worker need be intimidated by it.

Consistency of terminology is always a problem, particularly in a field of study which has spanned over a century and attracted such a diversity of concerns. The classification sequence idiot–imbecile–moron has given way, for example, to custodial–trainable–educable mentally retarded (CMR, TMR, EMR). Both sets of terms are used in what follows depending on the period under discussion and on which side of the Atlantic a given work originates. An exception is made of the label 'mongolism' where Down's syndrome (DS) is substituted in all but the quotations. However, one has misgivings; the objections to the original name were that it inaccurately allied the condition with one racial group and stigmatized the DS child in the community. The first consideration reflects a kind of condescension that Caucasians often inflict on others. The second concern panders to social prejudice. DS children do, after all, look 'mongolian' and a good diagnostic rubric is at least descriptive. A more fruitful attack on community resistance might be to capitalize on the unique physical configuration of the syndrome. It is not unattractive and the public is not deceived, in the long term, by masquerading nomenclature.

The contents of the book include just about all of the behaviourally relevant research including that which is interactive with the biological findings. Work more strictly in the areas of biochemistry, genetics, epidemiology and general pathology is not included where it does not touch upon behaviour – and most of it does not. The articles cited are predominantly in the English language, but not for chauvinistic reasons. It just happens that the primary concerns for the psychological dimensions of Down's syndrome have been heavily centred on Britain and North America. Other areas of research owe much to the French and German literature and more recently to Russian, Japanese and Spanish-language workers.

An integrative work necessarily suffers many stages of writing, often distorting the normal work schedules which pay the bills. The author is, therefore, grateful to the University of Calgary for its support. The author's research into the behavioural aspects of Down's syndrome and the completion of the present project were assisted by Federal grants (Canada) from Health and Welfare, Manpower, National Research Council and the Canada Council in the form of a Killam Resident Fellowship.

Special thanks are also due Mrs M. E. Clarke, Editorial Assistant to the *Canadian Psychological Review*, for her careful management of reference material and the many preliminary drafts; and to Kathleen M. Gibson, Reg.N., Dip. Speech Pathology and Audiology, for her critical appraisals of the language and management material.

D.G.

Abbreviations

A/G	Ratio of albumin to globulin
ANOVA	Analysis of variance
ANS	Autonomic nervous system
ATD	Palmar axial triradius angle
CA	Chronological age
CBS	Chronic brain syndrome
C–F	Cultural–familial
CHD	Congenital heart disorder
CMR	Custodial mentally retarded
CNS	Central nervous system
CVS	Cardiovascular system
DA	Developmental age
DIQ	Developmental intelligence quotient
DMA	Developmental motor age
DMQ	Developmental motor quotient
DQ	Developmental quotient
DS	Down's syndrome
EEG	Electroencephalograph
EMR	Educable mentally retarded
GSR	Galvanic skin response
HR	Heart rate
5-HTP	5-hydroxytryptophan
IQ	Intelligence quotient
ITPA	Illinois test of psycholinguistic ability
MA	Mental age
MBD	Minimally brain damaged
MR	Mentally retarded
POP-IN	Pivot-open practice instrument
RT	Reaction time
SA	Social age
SER	Somatosensory evoked response
SFF	Speaking fundamental frequency
SQ	Social quotient
SR	Stimulus response
TMR	Trainable mentally retarded
VSMS	Vineland social maturity scale
WAIS	Wechsler adult intelligence scale
WISC	Wechsler intelligence scale for children

I

Introduction

Rationale

In the USA alone, the maintenance and treatment of Down's syndrome (DS) commands between one and two thousand million dollars annually (*Time*, 19 April 1971) and the condition now represents over one-third of the severely to moderately retarded population. The prevalence of the disorder continues to mount because medical science can better ensure the survival of the high-risk DS infant. It is also a time when average maternal age is allegedly increasing and preventative measures are still not being widely applied. Consequently, training and habilitation programming for the DS population requires expansion on several fronts; to reflect the increasing number of cases at all ages, the growing proportion of adults to children, and the widening distribution of IQ levels regardless of age. There will be accelerating pressure on existing care facilities and a need to match advances in paediatric care with a better knowledge of psychological potentials at various stages of growth and decline for the syndrome. Some experts view preventative public health measures, based on cytogenetic screening and pregnancy termination, as an alternative to further elaboration of care services and techniques. Compulsory control measures, however, are slow to win legislative and taxpayer support. A final hope, absolute cure, is unlikely because the major structural and process disorders of DS are laid down embryologically and are developmentally prescribed, to a significant extent, from birth onward.

A predominant concern of this book is to give a critical overview of the mammoth behavioural literature on DS so as to identify links between biological and psychological phenomena; in the belief that improved care systems will require such a foundation. The task has not been previously undertaken, in any comprehensive way, because the best research evidence is recent. It is not unjust to suggest that most psychological studies before the 1950s could be discarded with no appreciable loss to our practical understanding. A second purpose of the book relates to the strong entry of parent organizations into the field of mental retardation (MR) management. These groups inherited a plethora of myths and half-truths about the nature of Down's syndrome. Contemporary behavioural images, perpetuated through the clinical literature, originated substantially from institutional data. We know a good deal less about how adjustment capacities, for DS, are expressed over years of home care and community life. It is because the 'mongol' is finally in our midst, the object of remedial rather than purely maintenance concern, that we must know if the classical stereotypes have substance and the extent to which they are alterable by physical and psychological intervention.

Historical considerations

Most authorities credit Langdon Down (1867) with the first comprehensive description of a disorder he called mongolism. His speculations on aetiology, prognosis and treatment included a genetic regression hypothesis about causation and a control programme designed to exploit the supposed imitative ability and good observational facility of the members of the class. The racial regression proposal of Langdon Down is a scientific nightmare but not totally outrageous in terms of our present understanding of the evolution of human chromosomes (Dobzhansky, 1955). Moreover, Down's ethnic classification of disorders of developmental origin, as proof of the unity of mankind, is ingenious for the period. Other physicians, too, were active in the search for order among the disorders of developmental origin. Guggenbuhl (Kanner, 1964) grouped cretins for treatment purposes because their appearance and conduct were relatively similar. Improved nutrition, fresh air and regular exercise were prescribed. Itard (1894), and later Seguin (Talbot, 1964), developed a training regime for children of imbecile-level intelligence (moderate MR) whose condition had an exogenous cause. Those designated in cultural–familial terms as feebleminded or educable MR were isolated early in the present century and taken to be the product of impoverished genetic stock. They were viewed, more or less, as homogeneous for socio-educational purposes. The clinical-genetic, traumatic, polygenetic and cytogenetic classes of developmental arrest comprise, collectively, the major components of what has come to be known as mental retardation. The various causal categories of MR are still not readily acknowledged as discrete for treatment and training purposes, even though they have little more in common than a general inability to cope with academic and productivity standards in the community.

There were several reasons for our failure to investigate the relationship between cause and consequence in mental retardation. The 'cure' movement of the nineteenth and early twentieth centuries had failed because the biological sciences were in their infancy. They could not then support effective treatment on a bio-behavioural and syndromic or causal basis. What remained was an amorphous group of intractable mental handicaps for which the economics of custody became the paramount concern. Industrial urbanization in North America and Europe had resulted in a concentration of poverty and crime which the average citizen came to see as associated with social and academic incompetence (Crissey, 1975). The emergence of compulsory schooling, in order to prepare a technically reliable worker population, served to expose large numbers of slow learners who were predominantly from lower socio-cultural levels of the community. The various categories of disorders of developmental origin were now easily assembled under one label; as those who couldn't learn or earn. The concern was to isolate afflicted individuals so as to protect private property and to ensure the integrity of the new education system. The popularization and misrepresentation of the precepts of biological evolution and a fear that genetic inferiority is replicated in the population at a disproportionate rate served as further supporting motives. The findings of the pioneer mental testing movement, that up to 25% of all school children have learning handicaps, served to reinforce the public case against the mentally retarded. Consequently, the fundamental dissimilarity of the many disorders making up the new MR category did not matter and routine custodial programmes prospered. In the context of control by disposal, the DS child merited no special attention.

The assembly of the numerous disorders of early development under one label had been a misfortune in other ways: medicine withdrew from active participation because the MR label had few implications for biological research or treatment. The new professionals in the MR field were educators and psychologists who presented a number of functionalist, environmentalist and quantitative views about the nature and management of the retarded. Their goals were to stratify degrees of learning handicap by psychometric means and to impose essentially traditional academic and vocational programmes, suitably diluted to correspond to abstracted mental ages. The relevance of the biological histories of handicap, for treatment purposes, was dismissed because these were poorly understood and, in any case, the new professionals were seldom trained to look behind the psychological presentation. The search for behavioural distinctions of a qualitative nature and the identification of interactions between damaged tissue systems and psychological potentials, among the various causal conditions which make up the MR category, languished as a result. Moreover, the studies resulting from a purely environmental approach to MR management have been disappointing. In the area of special education, at the primary level, there have been few durable gains (Dunn & Hottel, 1958; Cain & Levine, 1963; Guskin & Spicker, 1968; Kaufman & Alberto, 1976) with which to justify the effort. The effort continues because formal primary education is culturally sanctioned, professional services are self-renewing, and parents take comfort in them. This is not to say that special education cannot be useful. One purpose of the chapters to follow is to demonstrate that effective behavioural remediation can evolve to the extent that the distinctive somatic realities of DS and other disorders of developmental origin are understood. Accountability studies for the vocational habilitation of the mentally retarded, as a class, are similarly unconvincing (Windle, 1962; Cobb, 1967; Stephens & Peck, 1968; Gibson & Fields, 1970; Gold, 1973; McCarver & Craig, 1974). There is little to lose, apparently, by courting other styles of enquiry; in the present instance a bio-behavioural and syndromic approach to research and management. These approaches assume that behaviour is primarily a product of tissue systems and that quality of deficit varies systematically across the causal categories of developmental arrest. Down's syndrome provides the subject base of the present demonstration of the two viewpoints.

Organization

The major aims of what follows are:

(i) To trace the progression of events for Down's syndrome, from causal data to biological and behavioural outcomes.

(ii) To trace the developmental sequencing characteristic of the disorder.

(iii) To identify the behavioural research areas within DS most in need of additional attention.

(iv) To extrapolate, where possible, indications for the assessment of management.

With respect to the first of these goals, genetic flooding is observed in only two conditions where there is a relatively high frequency of occurrence and phenotypic outcomes which are not so muted as to preclude complex behavioural study. One is the XYY state and the other is Down's syndrome. The search for behavioural specificity of chromosome disorder has centred on the XYY group because of its association with maleness and the genetics of antisocial behaviour. The results of 400 investigations viewed to 1973 (Hoak 1973) show mild MR and above average height. The aggression component is most easily understood as a result of ineptitude, a spin-off of subnormality and a modestly distorted morphology. The identification of more reliable behavioural artifacts, of a given chromosomal nondisjunction, would require an accident of karyotype which (i) has a suitable intactness and complexity of expression in phenotype, ideally an autosomal phenomenon, (ii) is detectable early enough to chart developmentally and (iii) has within-syndrome variations of karyotype which would permit *post hoc* analyses of subtypes of chromosome disorder across behavioural outcomes (Jarvik, Falek & Pierson, 1964). Down's syndrome has these characteristics.

The search for a 'chromosomal psychology' has practical significance if the prognosis can be correlated with karyotype. There are theoretical considerations as well. Chromosomes are not merely containers for genes; they are transmitter systems governing the nature of gene interaction. Genes hold a given chromosomal position because they are compatible *in situ* and have mutual effects. Chromosomes are important, too, in evolution. Aneuploids advance evolution by adding genetic material through a process of nondisjunction and attachment, the initially surplus genetic load undergoing adaptive mutation more readily than established gene clusters. More important than the adding of genes, however, is the increasing complexity of chromosomal dynamics. Down's syndrome represents a research population which might advance our understanding of these dynamics.

The organization of the material is in ten units beginning with a concern for early development and the quantitative aspects of intelligence. Qualitative considerations appear more prominently in the chapters dealing with ability profiles, the origins of deficit, learning and arousal, personality, socialization and language. Management is viewed in two ways; the techniques developed by the practitioner, on a trial and error basis, and the indicators for treatment which grow directly from the biological and behavioural research literature. Within each chapter the plan has been to evaluate the stereotype for a given behavioural category, in the order of the clinical, statistical and experimental literature. Most chapters provide an evaluation of the degree of consensus from the three levels of enquiry and point to implications for management. The reader will appreciate that the clinical and research literature cannot be so neatly categorized with the result that there is an overlap in citation and discussion between units. The failing is unavoidable because the syndrome is a complex one with shifting somatic patterns and psychological outcome across the life span of its members.

2

Early psychological development

The tranquillity of the DS infant was first intrepreted by parents and professionals as a hopeful sign and these hopes were undisturbed in the first few months of infancy. As the child grew older the promise was not fulfilled, at least for the majority. As a result, the initial quiescence came to be viewed as a superficial attribute of little importance for later management; merely a clinical curiosity or a motivational prop for parents being counselled on adequate pre-institutional home care. Not until after 1950 was there sufficient evidence to present a more balanced account.

This chapter evaluates the mode and range of early development, beginning with a few historically important opinions about the motor and sensory equipment of DS children compared with normal and other retarded children. More recent studies assess the relative impact of exogenous, neuro-maturational, environmental and karyotypic factors on the developmental process. The possibility of building growth-forecast instruments, permitting the prediction of ultimate behavioural capacity for DS, is also considered.

The stereotype

The DS infant is perceived by parents and care workers as reasonably tractable. They are described as 'good' babies. Developmental studies of the DS infant have exposed, nevertheless, an accelerating motor lag and depressed reactivity levels (against the normal curve), from the beginning. Engler (1949) was among the first to describe the DS infant's response to nursing as mechanical and unenthusiastic, a passivity which can be easily mistaken for cooperation. During the very early months, motor capability can appear unimpaired but this is difficult to confirm since response to external stimulation and sensory acuity levels are reduced. The child is, shortly after birth, apathetic and lacking in reactivity except to stimuli of quite high intensity. Langdon Down (1866) thought them developmentally encouraging nevertheless. He claimed that 'Coordination facility is abnormal but not so defective that it cannot be greatly strengthened. By systematic training considerable manipulative power may be obtained' (p. 261). And again 'The improvement which training effects in them is greatly in excess of what would be predicted if anyone did not know the characteristics of the type' (p. 262).

To the acceptance of maturational promise was added the ingredient of uniqueness. According to Shuttleworth (1916) 'The physiognomy...are quite characteristic; and the mental condition equally so' (p. 101). Fraser and Mitchell (1876–7) stressed that the mental state is 'as distinct as peculiar and as steady as the physical'. The unqualified impression of relatively unimpaired early growth was short-lived. Wood (1909), attending the Australasia Medical Congress, described DS infants shortly after birth, as follows:

They do not stretch out their heads for the breast like normal children but lie passively on the arm until the nipple is placed in their mouths. They look happy and placid and do not take things in their hands until well after the sixth month. They are late in learning to walk; the earliest of my cases to walk has been 18 months, but as a rule from 3 years to 4 years is the usual time. (p. 40)

He further remarked

Regarding mental development, these mongoloids are by reason of their smiles and imitative faculties, all full of much promise as far as education is concerned, but unfortunately the realization of the promise never seems to be fulfilled. (p. 40)

Brousseau and Brainered (1928) agreed. Using both clinical and psychometric tools they denied any special developmental status for DS claiming that 'Mongol infants show no particular defect or perversion that distinguishes them from other aments; the development of their intelligence, however, lags in every respect behind that of the normal infant.' Initially, the DS infant is

inert, apathetic, and indifferent to his surroundings. Later, when he comes out of his torpid state he still remains unobservant; does not fix his eyes on objects about him but lies quietly in his cradle without crying or demanding attention. From time to time he smiles and wrinkles his forehead but these movements are apparently without meaning. Parents are often much pleased because the child is so good and gives so little trouble, not knowing that this placidity is not normal but is an indication of the existence of a cerebral defect. (p. 102)

There are some valid observations in this early work, but the dedication then to a uniform developmental process was little more than an extension of the compelling somatic stereotype. Because the biological features (the stigmata) are somewhat novel then so must be the developmental picture. Because the configuration of physical stigmata is relatively homogeneous, then so must be the early growth patterns. If these assumptions are true then an exclusive and more effective technology for DS should be indicated. Many of the studies which follow are unduly influenced by these suppositions.

Early expectations

Research on psychological development for DS has moved through single case descriptions, central tendency reports, and formal growth testing. The gains are not spectacular. More current research is directed at prediction and has been able to use newer evidence about the maturational process (Cowie, 1970) and its abnormalities (Thelander & Pryor, 1966).

Brousseau and Brainerd on sensory growth

The first reasonably complete empirical statement about development in DS was made by Brousseau and Brainerd (1928). But even here contradictions appear. The various sense organs were regarded as not seriously impaired maturationally and only quantitatively different from the normal. Sensibility to pain seemed normal and could be interpreted otherwise only because some DS infants are too retarded to register a sensibility. Self-abuse was thought minimal, possibly because many exhibit a slow reactivity and diminished motor output capacity. Brousseau and Brainerd observed the tactile senses to be diminished but they associated this with the inability of the DS child to give a reliable report. The more intelligent were able, nevertheless, to distinguish numerous tactile qualities on crude tests using sandpaper, glass, velvet and so on. Kinaesthetic and cutaneous sensory development was claimed to be slow due to central process deficiency rather than to any reduction of sensing capacity. They reported some DS children who were unable, however, to pass weight difference tests at even a 5-year mental level. Poor comprehension of instructions was identified as a contributing factor, as was a habitual clumsiness. Reduced facility for muscle contraction was said to be a function of disturbances in the sensory areas of the brain rather than representing any lack of ability for motor and kinaesthetic collation. The explanatory theme throughout is one of reduced behavioural outputs as a function of limitations in the central nervous system (CNS) of the sort found in any severely retarded child. Special inequalities of the peripheral systems were not apparent.

Certain other limiting factors were defined as specific to DS. Brousseau and Brainerd credited the DS child with a heat–cold insensitivity which they ascribed to an imperfect circulatory system. The sense of smell was reduced or absent. This deficiency was attributed to the presence of chronic catarrh and a 'defective condition of the olfactory mucous membrane'. Taste sense is diminished because of extensive tongue fissuring and hypertrophied papillae, in addition to defects of the central nervous system. The latter factor took precedence over secondary physical conditions. More intelligent DS subjects exhibited the usual taste ranges, albeit with less appreciation than normal children. Organic sensations were blunted, although toileting and other visceral wants were attended to by the brighter with some efficiency. These children adapted to a routine early and with little trouble. Sex drives seemed reduced but, judging from recent literature, are present.

Brousseau and Brainerd found perceptual deficiencies, across developmental stages of DS, difficult to separate from intellectual handicap. Inadequacy of attention process, they guessed, might provide a bridge between perceptual and intellectual handicap, but not in a way exclusive to the syndrome. Development of colour discrimination was slow for DS but was not an indication of a greater than normal frequency of colour blindness. Brousseau and Brainerd, testing DS subjects for perception of high saturation colours (red, green, blue, yellow), concluded that the failures were 'cortical and not peripheral'. Perception of size and shape was not especially unusual, developmentally. Their opinion was taken from casual observations of performance on Binet–Simon test items. They concluded that the DS individual fails in proportion to the degree of central process defect, and across all tasks, regardless of quality of task requirement. Deficiency of hearing was explained by poor attention, which was again attributed to central process deficiency. The belief that DS is unique for perceptual or sensory functioning is a current concern of the recent literature. Brousseau and Brainerd failed to uncover these peculiarities probably because of their inability to identify the distinctive mechanical, peripheral and central constituents of input–output circuiting for the syndrome.

Brousseau and Brainerd on motor growth

Brousseau and Brainerd's description of motor development in the DS child remains one of the most complete on record. Their pursuit of motor development trends began with observations of the spontaneous movements of the newborn. They claimed that response to general random stimuli (heat, light, sound, pressure), taking the form of generalized and diffuse muscular activity, is diminished or delayed in DS as compared with normal infants. Parents report, therefore, a placid child who does not as often squirm, wiggle, twist, cry or kick. They were of the opinion that 'The mongoloid infant is usually inert, listless, and there is a marked degree of muscular and tendon hypotonia; this may be noticed in the masseter and temporal muscles producing the dropping of the lower jaw, thus causing the mouth to remain open.' And further that ' If the arms are raised and released they drop of their own weight. This listlessness of the mongol infant is, for the most part, due to a lessened excitability of the neurones; and there is marked inertia of the brain and spinal cord' (pp. 109–110). Reflex actions were described as less vigorous than for the normal infant but not clearly in the defective range. Reflexive responses to a stimulus were only somewhat delayed or reduced in intensity. For instance, the finger grasp evident at birth in normal infants was reduced in many DS infants. There was a weakness of sucking movements and of swallowing for many.

Brousseau and Brainerd recorded the median ages and age ranges for the appearance of the traditional growth landmarks for DS. They contrasted Hellmann's (1908–9) description of a DS child creeping at 4 years and walking at 4½ years with a second case of creeping 13 months, sitting at 14 months and walking at 2½ years. These authors remarked further on a tendency for some to assume the intra-uterine position when in repose. The DS child suffering from a faulty circulation system might well affect this posture in drafty institutions. Their report of ages at which DS children are able to sit is summarized from single case studies by Shukowsky and Ainseberg (1912), Mickelthwart (1910) and others. A now commonplace observation, offered first by Mickelthwart, was the tendency of DS children to sit cross-legged, to rest the forehead on the ground, and to rock rhythmically for long periods. A combination of hypotonia, boredom and secondary neurological factors was thought to be responsible, although where the only institutional furniture is a bed, the comfortable 'tailor's' posture is practical. Delay in ability to stand erect, and unaided, was said to be due to nerve function deficit rather than to any 'muscular weakness'. Only anecdotal reports of single cases were given in support (Spicer, 1903; Degenkolb, 1906; Kellner, 1906; Van der Scheer, 1926). These reports illustrate little more than the wide age range of onset for various aspects of maturation in DS and certainly nothing which would justify a conclusion for syndrome-specific growth patterning.

Brousseau and Brainerd's own data on the onset of walking were based on a study of 167 cases; 110 boys and 57 girls. They tell of a DS girl whose motor laxity was so great that she walked on all fours with some agility. Qualitative observations on the nature of gait highlighted such features as poor coordination, legs widely spaced, knees bent, walking on the ball of the foot, pigeon-toed posturing, slowness, stiffness, jerkiness of locomotion and foot drag. The climbing of stairs was deliberate and careful. The growth rate and quality of hand and digital coordination would be both central and structural in origin. The DS child's hands are usually squared and the fingers short-ended so that sewing, catching, and other eye–hand behaviours would be more difficult. Degree of mental retardation, hypotonia, and sensory intake lag are among the other specific origins of delayed or distorted motor maturation.

The first crude estimations of the developmental parameters for DS, taken from the British and German clinical literature, have been partly confirmed by the statistical studies which followed. Their special value was to provide a sense of the complexity of growth events for the syndrome and to furnish hypotheses about the origins of sensory and motor lag or disability.

The statistics of growth

Engler's (1949) major contribution to the study of DS was methodological. He turned the literature from anecdotal descriptions of growth to sample based statistical observations which could be critically tested. Clinical reporters tended to collect the more bizarre aspects of growth and generalize from these to all members of the syndrome. The evidence was usually taken from institutions holding the older and more severely retarded. Engler was able to demonstrate an average age of onset of walking at 3 years with a range from 10½ months to 10 years. For 'beginning' to talk, his modal cluster was between 2 years 9 months and 4 years 6 months, with a range from 15 months to 14 years chronological age (CA). He thus exposed, statistically, the great variability of developmental progression for the syndrome. Engler observed that while 60% of his index cases were able to walk past 3 years CA, 16.5% of the older ones could still not walk. Two of his cases (of 200) achieved a form of walking only by the ages of 9 and 10 years. The general delay is claimed by Engler to be a result of deficiencies in 'will-power, initiative, and coordination' and possibly in that order. The quality of walking, once achieved, was poor. Respecting motor control, Engler concluded that they continue to walk on a wide base, to run in an awkward fashion, and to lack smoothness of movement throughout life.

Growth norms, derived from direct testing rather than from records searching, were first reported by Gesell and Amatruda (1949). These workers depicted the DS newborn as placid, inert and apathetic, though noting a pseudo-alertness in a few cases. They presumed some to have suffered secondary nervous system damage. The DS infant was described as displaying 'a general dynamic reduction with fragments of plausible behaviour'.

During the first 3–4 weeks of life the infant achieves, nevertheless, many near-normal landmarks. Past the 1st year of life the developmental lag becomes more evident. Gesell and Armatruda placed 'sitting alone' at 2 years, 'single words' by 3 years and 'toilet training' at 5 years. Quaytman (1953) indicated that the DS infant is able to sit alone at 1 year, walk without support at about 2 years, utter a few words by 3 years, and is toilet trained, on the average, by 41 months. Toilet trained means for Quaytman dry past midnight.

Despite a general consensus, most studies have not adequately defined the various markers or the standard for assessing developmental achievement. In any case, universal agreement on median development is of limited use in the face of the wide individual variation of timing of maturation for the syndrome. Thompson (1963) circumvented the latter problem by testing developmental progression on the basis of behavioural limits. Examining 29 DS children, she reported that all were able to walk, run, squat, climb, string large beads, pile blocks and were partially toilet trained by 5 years CA. Speech deficiency, and slowness of speech development, comprised the outstanding lag. Stedman and Eichorn (1964) demonstrated smaller intra-sample variability, across development markers, than have most others. Mean age of walking, for 30 DS infants, was 27.5 months and within a range of 18–37 months. Presumably, sampling deviation would be less for the usually early developmental markers. Fishler *et al.* (1965) observed that motor patterns in DS are almost normal during the first 6 months of life, with little variability evident between individuals. A gradual and growing discrepancy between the DS and normal child and from case to case, within the syndrome, appeared thereafter. By the time the child had reached 1 year CA he was often 6 months retarded developmentally, the gap widening with increasing years.

Confounding of growth judgements

Agreement about characteristic developmental timing is of little value for prediction or management if within-syndrome variability is high and its sources obscure. The syndrome is maturationally confusing because (i) we study polarized care systems (home versus large institution), (ii) we use measures of development which have been standardized on normal infants and are insensitive to the more subtle neuromotor deficits of the first months of life and (iii) we pay insufficient attention to the role of psychological and progressive pathological factors influencing growth. The following studies illustrate a few of these difficulties.

Stedman and Eichorn (1964) reported growth markers, e.g., age of walking, to be the same for hospital and home-reared DS children. Karlin and Strazzulla (1952) examined a community-based sample (clinic referred) finding that DS children sit alone at between 10.6 months and 14.7 months, walk unaided between 14.4 and 31 months, and use words somewhere between 34.5 months and 54.3 months of age. Gibson *et al.* (1964) examined 300 institutionalized DS children and recorded age of sitting at 11 months, walking alone at 2 years 5 months, single words at just under 4 years of age, and toileting by 3 years, on the average. In his study, however, institutionalization had occurred at 6 years of age or later. The group is thus distinct from exclusively home-reared or hospital-reared groups in that a reliable period of home care preceded institutional care. These gross developmental differences between care regimes are not large. While institutional groups demonstrate slightly slower early growth than home-reared samples, the practice of selective early hospitalization for the more severely handicapped could adequately explain them. A provisional conclusion is that early maturational variability within DS is biologically programmed, psychological factors having limited influence on release times.

The time of report of various comparative developmental statistics is also relevant. Nutritional and paediatric standards have improved dramatically over the past 2 or 3 decades. Kucera (1969) examined age at walking for three groups of DS children: those born in 1954, between 1955 and 1960, and between 1961 and 1966. His tabular material demonstrates a sharp shift of the mean and standard deviation for recorded growth landmarks across the three dated samples. DS children born before 1954 walked at 29.93 months, on the average, whereas those born between 1955 and 1960 walked at 22.31 months on the average. Kucera was unable to demonstrate similar differences for dentition. He attributed the pre- and post-1954 differences (for mean age of walking) to improved care methods (nutrition and training), and/or to the recall vagaries of mothers of the pre-1954 sample.

McNeill's (1955) statistical examination of developmental landmarks for DS was among the first to employ formal scaling devices. Grip strength was assessed using a hand dynamometer, coordination by use of the Moore eye–hand test, and non-language performance levels by the application of the Arthur adaptation of the Leiter international performance scale. He extracted a hierarchy of growth signs which seem to indicate that DS children are more heavy than tall; taller than strong; have muscle (grip) strength superior to eye–hand coordination; have social growth greater than vocabulary growth; and have vocabulary development greater than intellectual growth. The purpose of his study was to compare the effects of two treatment regimes on early growth rates in DS. Though his research supports no conclusion, in this regard, the proposed hierarchy of abilities matches Brousseau's central process deficiency hypothesis rather well.

A further suggestion for the cerebral origins of motor development in DS children has been made by Benda (1960 a, b) who held that the major growth indices may be more influenced by specific loci of damage, e.g., muscle hypotonia, than by a general cerebral agenesis. He concluded that while motor retardation does not begin to be generally obvious before the end of the first year of life, 'sitting up' behaviour is rarely established in most before 1 year. The DS child will not attempt crawling until significantly later. Nor do they attempt to walk much before 2 years and in most cases not before 3 years. The more retarded DS child will start walking as late as 5 years. Age at the onset of walking, according to Benda, is partly dependent upon degree of hypotonia and the related ability of the DS child to achieve and hold an upright balance. Early sitting behaviour evidently has some forecast value for early walking achievement even though the development of general motor stability, following the acquisition of erect motility, is slow. Gait remains infantile and quality of motor control, in leg and arm movements, often continues to be clumsy into adulthood. Benda thought that even a relatively high mental age would not permit good generalization about the eventual efficiency of motor control. Engler (1949), too, had assigned delay in onset of walking more to muscular hypotonia than to general maturational lag; but deduced that since the hypotonia subsides, as the child grows older, continuing delays in neuromotor development must be increasingly a function of primary mental arrest. It is not clear whether he considered the syndrome unique in this respect.

Kralovich (1959) compared 28 DS subjects with organic controls (matched both for mental age, and intelligence quotient), finding that DS children compared favourably for motor manipulation efficiency. The Cattell infant scale items were examined across all 113 subtests. Only five subtests separated DS children and organic controls, these items requiring 'simultaneous adductive and abductive hand movements' (p. 199). All significant items represented the first 22 months of mental growth (80 subtests in this period). The most obvious differences occurred between 5 and 10 months of mental development and indicated that (for the early stages of growth) DS subjects compared well with other mentally retarded subjects for overall motor development. An incidental finding was of more effective motor exploration for DS subjects, i.e., securing a cube, attempting to retrieve a pellet and covering a square box. Hypotonia in DS is probably less handicapping to the initiation of motor activity than might be the case for more centrally impaired organic controls.

Most statistical reports of developmental patterning for DS have indicated that very early motor development is not conspicuously distinct from that of normal infants but that later psychomotor and expressive growth tends to progressively greater lag. Recent opinion is that retarded development in DS is observable from the beginning. Standard measures of infant psycho-developmental progression, based on normal infant growth monitoring, may be too insensitive for use with the DS infant. Penrose and Smith (1966) claimed that 'some degree of poor head control and hypotonia may be present in normal newborn infants' but that, 'the normal infant quickly develops good muscle controls and head control while the mongoloid infant may remain hypotonic and show little evidence of being able to support his head' (p. 56). Similarly, Warner (1935) contended that the grasping reflex, evident in the normal newborn, is considerably diminished in the DS infant. Also late to appear is the ability to follow a light with the eyes. Perhaps the sensorimotor status of the DS infant is more deficient than the popular standardized measures permit us to believe and that the later 'deterioration' is an artifact of insensitive measurements in the early months of life.

A thoroughgoing examination of reflexive motor development, in company with retarded intellect, has been provided by Cowie (1970) in her monograph *A study of the early development of mongols*. Findings were for a growing connection, over time, between psychological and neurological indices, especially for developmental quotients as a function of variation in muscle tone. Up to 66 cases of DS, confirmed by chromosome analysis, were tested across a series of neonatal 'time zones'. Major neurological categories surveyed included muscle tone, traction response, ventral reflex, palmar grasp, plantar grasp, automatic stepping, the placing reaction and strabismus. Psychological indices included the Bayley developmental intelligence quotient (DIQ) and developmental motor quotient (DMQ) scales and the Piaget sensorimotor scale. Cowie's comments on the specific nature of early infantile reflexes in DS are extensive. Of primary interest is her evidence on the relation of behavioural response to infantile reflexes. Only by 16 to 32 weeks (time zone II) were the Bayley scores even minimally predictive for later development. The correlation of DIQ and DMQ between time zones I and III was 0.09 and 0.12, and between time zones II and III, 0.31 and 0.63. Hypotonia emerged as the single item most closely related to the neuropathological matrix. Marked or extreme hypotonus also co-varied with poor general development insofar as extreme hypotonia was correlated progressively, over time, with low psychological scores.

A second stage of Cowie's investigation subjected 24 of 40 study variables to a principal components analysis. The computer data supported a number of views, including

(1) That marked hypotonia is an essential part of a state in mongolism to which poor position in ventral suspension, a weak patellar jerk, poor traction response, and, in the early weeks of life, a partial or absent Moro reaction all add some weight. Strabismus seems to stand apart from the other variables in this complex, however, judging by the computer results. (Cowie, 1970, p. 60)

(2) Low scores on Piaget sensori-motor scales, low DMQ scores and low DIQ scores overlapped the main neurological effects.

(3) Three components of combined neurological–psychological development were identified. These were factor I involving hypotonia, DMQ, DIQ and Sensori-Motor item clustering with delayed dissolution of the early reflexes; factor II which isolated strabismus from the other variables; factor III which demonstrated independent variability and a changing balance of reflexive and psychometric indices. Cowie proposed that the 'placing' reaction is possibly exceptional among the early reflexive-motor behaviours for both consistency and strength of relation to degree of mental development. (The placing reaction is elicited by brushing the dorsal surface of the babies' foot against, for example, a table edge. The expected response is a knee and hip reflex and 'placing' of the sole flat on the tabletop). Finally, as the DS infant grew older, the neurological and psychological particulars became clearer, more stable, and more obviously correlated.

The importance of the Cowie approach is that later behavioural status might be anticipated on the basis of neonatal neurological measures. These findings are difficult to square with those of Woodward and Stein (1963) who reported no differences in locomotor development for DS children among the other forms of severe subnormality. Both conclusions might be warranted if a distinction is made between the qualitative and quantitative aspects of early maturation (see Coriat et al., 1967).

Fisichelli and Karelitz (1966) proposed an even more radical departure from traditional methods used for the early detection of developmental level in DS. They employed frequency and content spectra of infant cries. In a study comparing normal and DS infants, matched for age (6 months) and for sex, samples of tape-recorded crying were subjected to the panoramic sonic analyser. Frequency ranges were similar for each group but spectoral content showed the DS infants to be less active and more variable in sound level than normal infants. A second study by Fisichelli et al. (1966) analysed the gasps and whimpers of the DS infant. Subjects were compared with a like number of normal infants (21 children in each case) matched for age and sex. Significant differences were obtained for each of the audibles studied. These authors found that DS infants produced fewer sounds, sounds of shorter duration, and of less vigor than did normal infants of the same age. Dodd (1972) found no differences between DS and normal infants for patterns of vocalizaton and claimed that 'babbling does not reflect intelligence at this stage of development' (p. 40). Hearing loss and depressed arousal (motivational) thresholds have been mentioned by Lenneberg *et al.* (1962) and Lenneberg (1967) as potential points of confusion.

The Fisichelli approach, if confirmed, has the advantage of permitting the assessment of a motor behaviour (crying) which is sufficiently well formed at birth, sensitive to changes of somatic states or of impinging external environments, has a scalable energy output and arousal level component, and can be differentiated for duration, quality, intensity and appropriateness of response. Current methods of infant scaling are too crude for use with neonatal DS and can create a false impression of 'normalcy' during the first few months of life and of 'deterioration' thereafter as growth reaches more reliable test ranges. It is pure mischief for professionals to report normal developmental quotients (Gesell and Cattell scales) for DS infants only to find a developmental quotient (DQ) of 40 points or less on re-examination 6 months later. Parents should be made to understand that 'normalcy' in the DS infant might be largely a product of instrument coarseness and that their infant is aquiescent because of sensory immaturity and hypotonia of the musculature. These are related problems.

Sensory masking of early cognitive growth

It has been proposed that the DS child's motor performance is deficient because of a failure of the sensory system to activate motor responses. Brousseau and Brainerd (1928) preferred to place sensory intake handicap at the level of the central nervous system. Engler (1949) speculated that any delay in motor growth might be linked simply to the structural peculiarities of the syndrome. More recently, Benda (1960 *a*, *b*) remarked on the strength of even a 6 month old DS child, once aroused. He concluded that the immaturity of the nervous system demands more intense stimulus in order to penetrate the CNS apparatus and that when a sensory threshold is breached (in the very young DS individual) the motor reaction is vigorous and persistent. Assertions that the sensory system of DS infants is at a greater disadvantage than the expressive-motor potential, might have merit; although the ongoing and chronic postural clumsiness of the child also implicates central neurological factors in psychomotor maturation. Proper separation of the influences of central, expressive and receptive variables will be required for a fuller appreciation of the developmental processes peculiar to DS. Purely structural factors (related to the skeletal, respiratory and circulatory systems) might also be important.

Benda (1960 *a*, *b*) reviewed the sensory status of DS in some detail. He suggested that members of the syndrome share a poor sense of smell, poor tactile ability and reduced heat–cold discrimination but agreed that some of these handicaps were artifacts. Sensory development, for instance, can be complicated from the very beginning by the presence of strabismus. Estimates for frequency of strabismus in DS vary widely (Oster, 1953; Gibson & Frank, 1961). Brushfield (1924) had claimed that 100% of DS infants display convergent strabismus. Benda thought that the poor visual reception of the DS child might be due, as well, to a lack of myelinization of the optic nerves. The auditory and olfactory sensoria exhibited low discriminatory powers when compared with other types of mental retardation or with the normal infant. Structural deformities of the ear, nose and tongue, and the frequent upper respiratory complaints of the DS child have been thought responsible for reduced auditory and olfactory functioning. Gordon (1944) questioned the behavioural importance of these specific sensory deficiencies because he was unable to demonstrate a correlation between the performance of young patients on simple sensory tests and subsequent Binet IQs. He conceded, however, that sensory efficiency is generally depressed for all psychometric performance areas of DS, as compared with normals of a similar age. An interesting incidental observation was that while normal children often show tactile discrimination facility superior to visual discrimination efficiency, particularly in the early years of life, the DS child tends to display higher visual than tactile efficiency at similar mental ages. The presence of hypotonia and associated cerebellar immaturity probably account for these differences. Even so, the visual-perceptual facility of DS infants, compared with normal infants, is reduced. Miranda and Frantz (1973) subjected 20 DS infants and normal controls to 13 pairs of visual targets. The DS infants looked longer but made response differentiations for only three of the stimulus pairs compared with eleven pairs for the normal infants. Form contour elicited the most marked group differences, suggesting to these authors that visual-perceptual and attention gradients in infancy might have forecast value for later cognitive status. More to the point, reflexive, motor, sensory and central deficiency are all evident at or shortly after the birth of a DS child. These disputes are treated more fully in the chapter on learning and arousal.

Developmental variability: primary sources

Some of the factors contributing to a surprising degree of biological and behavioural variability for the syndrome during early maturation have been mentioned. Summary landmarks for DS cannot, therefore, be used indiscriminately to counsel parents or plan educational and psychological management regimes. Physical growth patterning is no less variable than is psychological growth. Oster (1953), Gibson and Frank (1961) and Levison, Friedman and Stamps (1955) have provided data concerning the inconstancy of the cardinal physical stigmata of the syndrome. The latter authors showed age of sitting (without support) to range from the normative 6 months to as late as 3 years. Onset of walking shows a spread from a normative 12 months to 4½ years. A finer appreciation of the directions of maturational variability, and some of its primary sources, might permit eventual prediction and planning applicable to individual cases. The major origins of developmental differences are likely to include the variable effects of karyotype, secondary organic process, physical nurture, stimulation level, health status, sex and the structural factors peculiar to the syndrome.

Information about sex differences and developmental variability in DS, is not abundant. While observing no significant sex-specific growth difference (e.g., onset of walking) Engler (1949) does reinforce the institutional behavioural stereotype, e.g., that DS females are good dancers and presumably better coordinated at early ages than males. Oster (1953) reported that while most of his sample talked between 3 and 5 years CA, the girls began somewhat earlier than the boys. Sex-separated training techniques, evident both in home and nursery school practice, could account for a portion of these dissimilarities. Mortality rates, thought to vary by sex, provide an additional source of sex-specific behavioural distinctions, especially among the older. Otherwise, the prospect is that sex differences in growth and behaviour are less divergent for DS than for normal children, or for other forms of mental retardation. The impact of the aberrant karyotype is a massive one and could conceivably obscure normal sex differences.

Subtype of chromosome anomaly is another probable source of growth variability. Gibson (1965) reported that translocation DS subjects achieved a mean CA of 10 months for eruption of the first tooth, sat by 11 months, walked by 25 months and were toilet trained by 34 months. The standard trisomy child teethed at 10.5 months, sat alone at 16.6 months, walked at 26 months and talked (first words) at 35.1 months CA, on the average. These differences are not remarkable but do consistently favour the translocation variety of DS. Dispersion of growth markers was less for the translocation than for the trisomy sample. A more pronounced spread of developmental indices, for standard trisomy infants, was documented by Dicks-Mireaux (1966). Developmental deviations have also been found between mosaic and other chromosomal categories of DS (Johnson and Abelson, 1969 a, b). Eventual support for developmental scheduling linked to the chromosome aberration is likely providing the intervention mechanisms can be identified. In this regard, Pueschel, Rothman and Ogilby (1967) have found a smaller than expected birthweight for DS infants compared with their normal siblings. The difference survived the search for external factors, such as mothers habits and health to presumably strengthen the explanatory role of karyotype variation. Reduced birth weights might provide a base for a host of other developmental departures within DS.

The preceding citations on the origins of developmental deviation for DS are not comprehensive, much of the evidence being interwoven with topics covered in other chapters. They serve here, chiefly, to identify the problems of measuring early development for the syndrome.

The measurement of development

Human development can be scaled so as to provide comparisons of growth rates and styles between individuals, to identify specific growth lags, and to give clues to direction and quality of further growth. There are two preliminary observations of importance in scaling and developmental forecasting for DS: (i) general growth and behavioural increments do not reliably parallel increasing CA, (ii) early developmental markers for DS may have greater forecast value for later growth rate and level than is true for the normal infant. The contradictions can be reconciled.

Non-linearity of psychodevelopmental indices

A test of the linearity of development for DS was first conducted by Share, Webb and Koch (1961). Growth rates slowed markedly as age advanced. Ordinarily, a given developmental progression in the first year of life (be it for a normal or a handicapped child) might presage a similar developmental rate into the second and third years. Not so the DS child for whom, increasingly, data points to a distinct maturational time-table. Psychodevelopmental curves for the syndrome have been described more fully by Zeaman and House (1962) and by Gibson (1966). These will be explored in the section dealing with predicting growth.

Initially, both Gesell and Amatruda (1941) and Benda (1949) observed a progressive slowing of developmental rates for DS children, with advancing CA. Gesell was able to chart (by item analysis of infant scales) the rate of the deceleration. He reported that developmental quotients (DQ) for 1-year-old DS subjects are not infrequently in the borderline range of intelligence. The picture quickly changes with psychometric intelligence stabilizing, typically, at the low trainable levels by approximately 11 years CA. Share, Webb and Koch (1961) examined 16 DS subjects over 3 years of life. They concluded that developmental quotients, for the first 13 months, are not reliable predictors of developmental quotients taken later. Yet, the Gesell scores of the 15–24 month old group were predictive of later developmental quotients. These authors anticipated that such DQs would lose their forecast power beyond 4 years CA. While their data support the notion of developmental regression with age, the small sample used cannot be reliably apportioned across three age groups.

The predictive value of very early developmental markers, of the classic sort, is even less certain. Age at first tooth was correlated 0.21 with later IQ whereas age at walking (seen usually in DS by 3 years (CA) was correlated 0.54 with later Binet IQ (Gibson, 1966). It is likely that sufficient growth patterning dissimilarity exists between normal and DS babies to impair the validity of any formal infant scaling for the latter. Fishler, Graliker and Koch (1965) examined the comparative predictability of the Gesell scales for different types of mental retardates, including DS. Their study was motivated by the continuing debate about the possibilities of predicting from infant scaling in general (Illingworth, 1961, 1962; Bayley, 1955). Five diagnostic categories were examined: cerebral palsy, congenital cerebral anomalies, DS, pseudo-retardation and hypothyroidism. There were 28 cases in the DS sample. Each infant was tested at intervals of from 3 to 6 months, over the first 3 or 4 years of life. Thereafter, the child was examined annually using the Binet test of intelligence. Correlation coefficients were then obtained for both sample and subject comparisons of DQ and IQ. Correlation coefficients, between DQ and later IQ scores, were plotted across DS test age levels. At test year I, the between-measures correlation coefficient was 0.50; by year II it was 0.64; by year III, 0.85; and at year IV, 0.82. All coefficients were statistically significant. Their results support the proposed phenomenon of regression of development for DS through infancy to 4 years CA, and as distinct from the other disorder categories tested. Fishler *et al.* (1965) were impressed by the number of DS infants who showed borderline developmental quotients during the first year of life, while displaying IQ scores between 30 and 50 points in later childhood. These decelerative growth trends have been noted to extend into the later years. Thompson (1963) examined 29 post-infancy DS subjects having CAs of 5 and 6 years. She recorded a mean mental age of 2 years 6 months for the 5-year-olds, and 2 years 9 months for the 6-year-olds. The IQ drop would represent a mean decline of 4 points over 12 months.

Most studies of the regressive quality of early development for DS have been undertaken to demonstrate the role of nurture. Carr (1970) has contested this approach. She compared a control group of normal infants with samples

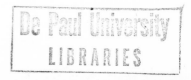

of home-reared and boarded out DS infants. The Bayley infant scales of mental and motor development were employed. Indications are for a non-linear regression of development for the two treatment groups of DS infants, and more especially for those between age 6 weeks and 2 years of age. The normal infant controls showed the expected linear progression of growth across the same time span. There can be little doubt that DS growth is decelerative, with time, and that environmental explanations, such as institutional effects, are possibly necessary but seldom sufficient (Melyn & White, 1973). A further study by Carr (1975) reported the major developmental regression for DS infants to be between 6 weeks and 10 months of age. Other later sources of regression of test intelligence (e.g., the failure to master speech skills and progressive neuropathology) seem less relevant. To test the point Carr removed the verbal items from her examination only to find that the DS children fell even more significantly behind the controls. Standard infant tests are apparently not attuned to the insidious general growth lag of DS infants so that intellectual decline is not easily observable until 3 or 4 years of age, at which time the traditional mental test includes discrete cognitive and verbal material.

Developmental uniqueness in DS

Brousseau and Brainerd's (1928) review of the sensory and motor equipment of the DS neonate had disclosed a number of growth features not well represented on contemporary infant schedules. All the same, Fishler and her colleagues were able to show relatively good prediction of Gesell infant schedules for later intellectual development in DS; especially when compared with forecast efficiency using normal samples of the same ages (Bayley, 1955). Fishler *et al.* (1965) considered that there might be sufficient stability of development in DS (between 3 and 4 years CA) to permit reliable IQ prediction from DQ scores. Other DS infant growth studies have supported this hope. Kostrzewski (1965) reported a mean Cattell DQ of 34.52 ($N = 46$) for a young sample and a mean Binet IQ of 33.94 ($N = 109$) for an older group. He concluded that Cattell developmental scaling, past early infancy, can provide a good estimate of IQ scores in later childhood. The narrow competency range and continuing dominion of sensorimotor over cognitive indices for the syndrome, even into early adulthood, gives standard infant scales a greater predictive potency than would be expected.

The decelerative feature of early development in DS is widely appreciated. Whether quality and patterning of growth are peculiar to the syndrome, is not. Fishler, Share and Koch (1964) inspected developmental achievement

Table 1. *Syndrome samples for selected developmental landmarks in months chronological age (CA)*

Landmarks	DS (N)	DS CA range (months)	DS median CA (months)	Normal median CA (months)	Difference in normal and DS median in months and percentages
Holds head erect	170	1–50	5	3	2 (60%)
Rolls over	165	2–50	7	5	2 (71%)
Transfers objects in hands	95	5–30	10	7	3 (70%)
Sits unsupported for 1 minute erect	149	5–50	11	8	3 (73%)
Crawls and pivots	123	5–50	13	8	5 (62%)
Pulls self to standing position	104	7–50	17	10	7 (59%)
Creeps	80	9–45	17	10	7 (59%)
Walks with support	96	9–55	20	13	7 (65%)
Stands unsupported	84	13–56	23	14	7 (61%)
Walks unsupported	88	14–66	24	15	9 (63%)
Walks upstairs with support	60	18–61	30	18	12 (60%)
Able to seat self in chair	66	15–49	28	18	10 (64%)
Walks downstairs with support	43	15–65	31	21	10 (68%)
Draws or imitates a circle	23	31–67	48	24	24 (50%)
Stairs up and down alone	28	24–56	40	24	16 (60%)
Dresses self simple garment	25	24–60	48	24	24 (50%)

After Share and French (1974).

levels for 30 items of behaviour taken from the Gesell developmental scales. They examined 71 DS infants over a 7-year time span. Later Binet IQ scores were calculated for the 28 children still available. Comparisons with normal children, for motor growth, were possible up to an age of 2½ years. Test items yielded little discrepancy (between the DS and normals) during the first 6 months of life, but a non-linear growth lag became evident for the DS children by the developmental age (DA) of two years. Communication ability was the most reliable deficiency, typical cases (CA over 2 years) showing vocalization of the 10-month-old level. Personal–social growth patterns, when contrasted with the normal child, were similarly disadvantaged. Only for ease of toilet training was the time discrepancy between the DS and the normal infant relatively small. Share, Kock, Webb and Graliker (1964) were surprised by the successful training of DS in self-help routines, compared to normals and to other types of mentally handicapped of similar ages. A prolonged period for imitative behaviours and an apparent lack of motor tension associated with self-care habit training has been suggested as an explanation but is not clearly established. However, Share and his colleagues were disappointed that none of the sample of 71 DS children were able to dress themselves completely. The delay of finer coordination for DS might favour some aspects of early habit training and not others. Share and French's (1974) later comparisons of growth landmarks, for DS and normal children, are shown in Table 1. The ability to manage single garments occurs at a median CA of 48 months for DS and 24 months for normal children – whereas only 2 months separate DS and normal infants for 'holds head erect' or 'rolls over'. With regard to quality of development, Share (1975) argues that motor patterns are relatively normal up to 6 months and that later, motor maturity (walking, running, squatting, climbing, etc.) continues to be superior to other developmental areas. Lesser discrepancies of development are found in areas of personal habit training, toilet training especially. The greatest lag was found to be in the speech area, more so with receptive speech than with expressive language. These developmental priorities also hold for normal children.

The approach of Dicks–Mireaux (1966) to developmental uniqueness for DS, is similar to that of Share and his colleagues. Dicks–Mireaux dismantled the Gesell scale and grouped the items in terms of motor, adaptive, social and language development. His sample comprised 12 standard trisomy DS infants living at home. The babies were tested at intervals up to 82 weeks CA, the testing points being designated as 'focal' by Gesell. Test control conditions for the study appear to have been satisfactory. Mean developmental quotients, for each of the three behavioural areas and for each key age range, were calculated. The findings indicate that:

(1) With the exception of motor behaviour, there is *reduced* variability of scores, especially for adaptive and social behaviours, with increasing age.

(2) Index of slope calculations expressed a significant decline for motor development but not for adaptive and social behaviours, with increasing age. Dicks–Mireaux concluded that the median developmental quotient for DS is firmly in the 'defective' range by three months CA. A later study (Dicks–

Mireaux, 1972) of Gesell norms, compared DS infants of between 16 weeks and 18 months against a normal sample. Comparisons were made for motor, adaptive and social behaviour. The DS infants showed a lower DQ score than normal infants and progressively so. Motor retardation was the area of major decline and social–behavioural status the area of least decline.

Fishler *et al.* (1964) had previously stated that motor growth for DS children was close to normal during the first 6 months of life. Considering the small samples used in most studies, variations in outcome could depend on nurtural history, cytogenetic status, sex, time of institutionalization and extent of secondary handicap. Carr's (1970) more recent examination of motor growth for the DS infant uncovered a sharp decline of Bayley motor scale quotients (home-reared) from 6 weeks to 2 years of life. The mean DMQ of her sample was 90.24 at 6 weeks of life and 25.38 by 15 months. The range and comparative decline of DIQs, for the same life period, was significantly less. Instability of motor status appears to be a peculiarity of the syndrome and not necessarily accompanied by variation of intellectual standing. The conclusions are different from those of Cowie (1970) who assumed that motor performance corresponded approximately with degree of intellectual development in DS. According to her, the sources of early developmental uniqueness for DS depend ultimately on the interaction of central and peripheral physiological processes.

A further hint of a special developmental status for DS is found in the Dicks–Mireaux scattergram analysis of Gesell age-specific items. These data indicate that maturation in DS is faster between 3 and 9 months than between 9 and 18 months CA; although the effect might be merely a product of the standardization of infant schedules using normal populations. In this regard, Carr (1970) had observed a fair consistency of developmental trends between her normal infant control series and home-reared DS infants. Perhaps commercial infant schedules have more useful predictive value for community than hospitalized DS subjects. McNeill (1955) examined a number of qualitative growth differences for DS. His item analysis of developmental markers indicated most rapid early growth for the physical, and least rapid growth for the intellectual–symbolic test items. By 21.11 months of mental age (MA) (representing a sample of mean CA 6 years) motor coordination was found to occur, on average, at 30 months, grip strength at 41.22 months, and social growth at 22.56 months. Similar findings were reported by Stedman and Eichorn (1964). These workers compared symbolic development with neuromotor development for DS as part of an examination of the relative efficiency of home and institutional care systems. Even within the areas of symbolic functioning, a syndrome-specific hierarchy seemed to emerge. Cornwell (1974), comparing language and number skills, found number concept management, markedly poor at all MA levels, whereas rote counting developed adequately. These questions are explored more fully later using samples of older DS subjects.

The foregoing infant scale studies have tended to compare the development of DS children against themselves and normal infants. Murphy (1956) dismantled several developmental schedules to examine comparative growth across distinct diagnostic groups of the mentally retarded. These included familial MR, brain damaged MR and DS (sample sizes; 40, 38 and 40 cases respectively). Tests selected were the Cattell, Stanford–Binet, and 'draw-a-man'. The three aetiological groups were CA matched. Appropriate Binet and Cattell tasks were collected as a general index of verbal development. The 'draw-a-man' test was treated as an indicator of concrete performance style, neuromotor growth level and eye–hand coordination proficiency. Murphy concluded that development for DS subjects appears to be restricted to a narrower range than for the other two groups in both verbal and performance areas. She also asserts that cognitive growth patterns in DS are quantitatively (in terms of lower general potential) like the exogenous mentally retarded and qualitatively (in terms of being less variable) like that of the endogenous mentally retarded. The Murphy study was designed to support an 'injury' hypothesis for the aetiology of DS and was only incidentally concerned with comparative growth across causal subgroups.

The uniqueness of early development for the syndrome is uncertain. Quality and range of motor growth is not precisely like the normal infant or other retarded infants, for some studies and under some conditions. The relation of motor maturation to later facets of developing behaviour also varies across studies. The confusion has several sources: (i) the magnitude, quality and range of development depends on how it is measured, none of the conventional scales being especially suitable for the DS infant; (ii) the evidence for distinctiveness of early growth is better for the few empirical than for the many psychometric studies and provides additional evidence of the inadequacy of standardized infant scaling for the syndrome; (iii) DS is more quiescent in infancy than are other groups of trainable mentally retarded (TMR), there being apparently less to observe and record behaviourally. Clearer evidence of distinct developmental patterning is more readily available for the older DS child. This material is held to later chapters because it tends to be thematic, e.g., social, personality, cognitive, language and special abilities development.

Forecasting development

The research reviewed thus far supports the proposition that reliable growth forecasting for DS might be feasible if the maturational dimensions of the syndrome are incorporated. Difficulties mentioned have included the non-linear and regressive nature of intellectual and motor indices, the inappropriateness of most traditional test norms and some measurement distortions resulting from the considerable developmental scatter evident for the DS infant. Other difficulties to be considered include (i) our poor appreciation of developmental regression rates and their consequences for prediction, (ii) the uncertainty about growth termination ages, (iii) the relation of cytogenetic status to growth patterns, (iv) the influence of progressive physical degenerative processes (both primary and secondary) on growth trends, (v) the effects of different nurtural processes on development, and (vi) the impact of high early mortality rates on cross-sectional sampling. In support of a degree of predictive efficiency for existing infant scales is the fact that they are based on sensorimotor growth events which, for DS, continue to be paramount in later childhood (Shotwell, 1964). Moreover, developmental reach (across a given CA period) is only about one-third of the normal rate. The prediction of developmental events for the syndrome would thus engage fewer growth events in a given time, than is the case for normal children, and might invite less error of measurement.

Predicting growth from infant schedules

The forecast power of standard infant scales for DS has been widely debated and poorly researched. Dameron (1963) examined 12 DS infants between 2 and 5 months of CA. A control group of three normal infants was included. All subjects were tested on the Bayley California first-year mental scale. Results were compared with the Berkely growth study norms at six growth stages, ranging from 3 to 18 months. Dameron found that the intellectually typical and the brighter DS child do not obviously differ, in terms of magnitude of development quotient, at 3 months of age. Only the most severely retarded displayed depressed developmental quotients at between 3 and 6 months CA. Dameron concluded that formal infant growth schedules, used in the first months of life, are of value merely for confirmation of the clinically obvious. The study is difficult to evaluate, for present purposes, insofar as Dameron credited all non-passed items preceding a passed item. Previous discussion postulated distinct deficiencies of psychological growth and considerable variability between cases for DS infants. Pro-rating of test items would tend to obscure these two phenomena and reduce the likelihood of successful scaling for prediction purposes.

Shotwell's study (1964) of early developmental prediction from tests is more encouraging. She used the 1922 Kuhlmann–Binet scale to determine the stability of correlations compared with other scales of psychological development, e.g., the Vineland social maturity scale. Two samples of DS (35 and 37 cases) were selected and compared for developmental achievement with samples of post-traumatic, familial-undifferentiated and a causally mixed group of mentally retarded subjects. While item analyses indicated no distinct success–failure pattern for the DS subjects, there was evidence that a number of Kuhlmann–Binet infant scale items shifted in order to age-graded difficulty. The shift occurred across individuals, samples and diagnostic categories. Sequence of development appears to be different for the retarded than for normal infants, although not significantly so across diagnostic categories. Shotwell concluded that 'infant tests assess, at least in retardates, a most important if not the most important predictive factor of intelligence. We refer to sensory motor functioning and its underlying neural integration' (p. 760). Reliability coefficients (test–retest) for the early sample (first test at between 2 and 5 years of age and second test after 5 years) were also determined. The mean CA for the first test was 3 years 4 months and at time of retest was 7 years 4 months. The correlation coefficients were 0.70, between first and second mental stage, and 0.72 between first and second set of IQ scores. Correlation coefficients were not reported separately for aetiological categories and there is no way of assessing the forecast efficiency of the procedure for the DS subjects alone.

Quaytman (1953) observed that most investigations of the nature of developmental staging for DS have been based on hospitalized samples. This continued to be true. Institutional cases frequently differ from community cases by mental level, socio-economic and ethnic status of the parents, age of the parents, and possibly, therefore, by cytological subclass of DS. Quaytman contended that only up to 20% of all Down's cases are hospitalized. Thompson (1963) compared growth indices for home-bound and hospitalized DS showing hospitalized samples to be 'selected'. By 5 years of age, all of the community series were capable of walking, running, squatting, climbing, stringing beads and were partially toilet trained. Speech development was the outstanding limitation, both in absolute terms and in comparison with each child's mental age. Meindl, Barclay, Lamp and Yater (1971) recorded marked differences of mental growth curves for institutional and non-institutional subjects, especially in respect to mental growth after 9 years of age.

well-considered group care is inherently inferior to nuclear family care, or that conventional community infant and child care provides the ideal adjustment base for the mature DS individual.

(3) The distribution of IQ for DS seems to centre at mid-imbecility (TMR), with a large minority grouped in the custodial category and a not-so-large minority within the educable class. Precise agreement is difficult to obtain insofar as classification ratios shift with advancing age. Furthermore, the problem of defining neuro-maturational 'majority' for DS is a thorny one. There is evidence that mental growth continues for some well into the twenties yet terminates for many others, perhaps the majority, by as early as 11 or 12 years CA. Study of the quite disparate rates of erosion of IQ for DS might identify those variables which help to 'hold' IQ levels, against those associated with deterioration, at various mental and physical ages. Meanwhile, continued bickering about the 'typical' mean and range of IQ for DS is of little practical or research value.

Qualitative aspects of intelligence

Many of the investigations of the quantitative features of intelligence for DS have recorded qualitative oddities. Some have undertaken item analysis and scatter analysis to determine the influence of these qualities on the structure of intelligence for the syndrome. They are of interest here because they restrict free interpretation of the aggregate data. A fuller consideration of cognitive uniqueness is contained in later chapters.

The case for distinctive intellectual parameters

A first rudimentary psychometric profile analysis was offered by Brousseau and Brainerd (1928). They concluded 'that the mental (test) characteristics of this group do not differ in any marked degree from those of feeble-minded children of other types' (p. 133). They described Binet test scatter for seven mature DS subjects of middle- to upper-trainable level intelligence. The pass–fail distribution of the test items is remarkable for its spread across as many as five mental age years. A simple sign–test re-analysis of their pass–fail pattern data reveals potentially significant trends for type of item failed early, as against more time resistent items. Much later, Pototzky and Grigg (1942) argued that the qualitative characteristics of intellect for DS are not especially different from those of other retarded children. They claimed that 'Arithmetic, always the most difficult subject for all retarded children, is not more difficult for the average mongoloid than for other retarded children' (p. 509).

Gordon (1944) arrived at quite a different conclusion. Comparisons were made between DS and normal subjects, equated for mental age, on visual discrimination performance (size, pattern, 3-dimensional form, visual texture, brightness and saturation) and tactile discrimination for the same qualities. Individual differences were recorded which could not be explained on the basis of gross intelligence. Whereas tactile discrimination was easier than visual, for the normal, the reverse was true for DS. The case rested there for two decades; until the work of Kostrzewski (1965) and Thompson (1963).

Kostrzewski undertook the analysis of number-sense development for 120 DS individuals. Test tasks included memorizing and repeating a sequence of two, three, and four digits, imitating a number of taps, and other graded items including the performance of simple number exercises. He argued for a close correspondence between the development of these numerical abilities and growing mental age, independent of CA. Pototzky and Grigg (1942) had previously said that 'Critical analysis of the arithmetic testing revealed that among our children there is no high correlation between mental age and score on the test.' (p. 509.) The Kostrzewski data were further treated by a process of developmental grading. Phase I of numerical development in DS occurred between 2 and 3 years of mental age and consisted of such rudimentary number concepts as 'more', 'less' and rote counting for up to four objects. Phase II, he said, appears at a mental age of between 3 and 4 years and encompasses memorizing and repeating four numbers, recitation of from five to ten numbers, etc. Number concept growth for the majority at this mental age was limited to the abstraction 'one'. At phase II he asked the child to give up one object on request, to imitate one tap, and so on. Phase III included the appearance of number sequencing facility which is said to be evident at a mental age of between 4 and 6 years, but for his sample, at close to 6 years. The majority could give, on request, from three to seven objects, recite up to twenty-eight and count between eight and twenty-one objects. His terminal phase IV represented the sixth to seventh years of mental development, including such skills as simple addition and subtraction (up to ten), but only in concrete situations. Kostrzewski reported a few cases at a mental age of 7 years who, he claimed, were able to understand the concept of fractions. In all, only 2% of this sample reached level IV for number concept development. He suggested that number development for DS might be associated with speech lag and/or specific auditory-perceptual difficulty, but that fundamentally, the failure of DS to evolve an abstract attitude is the primary factor.

It was also Thompson's (1963) belief that the abstract attitude in DS is developmentally arrested as a partial result of language growth lag, although clearly the obverse could be true. Thompson examined the results of Stanford–Binet tests for 5- and 6-year-old DS children. None of her children enjoyed speech on a par with their mental age. Thompson reasoned that the verbal communication deficiency was not merely a function of general mental retardation because relatively bright DS children compensated, often quite ingeniously, with gesticular and posturing communication. The duller, having similar speech deficit, did not employ these compensatory devices. Since thinking and language are interactive developmentally, the abstraction deficiency is possibly a consequence of faulty speech mechanisms rather than primarily of central or sensory circuiting systems limitation.

The method of her study is of special interest. Thompson's demonstration involved the clustering of Stanford–Binet test items from Binet year II through to year IV, according to the language content of each (both request and response). The four classes used were:

   (i) Little or no language, e.g., form boards.
   (ii) Verbal direction and non-verbal response, e.g., pointing to objects.
   (iii) Verbal direction and verbal reply using concrete materials, e.g., picture vocabulary.
   (iv) Verbal direction and verbal response, e.g. repeating numbers.

DS children of 5 and 6 years old (mean mental age 2 years 9 months, and mean IQ 45 points) were examined. Items requiring non-verbal response were performed consistently at the overall mental age level of the child. Directions were repeated to ensure maintenance of attention insofar as failure was often a function of the child's lack of experience with the vocabulary used in instructions. Responses requiring verbal reply and using concrete materials were passed appropriate to the child's mental age, even though responses were frequently deficient in quality of verbal content, e.g., fewer sentences being used. Purely verbal input and output situations were failed consistently at the child's mental age level, e.g., repeating two digits. A more direct test of the relative independence of thought and language deficiency in DS (Thompson's level D items) would require the separation of number comprehension from its memory components. Intellectual growth for DS, past 4 years MA, evidently requires a capacity for language and the ability to generalize, group, or relate, i.e., to display the abstract attitude.

Stickland (1954) argued that mental test similarities among DS subjects help to shape the impression of intellectual uniqueness. His Binet (Stanford–Binet form L and M, 1939) patterns for relatively bright home-reared adult DS showed similar congruence of pass–fail scatter. One could conclude that mature DS is intellectually more homogeneous than other forms of MR.

Stickland explained these similarities as (i) an inability of DS to use words at a conceptual level, (ii) the effect of intensive and uniform care regimes and (iii) a relatively intact rote memory.

Despite the *post defacto* nature of the data it is fair to conclude that secondary factors – sensory thresholds, and speech capacity being two – have played some part in moulding the clinical and psychometric image of intelligence for DS. The main body of the 'intellectual uniqueness' research is concerned, however, with various central process hypotheses. These require testing against other aetiological groups of MR.

Cross-aetiological comparisons of intelligence

Hermelin and O'Connor (1961) failed to support a special intellectual status for DS. They were unable to detect visual-perceptual anomalies for DS, compared with normal children of similar mental ages or to find recognition or matching differences between DS and other mentally retarded. The Down's syndrome group, however, did not perform as well for copying from memory, making finer motor discriminations and for psychomotor control as either the non-DS retarded or normals of equivalent mental age. Gordon (1944) had previously reported DS individuals to be inferior for tactile discrimination when compared with normals equated for mental age. O'Connor and Hermelin (1961) attempted unsuccessfully to replicate this finding for DS and non-DS retarded. Differences in visual discrimination performance, between mental retardation subgroups, were unimpressive; despite Thompson's point that DS children seemed frequently to have impaired vision contributing to classroom difficulty.

Nakamura (1965) undertook Binet scale item analysis for a severely retarded group of older hospitalized DS patients, comparing their test profiles with those obtained for an aetiologically undifferentiated mental retardation sample. He expected, given the specificity of the chromosomal aberration. that DS 'would illustrate greater intra-class ontogenetic similarity in characteristics among its members than members of other populations' (p. 661). Sixty-four institutionalized DS cases, older than 16 years, were matched with aetiologically mixed mentally retarded subjects for age, sex, and IQ. Analysis included the pass–fail percentages for test items from the Binet, years II to VIII. A test of differences was also made for all Binet items which could be grouped as 'memory' and 'low-verbal' in content. Significant differences were reported in favour of the non-DS group for repeating three digits, and in favour of the DS patients for formboard performance, block-bridging and circle drawing. No cross-aetiological differences were recorded for the Binet memory item cluster or for the low-verbal item cluster. Interpretation of these findings is difficult because of the heterogeneity of the various exogenous aetiologies represented in the so-called 'undifferentiated' control series. The superiority of the DS subjects on Binet material involving perceptual-motor proficiency is possibly a function of deficit patterning in the control series and need not indicate intellectual specialization for DS.

Accordingly, Brousseau and Brainerd's (1928) original assertion that DS subjects are intellectually like other mental retardates is not fully consistent with the modern psychometric and experimental evidence. On the other hand, these pathfinding studies have failed largely to engage suitable comparison groups, to control or randomize those variables known to confound test results, or to use optimal data analyses. They have been studied here because they served to shape the issues debated in the later multi-dimensional psychometric (see Ability Profiles) and experimental literature (see Learning and Arousal).

The sections to follow sketch and broader dimensions of intelligence for the syndrome (limits, timing and deterioration effects) and explore these in the context of the somatic events.

The shape of intelligence
The upper limits of intelligence: traditional views

Defining the proper boundaries of intellectual expression for DS, and thus its plasticity, is an ongoing debate. Past opinion has ranged from a trainable level (below IQ 50) upper limit in adulthood, to claims for intellectual normalcy in a few instances. The variety of conclusions can be attributed to sampling differences across studies, especially with respect to age at examination and nurtural conditions. Most DS adults who have spent some time in an institution, are generally of low TMR status. For a random sample of 100 physically mature institutional cases (Gibson, 1960) an IQ of 53 proved to be the highest score. Only 4 of the 100 scored an IQ of 50 points or more. Yet, there is an increasing recognition that educable mentally retarded (EMR) ratings, and even borderline to 'normal' infant scale scores, are not unusual for the DS child. These reports may be deceptive. The failure of standard developmental schedules to identify growth lag in DS infants, the tendency towards considerable deceleration of intellectual growth with advancing age, and especially the uncertainty about the physical maturity limits of intellectual growth have contributed to the confusion about the ultimate performance expectations for the syndrome.

Loeffler and Smith (1964) examined the upper limits of intelligence for DS children under 3 years of age and for those between 3 and 9 years CA. Of the younger children results were 47% EMR and 23% borderline (IQ 70 points plus). Of the older sample results were 60% TMR and 29% EMR. There was no case of borderline intelligence in the latter group. Penrose (1949 a, b) set the realistic upper limit of mental age for DS at 7 years. Durling and Benda (1952) considered the upper mental age limit to be 7 years 11 months. Pototzky and Grigg (1942) observed that DS reaches intellectual maturity somewhere between MA 2 and 8 years. Nakamura (1961) reported that a Binet mental age of 7 years represents the substantive upper limit. Sternlicht and Wanderer (1962) proposed approximately 6 years MA as the upper limit for DS adults in institutional settings. While most studies have settled on mental age limits of between 2 and 7 years, Pototzky and Grigg (1942) recorded upper mental ages of almost 11 years for their institutional sample of 21 cases. The majority had achieved mental ages in excess of 6 years. What is equally remarkable was a mean IQ of 46 points for their hospitalized adults. The Bancroft school was said by Pototzky and Grigg to be highly selective of its students and to offer a beneficial educational and treatment programme. Still, in order to reach a mental age of almost 11 years, and in view of the usually wide psychometric scatter and the early erosion of intellect noted for the syndrome, it would be necessary to achieve 'adult' success for a number of Binet scale items, a rare event in view of most other evidence. Whatever the inconsistencies, the Pototsky and Grigg paper has helped to shatter a previously too narrow concept of intellectual growth expectation and was the beginning of a concern for the karyotypic, somatic, situational and age variables associated with the upper limits of IQ for the syndrome.

Wallin (1944) anticipated a number of the foregoing complexities, including the question of upper limits and the influence of nurture. He wrote,

'The writer has never known more than one mongol who tested as high as 7–8 among over 15000 examinees in five psycho-educational clinics in five states. In Delaware the highest rating is 4–5, IQ 67, based on Form L, for a boy whose chronological age was only 6–7. This is the highest Binet IQ of any of the writer's cases. But this child was diagnosed as a mongoloid on the basis of slight mongolian finger, head, and eye characteristics. He was not a decided case.' (p. 108)

Wallin's work on home-reared DS indicated a higher upper limit of intelligence, at maturity, than is usually projected from institutional samples. The Cornwell and Birch (1969) data is also derived from home-reared cases, some of whom were as old as 17 years. These data supported no unusually elevated IQ scores or mental age levels for the adults. Particularly apparent were (i) the substantial social quotients achieved in some cases, one as high as 83 points, and (ii) the rather minor changes of psychometric (Binet) basal rates, over time in contrast with the increasing upward scatter of a few specific test items passed as a result of special training and life experience. Basal test age changed little past a mental age of 4 years; yet the older DS subjects continued to make spotty and isolated gains on mental tests. Psychometric successes for the young adults proved to be in the area of social responses; or were based on progressively stabilizing attention; or were related to specific skill acquisition where training was ongoing and intensive. By way of illustration, Dunsdon, Carter, and Huntley (1960) selected cases from among the brightest of a group of 390 community resident DS individuals who had been attending a hospital clinic. Of these brighter children, 44 were available for further study. They were subjected to the Stanford–Binet (1937 revision), the Vineland social maturity scale, Burt's reading-accuracy scales and a number of oral arithmetic tests. Most of the children were attending community schools for the educationally subnormal, or private schools. The highest IQ recorded was 68 points, 20 of their cases displaying IQs of 45 points or over. The IQ of 68 points was for a CA of almost 18 years. Dunsdon *et al.* concluded that up to 7% of community-based DS is potentially 'educable'. Definitions of the upper limits of intelligence for DS appear, therefore, to differ depending on whether or not the sample has been derived from hospital or community populations. Exceptions apart, the great majority of DS individuals in home or hospital achieve peak mental ages of less than 4 years and IQs usually in the 30 to 40 point range. Community-reared DS often attain somewhat higher adult MA levels, an advantage which can be assigned to the more test-appropriate socialization and schooling opportunities available to them, to the probability that those cases most in need of intensive care are placed in institutions as soon as eligible, or to genuine nurtural advantages.

Vigorous and appropriate training, started early in life, will quite probably influence IQ scores at maturity, but unevenly across cases. DS individuals differ in neuromotor and sensory system status at birth and in the subsequent unfolding of these systems during childhood. Regression rates are variable across individuals with respect to intellectual development. It is for these reasons that DS children, raised in equally good environments, can achieve widely ranging terminal mental ages and at different times in their life span. Differential expression of karyotype and the degree of secondary pathology in individual cases are two explanations. Some of these complexities are examined now for standard trisomy DS. The intellectual status of partial states, mixed karyotypes, low abnormal cell frequency mosaicism and the superficially stigmatized trisomy 'carrier' is explored elsewhere.

The timing of majority mental age

Throughout the literature on test standardization is the assumption that intellectual maturation is complete for DS, as for most normals, at about 15 years of CA. Admittedly, there are many exceptions to the rule (Bayley, 1955). The problem of defining neuro-maturational majority for DS is doubly difficult because capacity peaking is influenced by the early onset of CNS deterioration. Other cases display a superficial advance of mental age into adulthood. For most, a maximum mental age has been achieved by 10 or 12 years of CA.

The following studies illustrate the problem. Durling and Benda (1952) found 'custodial' DS to be neurologically mature by 11 years CA: usually with no more than 3 years of mental age then reached and typically only 2 years. Another much smaller group of initially brighter DS children displayed a mental age growth-curve peaking at 18–20 CA. Almost half of these latter cases gained in mental age past 20 years CA, and a few even into the fourth decade of life. A comparison group of familial retardates peaked reliably for mental age before CA 18 years. Durling and Benda observed that mental growth for DS appears to arrest at the point 'senility' begins, albeit a premature senility. Thus, whether mental growth has ceased by 10 years or by 30 years, there is no substantial time span of stable intellectual majority for most. In fact, intellectual maturity is evident at about the time deteriorative processes are clinically visible, a congruence suggesting that the staging of neuro-maturational maturity is tied less to growth or releasor events than to the timing of cytopathological suppressor events. Owens, Dawson and Losin (1971) have recorded the appearance of symptoms of pre-senile Alzheimer's disease in many older DS children. Gibson (1966) found most of his institutional sample to achieve maximum MA between 9 and 11 years CA. A few continued to show mental growth into the young adult years. Ross (1962) reported a maximum MA between 10 and 11 years CA, while noting several examples of slight MA advance into the third decade of life. These substantial individual differences, for timing of majority MA in DS, had puzzled McNeill (1955).

Ross (1962) replicated the Durling and Benda study using 319 cases and 520 test scores taken from the Stanford–Binet, Wechsler, Kuhlmann, and Cattell scales. While the study suffers from many of the problems inherent in any cross-sectional analysis of developmental data, the large sample used is reassuring. Ross charted mental age scatter to approximately 40 years CA, as against both Benda's 1949 data and a theoretical normal. Growth of mental age in DS appears to progress in linear fashion between 10 and 15 years CA.

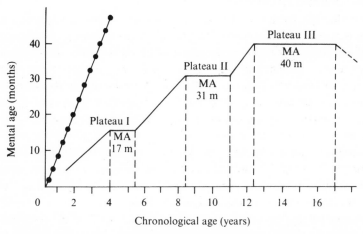

Fig. 1. Schema of mental age against chronological age in Down's syndrome (N = 303). (From D. Gibson (1966). *American Journal of Mental Deficiency*, **70**, 24.)

Thereafter, a marked deceleration develops. Ross acknowledged the potential sampling problem created by the effects of differential mortality on the IQ distribution of samples taken cross-sectionally. Useful gains might be made for an understanding of typical, terminal and potential intelligence in DS by examining comparative IQ levels of expired and surviving cases, matched for CA, and with environmental control.

Gibson (1966) examined psychometric test records for 303 hospitalized cases of DS, ranging up to 44 years of age. The relation of CA to MA was plotted for all cases, as shown in Fig. 1. and is a schematic representation of the staging of mental growth for the syndrome against a theoretical normal. The acceleration of mental age appears progressively less marked as CA advances, with successive developmental plateaus spanning greater CA ranges. These are, of course, inferences based on cross-sectional data and are subject to the usual criticisms. Stage I of MA growth begins to level at about 4 years of CA, representing approximately 18 months of MA. The first stage resembles closely that proposed by Fishler *et al.* (1965). Stage II mental growth accretion begins at about 5 years of CA, levels again at approximately 9 years of CA and represents a median mental age of about 31 months. The plateau spanning 9–11 years CA is, for many, a terminal growth stage. A significant number display a third growth spurt levelling at over 12 years of age and representing a final MA of 3–4 years. Over 17 years CA, a general decline in mental age values was obvious. These projections are consistent with reports by Jervis (1948) and Nakamura (1961) concerning onset of 'premature' aging in DS.

One could conclude that the majority of institutionalized DS individuals show little MA increment past 10 or 11 years CA. We do not know the extent to which early MA peaking is a maturational phenomenon for DS or whether or not continuing neuro-maturation is attenuated by the onset of pre-senile events, or if maturational timetables differ by quality of nurture and pre-selection for type of care. Apart from the Benda and Durling suggestion that the most retarded exhibit the earliest MA peaking (in terms of CA) little is known about the origins and distribution of majority timing for the syndrome. Study should be made (i) of the clinical, cognitive and aetiological charac-teristics of late versus early mental maturation in DS and, (ii) of the relation of secondary deteriorative processes to both the staging and quality of mental maturity for the syndrome.

Ageing and intelligence

The early and often rapid 'deterioration' of intelligence for DS has been claimed as environmentally induced. Down's individuals who are reared in high-expectation school and family situations might drop IQ points on being transferred to low-intensity group care regimes, particularly in later life. Those moved from individual care to group custodial programmes do display deterioration of intellectual performance (Nakamura, 1961) and apparently more so than for other clinical types of mental retardation. It is unclear, though, whether or not the erosion of IQ, following institutionalization, is somehow a result of organic decline which led finally to a decision to hospitalize. Cross-sectional sampling bias, differential mortality effects, moti-vational changes and timing of institutional placement are all factors to be evaluated. A consideration first of progressive pathogenesis for DS might serve better to isolate the other variables mentioned.

Senile-like changes for the syndrome were first studied by Jervis (1948). He attributed much of the early intellectual and emotional decline in DS to such changes. Jervis described three cases, age 35, 42 and 47 years. In one case there was a flattening of motivation, depression, loss of vocabulary and reduction of self-care habits. Histological examination showed senile plaques throughout the cerebral cortex and numerous other structural and cellular alterations. A second case displayed a marked behavioural change at the age of 38, including noisy excitement, deterioration of speech, indiscriminate eating and IQ loss. Post-mortem examination uncovered the classical physio-logical evidence for senile dementia. The third, a man of 34 years exhibited increasing hostility, restlessness, food refusal and untidiness. On autopsy, the usual organic concomitants of senile dementia were observed. By 1970, Jervis had examined 23 cases with findings similar to those of his early paper. Cooke (1970) noted degenerative changes in DS occurring at even earlier ages. These alterations included cataracts in 92% (by 14 years CA) and skin pigmentation associated with advanced age in normals. Kaback (1970) speculated that the ageing process begins at the cellular level before birth and represents a derangement of cellular regulation which is typical for the syndrome. Jervis (1970a, b) postulated that 'cells with an extra G-group chromosome (characteristic of mongolism) may require a longer period of DNA synthesis indicating a "cellular ageing" phenomenon' (p. 1). He recorded a 20 to 30 point IQ decrease, despite initially low IQs, suggesting to him that a slow and progressive deterioration must have been long-standing despite the apparent suddenness of representative behavioural changes. Similar case studies had been published by Struwe (1929) for a 37-year-old, and by Bertrand and Koffas (1946) for a 42-year-old DS individual.

Jervis's opinion has been recently strengthened by the investigation of Owens, Dawson and Losin (1971) of Alzheimer's disease in DS. The disease is taken by many to be a pre-senile dementia differing from true senile dementia largely by its earlier onset. Owens et al. examined 43 institution-alized DS subjects over 35 years of CA. Excluding those exceeding the age of 50 and others with evidence of birth trauma, congenital defect of the spine, gross neurological or sensory defect, or IQ less than 25 points, the sample narrowed to 19 cases. A second group of 16 DS adults, of between 20 and 25 years CA, were equated for IQ with the foregoing series. Criteria for orientation, object relationships, memory, neurological status and EEG tracings were established. Although no case of clinical Alzheimer's disease was evident in either sample, the older group revealed a significantly higher incidence of aphasia–agnosia (object identification), frontal lobe dysfunction and diffuse cerebral dysfunctions in general. The findings are claimed to be consistent with a diagnosis of Alzheimer's (Blackwood et al., 1963). The importance of the work of Owens et al. centres on the evidence for organic deterioration, in DS youth, of the sort usually associated with much older people and not found in other forms of mental retardation to the same extent. Support continues to accumulate. Little and Masotti (1974) examined the palmo-mental reflex in normal and mentally retarded adults. The Down's group, while comprising 44% of the retarded sample, disproportionately retained the reflex. They concluded that it is 'a primitive reflex which persists in cases of developmental delay or may re-emerge in acquired brain disease'.

Neuropathological changes, usually tied to senile dementia, have been examined by Solitaire and Lamarche (1966) for five cases of DS. All were significantly below the age at which senile dementia is seen in the general population. The occurrence of senile plaques and neuro-fibrillary alterations in the brains of the five were consistent with the identification of senile dementia or pre-senile Alzheimer's disease. Richards and Sylvester (1969) wrote that 'risks to life connected with ageing occur early in mongols whereas non-mongol imbeciles do not differ in this respect from the general population' (p. 286). Their curve, for death rate per 1000, has its steepest climb in the 40–49 year age range. Richards and Sylvester observed that only a few of the older DS patients were of idiot grade, more of these perhaps having expired earlier in life.

Ageing rates in DS can also be monitored by the study of the skeletal system. While Engler (1949) first contended that bone maturation among DS approximates the normal rate, Benda (1960 a, b) claimed that the appearance of ossification centres is frequently retarded and irregular among DS children, as compared with either normal or other retarded children. Pozsonyi, Gibson and Zarfas (1964) examined these and other conflicting findings and concluded that this might be caused by different CA ranges for the various samples. The investigations by Pozsonyi et al. of the syndrome, reported a maximum delay in bone age up to 4 years CA, an approximation with the normal curve of skeletal development up to about 8 years CA, and an acceleration of bone age in advance of CA beyond 8 years of age. Termination of skeletal growth appeared to occur in DS before 15 years CA, fully 3 years or more in advance of normal expectation. Longitudinal data, treated by Rarick and Seefeldt (1974) is partly in agreement. They rated DS as markedly inferior in stature and sitting height during the circumpubertal years. Age of maximum growth after 10 years did not differ from normals. Pozsonyi et al. had concluded that while the bone evidence is uncertain, there are clinical indications of premature ageing (Fig. 2). By the third decade of life DS cases often exhibit the posture and life style characteristic of the normal in the fifth or sixth decade of life. They say, 'it had been widely assumed that the picture of mild debility, common in mongolism past early childhood was a consequence of poor habits of self-care, e.g., nutrition and hygiene, or of the sometimes impersonal institutional regimes, etc.' (p. 78). The findings implicate instead a rate of early ageing which is intrinsic and particular to DS. Rundle et al. (1972) agree to a point but warn that cross-sectional surveys are not sensitive to the effects of differential mortality rates in relation to degree of mental handicap. Roche (1964) claimed that the acceleration of bone growth, between birth and about 8 years, is not due to

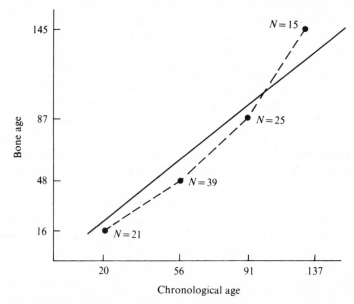

Fig. 2. Bone age as a function of chronological age expressed in mean months against a theoretical norm. (From J. Pozsonyi, D. Gibson & D. E. Zarfas (1964). *Journal of Pediatrics*, **64**, 75–8.)

selection by death but gives no evidence supporting this. Further research into rates of physical and psychological changes with increasing age, and of the aetiological and environmental correlates of such change, would help to anticipate the rise and fall of competence for the syndrome.

DS and intellectual normalcy: general considerations

Knoepfelmacher (1926, in Engler, 1949) claimed that DS can achieve normal intelligence. Crookshank (1925) postulated a non-clinical form of DS with intellectual normalcy. Support for these beliefs has been reported by Cant, Gerrard and Richards (1953) who described a female with an IQ of 116 (Stanford–Binet). She displayed many of the superficial physical stigmata of DS and was so diagnosed. They cite Sutherland's (1907) pioneer report of intellectual normalcy for an 8-year-old DS girl and also referred to an opinion by Weber (1917) that DS need not be accompanied by any serious mental retardation. Two instances of high (but still retarded) mental status for DS were described by Stickland (1954). His first case, a male, was raised at home under good care conditions. He achieved a Stanford–Binet (form

M) IQ of 46, a Porteus Maze IQ of 73 and a Passalong IQ of 79 points. The normal siblings tested as high as 139 IQ points. Stickland observed well-developed rote memory, advanced socialization, and excellent nurtural conditions. A second case, that of a 27-year-old DS female educated in a private school, exhibited highly developed social patterns, could play a few tunes on a piano, ride a cycle, embroider and so on. This girl subsequently became anxious, delusional and violent. She achieved a Binet IQ of 44, a Porteus Maze IQ of 53, and a Passalong IQ of 77 points. Buck (1955) describes a DS youth with a Binet IQ of 70 and basal MA of 6 years. Upper level successes were in sentence building at the superior adult level I. His wide range achievement test scores were grade 8.7 for reading, 6.7 for spelling and 4.1 for arithmetic.

The results from the test on these individuals exhibit the effects of compensatory training built on unimpaired rote memory and a careful shaping of motivation and personality properties. Test profile disparities are common enough in all types of mental retardation, especially when unidimensional and specialized ability measures are compared. They should be interpreted with caution. The exploitation of unimpaired ability parameters to mask specific deficiencies is especially common for DS children. Otherwise, there is no evidence that members of the syndrome can transcend the more fundamental conceptualization and communication deficiencies.

The question of whether 'normalcy' should be narrowly defined as cognitive ability is raised by Butterfield's interesting anecdotal account of a 'provocative case of overachievement' for DS. He described a community-based adult who had received quite adequate training and care. The subject was 36 years of age with a mental age of 5 years (Binet), a Peabody picture vocabulary test score of 54 points and a Vineland social maturity scale rating of 44 points. He managed his mother's house relatively independently, paid the bills, made and sold various items in the community, played the piano and wrote legibly. Despite his limited psychometric ratings, he earned a reading grade level of 5.6, a spelling grade level of 5.0 and an arithmetic grade level of 2.2. Oral reading was at the grade six performance level. These findings raise a number of questions bearing on the psychometric definition of upper performance limits for DS. A most obvious interpretation would be for over-training or for some sort of 'idiot savant' phenomenon. The absence of psychological pressure signs, along with the general life-style of this man, tends to discount these explanations. Life success need not, of course, be largely or even significantly rooted in intellectual process. Both Liverant (1960) and Rotter (1960) urged that life adjustment prediction tests for DS should incorporate motivational and situational variables. Down's syndrome is a particularly cogent example of this need insofar as the practical items are omitted from mental tests as age increases. The effect is for most global IQ tests to sample increasingly the behavioural deficits of DS at the expense of its assets. Reports of high test scores achieved by DS individuals for such specialized measures of intelligence as the Porteus Mazes and other tests which include no language and limited conceptual content, can be understood in this context. The alternative is a special abilities hypothesis.

The cases of Nigel Hunt and Bernard are instructive in regard to separating general ability, special abilities and compensatory training effects in relation to the upper performance limits of the syndrome. *The world of Nigel Hunt: the diary of a mongoloid youth* (1967), given Nigel's good nurture and command of the written language, permits an examination of the more subtle aspects of real-life perception and cognition for the syndrome. Nigel Hunt wrote and typed the 12 000 word diary himself. His father, a retired head-master, has added only some necessary punctuation. An obvious conclusion is that an intensive training regime can produce a much higher functional output than would ordinarily be achieved. Such a deduction would assume that DS individuals are, in the main, born with about equal capacities and that environment creates all or most subsequent performance variability. The various genotypic and secondary exogenous (organic) variables, which influence individual behavioural differences for DS, are described in the chapter to follow. What is impressive about Nigel's account of himself is evidence of a pleasing personality, sound social preparation, well-nurtured rote memory, emotional integrity and a carefully developed observation facility. Yet despite an extensive vocabulary, Nigel's cognitive expressions are entirely concrete. He shows no interest in concepts and abstractions and makes no generalizations. He relates events and things only in an ordinal sense and does so by rigidly compartmentalizing each. Thus, he verbalizes and arranges numbers but fails to use them in simple addition and subtraction operations. Otherwise, the narrative is purely descriptive of sights and sounds. Nigel has benefited both from a careful upbringing and a compara-tively advantaged physical status within the syndrome.

There is no evidence in *The world of Nigel Hunt* or in any of the 'bringing up our mongol' books that the fundamental performance limits of the syndrome have been surmounted or that nurture can influence these per-formance limits. These accounts include *Yesterday was Tuesday* by M. Y. Seagoe (1964); *Elizabeth* by Mary Green (1966); *David* by Nancy and Bruce Roberts (1968); *Slant-eyed angel* by J. Van der Hoeven (1968), *Small ship, great sea* by T. de Vries-Krutt (1971); and *Bernard* by John and Eileen Wilks

(1974). Where intellectual 'normalcy' is convincing, the accuracy of the diagnosis is usually questionable.

Intellectual normalcy and the diagnosis of DS

The traditional diagnostic approach, which pre-dated identification by cell analysis, was to count pathognomonic physical signs. Three or more, of seven to ten such signs, was taken as evidence for DS. The unreliability of this method is now well established. Gibson, Pozsonyi and Zarfas (1964) demonstrated that certain cardinal signs (the traditional major physical features used in confirming a diagnosis) are more diagnostically important than others and thus diagnosis by stigma counting can be a dangerously elastic procedure (see Table 2). There is little agreement about the proper definition of many indicator symptoms or their distribution over independently derived samples (see Table 3). Gibson and Frank (1961) illustrated a significant variability of diagnostic signs, with CA, especially for the traditional signs founded on skeletal system anomaly (see Tables 4 and 5). So-called dermatoid diagnostic signs proved to be more stable, with changes in age, and thus provided a more reliable identification index. Walker (1957) is credited with establishing formal statistical cutting-points using dermatoglyphic norms. Unfortunately, the palm and sole print method produces an appreciable overlap group between DS and normals. Diagnosis cannot, in these cases, be statistically confirmed. The Cant, Gerrard and Richards (1953) report of normal IQ in a DS child was subsequently questioned by Dunsdon, Carter and Huntley (1960) on the grounds that the dermatoglyphics, especially the palmar axial triradius (ATD) angle, did not support, even equivocally, a diagnosis of DS. Another instance of exceptional intelligence, for translocation DS, was reported by Finley et al. (1965). Follow-up by Rosecrans (1971) showed a WISC performance IQ of 68 and a psychometric finding of 'chronic brain disorder'. The child was 10 years CA at re-examination and had enjoyed a Binet IQ of 86 points some years earlier. While the diagnosis of DS is now taken from cytogenetic analysis, many previous reports of intellectual normalcy in DS were not so confirmed. Cases of apparent normalcy were usually very young and borderline for the clinical markers.

Penrose and Smith (1966) found a wide distribution of the superficial microsymptoms, identified with DS, in the normal population. Many normal individuals exhibit a few such signs and a number quite a few. The distribution of these DS-like physical minutae in normal populations has been claimed to vary with ethnic and familial origin, although there is some

Table 2. *Correlation matrix of the common cardinal anomalies of mongolism*

	Abnormal nostril direction	Abnormal toe spacing	Short 5th digit	Curved 5th digit	Squared hand	Epicanthic fold	Fissured tongue	Simian crease	Single 5th flexion	Abnormal ear	Adherent lobule
High cephalic index	-0.01	-0.09	-0.07	0.00	-0.12	0.14	0.03	-0.09	-0.17*	0.06	-0.02
Abnormal nostril direction	—	-0.16	-0.05	0.17	0.11	0.20*	-0.03	0.15	-0.05	0.02	-0.14
Abnormal toe spacing		—	0.04	-0.09	0.08	-0.09	-0.01	0.02	0.11	0.17	0.02
Short 5th digit			—	0.22*	0.04	0.05	-0.18	0.05	0.45*	-0.01	0.04
Curved 5th digit				—	0.03	0.03	0.15	0.03	0.36*	0.07	0.16
Squared hand					—	0.06	-0.06	0.25*	0.10	-0.04	-0.09
Epicanthic fold						—	0.00	0.17	-0.07	0.15	0.03
Fissured tongue							—	-0.03	0.14	0.00	0.06
Simian crease								—	0.12	0.11	-0.02
Single 5th flexion									—	0.05	-0.02
Abnormal ear										—	0.03

After Gibson, Pozsonyi and Zarfas (1964).
* Indicates statistical significance by chi-square (0.05 level or greater).

Table 3. *Comparative stigma occurrence by percentage for 100 mongoloids*

Stigmata	Gibson and Frank	Oster	Gibson and Gibbins	Newman	Levinson *et al.*	Johnson and Barnett	Means (%)
Cephalic index	42	—	34	53	—	62	48
Nostril direction	52	28	56	55	—	75	53
Toe spacing	44	47	66	95	44	—	59
Short 5th digit	41	57	50	48	66	—	52
Curved 5th digit	55	48	28	60	68	74	56
Squared hand	66	67	47	73	74	—	65
Epicanthus	66	28	44	100	50	46	56
Fissured tongue	82	59	75	95	44	90	74
Simian crease	58	43	56	43	48	36	47
Single 5th flexion	17	31	25	10	10	3	16
Abnormal ear	30	49	41	—	48	57	45
Adherent lobule	49	82	50	20	80	46	55
Abnormal heart	22	11	—	—	28	—	20

After Gibson, Pozsonyi and Zarfas (1964).
The stigma frequencies are treated arithmetically as if scores so as to preserve the
identity of the smaller samples. Total $N = 836$.

dispute (Buck, Valentine & Hamilton, 1966). Nor has cytogenetic evidence
been accepted as irrevocable. There have been reports of classical clinical
DS having a normal set of 46 chromosomes (for example, Schmid, Lee Chi
Hao & Smith, 1961). These accounts have since been discredited. Work by
Clarke, Edwards and Smallpiece (1961) demonstrated that atypical DS can
be a product of cell mosaicism, a phenomenon in which perhaps a minority
of body cells show the supernumerary chromosome. The aberrant cells could
easily be missed. Clarke *et al.* says that the mosaics may sometimes be
phenotypically normal but produce a high proportion of affected gametes.
The child examined by them had an IQ of 100 points at CA 2 years 3 months
and after her fifth birthday could count to 40. Laboratory analysis disclosed
an extra small acrocentric chromosome and 38% trisomic cells. Details of
dermatoglyphic analysis for this case were reported in *Nature* by Penrose
(1963a), who found 'some of the features of the mongol stereotype' (p. 935).
The clinical evidence supporting a diagnosis of DS is not convincing and the
dermatoglyphic evidence was not based on standardized (Walker, 1957)
techniques. Cellular irregularity can occur benignly in normals having otherwise healthy physical and psychological characteristics. A section to follow

Table 4. *The age stability of seven indices of mongolism; biserial correlations of chronological age (at time of stigma assessment) with stigma severity*

Stigmata	Number total	Number (severe)	Number (moderate)	Mean CA (severe)	Mean CA (moderate)	Difference	Standard deviations	Biserial correlations	t-Level
CI (+/− mean 0.876)	43	25	17	6.98	8.91	1.93	3.29	0.36	0.05
Fissured tongue	82	33	49	13.75	11.23	−2.52	3.55	−0.44	0.01
Four-finger furrow	58	26	32	10.82	12.02	1.20	3.65	0.20	—
Nostril direction	52	14	38	10.64	10.92	0.28	3.26	0.05	—
Single 5th flexion	17	14	3	10.93	15.00	4.07	3.88	0.59	0.05
Short 5th flexion	41	31	10	10.18	11.95	1.77	3.49	0.29	—
Curved 5th digit	55	44	11	11.30	10.90	−0.40	3.93	−0.06	—

After Gibson and Frank (1961).
Positive correlations denote decreasing severity with CA.

Table 5. *The age stability of thirteen indices of mongolism; biserial correlation of chronological age (at time of stigma assessment) with stigma occurrence*

Stigmata	Number normal	Number arrested	Mean chronological age (normal)	Mean chronological age (arrested)	Difference in mean age	Standard deviation	Biserial correlation	t-Test (Wallace Snedecor tables)
CI (+/− mean 0.82)	58	42	8.22	7.35	−0.87	3.33	−0.160	—
Nostril direction	48	52	12.40	10.85	−1.55	3.82	−0.248	0.05 level
Toe spacing	56	44	11.27	12.02	0.75	3.82	0.124	—
Short 5th digit	59	41	12.28	10.61	−1.67	3.82	−0.255	0.05 level
Curved 5th digit	45	55	12.04	11.23	0.81	3.82	0.130	—
Square hand	34	66	11.96	11.41	0.55	3.82	0.087	—
Epicanthic fold	34	66	12.74	11.00	−1.74	3.82	−0.273	0.01 level
Fissured tongue	18	82	8.61	12.25	3.64	3.82	0.535	0.01 level
Four-finger line	42	58	11.75	11.48	0.27	3.82	0.043	—
Single 5th flexion	83	17	11.53	11.64	0.11	3.82	0.020	—
Abnormal ear	70	30	11.50	11.80	0.30	3.82	0.050	—
Adherent lobule	51	49	11.80	11.37	0.43	3.82	0.070	—
Abnormal heart	78	22	7.88	8.14	0.26	3.33	0.035	—

After Gibson and Frank (1961).

examines more closely the likelihood of graded and partial DS and of *forme fustes* for the syndrome.

The search for intellectual normalcy in DS has raised a number of questions. These include (i) the reliability and predictive value of early high IQ scores for the syndrome, (ii) the variety of 'partial' karyotypes, karyotype overlaps and other cellular peculiarities which confuse the certainty of diagnosis and the precise definition of behavioural limits for the syndrome and (iii) the diagnostic significance of superficial stigmatization in otherwise normal individuals. Carter's (1967) male of 22 years, with IQ 80, and the Giraud *et al.* (1963) female of 17 years, with IQ 85, can probably be understood in these terms. A better appreciation of the interaction of somatic and behavioural artifacts would, presumably, aid in defining the dimensions of intelligence for the syndrome.

Biological aspects of intelligence in Down's syndrome

Research into the relationships between the mental and physical attributes of DS has taken two forms. One seeks a systematic link between the occurrence, severity or frequency of DS stigmata (in particular the traditional diagnostic signs) and measured intelligence. The second proposes a connection between IQ gradient, temperamental status and general body configuration for the syndrome. Interest in these two questions has been variously motivated.

(1) Prior to the discovery of the role of genetic over-sufficiency in the aetiology of DS, numerous possible causes were debated. The view that DS was caused by multiform factors led to some expectation of multiform clinical consequences, prompting attempts to identify symptom subtypes which could be made to correspond to the various postulated causes. Among the most likely of the aetiological positions were the effects of advancing maternal age, uterine exhaustion, irradiation of the mother, nervous disorders of the mother, nutritional variables and a host of imagined genetic mechanisms. Butler (1960) elaborated the multi-causal hypothesis. He found that the factoring of a large number of stigmata (78) for DS could be made to yield four classes, or a general class and three subgroups. Future work on the clustering of somatic and behavioural artifacts for DS might show the Butler solution to correspond to some extent with aberrant chromosomal subtypes.

(2) Some workers undertook stigma frequency-IQ studies to determine the clinical-phenotypical boundaries of DS and to establish the existence of *formes fustes*; especially they anticipated borderline occurrences where high

IQ was accompanied by less typical somatic features. For others, the aim was to establish a bridge between DS and clinically similar (e.g., cretinism) or undifferentiated forms of severe mental retardation. The attempt was to expand the range of explainable mental retardation by demonstrating clinical continuity between retardations of known and unknown cause.

(3) There have been efforts to test predisposing conditions using 'severity' gradients of DS (both for degree of mental defect and degree of physical expression) as the hypothetical dependent variable. The considerable literature, comparing the clinical artifacts of DS with advancing maternal age, provides an example of this approach (Penrose & Delhanty, 1961; Gibson & Frank, 1959; Kaariainen & Dingman, 1961; Rowe & Uchida, 1961; Coppen & Cowie, 1960). Gibson, Pozsonyi and Zarfas (1964) reported no connection between maternal age and type or frequency of microsymptoms, but did find a tenuous connection between severity of several microsymptoms and advancing maternal age. The search is complicated by the evidence that standard trisomy DS occurs more usually in older mothers and that standard trisomy DS might be more clinically typical than translocation DS (Gibson & Pozsonyi, 1965; Pozsonyi & Gibson, 1965).

(4) The prediction of learning capacity in DS is made uncertain by the non-linear nature of intellectual growth and by the capricious eroding of intellectual potential during the early years of life. Thus, the tailoring of ongoing behavoural, educational and other care styles for individual cases is still largely an intuitive procedure. One remote hope for the stigma frequency-IQ studies has been that they might permit eventual assay of the long-range behavioural capacity of a given DS child on the basis of his physical stigmata and karyotypic subclass.

Intelligence and the physical particulars

Hypotheses and problems

Students of the relationship between intellectual and physical status in DS have proposed (i) increasing intelligence with increasingly typical clinical configuration, (ii) decreasing intelligence with increasingly typical clinical picture, or (iii) no connection whatever between physical and intellectual indices. These observations have been of two general sorts, clinical and statistical.

The earliest naturalistic observations on the subject were those of Fennell (1904) and Shuttleworth (1909). Fennell remarked that 'the more marked the physical stigmata the deeper has been that amentia' (p. 34). The expression 'marked' may refer to frequency or severity (or both) of the usual diagnostic signs. Shuttleworth subscribed to Fennell's view. Of the mental peculiarities of DS, Shuttleworth said, 'These vary with the degree of mongolism which may be superficial or profound' (p. 664.) A similar position was taken by Engler (1949) who offered that the learning and development rate of DS is greatest in those with relatively few traditional physical signs. Another early opinion was presented by Sherlock and Donkin (1911). They claimed that, 'as with other diseases there is an inverse ratio between the severity of the symptoms and the duration of life...we find that idiots die young, the imbeciles probably break down before reaching middle life while the weak-minded, if suitably cared for, may attain a fairly advanced age' (p. 211). The sense of the observation seems to be that the relatively bright DS child has fewer somatic symptoms, especially of the sort that are apt to contribute to early death. Tredgold claimed (seen in McNeill, 1955) that 'there is a distinct relation between the degree of defect and the severity of the physical signs' (p. 218)

Later opinion was more varied. Spuehler (1929), Fanconi (1939) and Oster (1953), held that any systematic connection between symptom configuration and mentation in DS would be unlikely. Oster claimed 'no correlation can be demonstrated between the number of mongoloid stigmata and the degree of mental deficiency' (p. 55). Oster offered no statistical evidence for this conclusion. Curiously, he does claim later that 'the stated tabulations show furthermore that among the mongols with particularly few cardinal signs only a small number had a relatively high intellectual standard' (p. 70). This would indicate that lightly stigmatized DS individuals are especially amented; a similar clinical opinion has been offered by Donaldson (1961). Jones, Croley and Levy (1960) examined the relation between physical and mental retardation but with inconclusive results.

Statistical studies of the doubtful relationship between stigma frequency and amentia level for DS began with Tennies (1943). He said, 'not all mongoloid defectives had the same degree of physical stigmata and that those with the fewer signs of mongolism appeared to have a higher mental age' (p. 48). Tennies referred to a supporting opinion by Ward (1941). Considering hypotonia in DS to be especially representative of the clinical stereotype, Tennies reported joint flexibility or marked hypotonia in 129 of 188 idiot cases, 156 of 256 imbecile cases and three of eight morons. Expressed as percentages (68%, 61% and 38% respectively) it appears that the more amented are also the more physically afflicted. Tennies explained his IQ-stigma data in terms of differential mortality effects, thus,

When it is considered that the MA increases with the CA and that a high CA shows a lack of stigmata it seems reasonable to assume that on the whole the fewer the stigmata and the fainter their characteristics the better chance the mongoloid has of living longer and showing a higher intellectual level than his more unfortunate brothers. (p. 53)

The first large scale statistical treatment of the problem was made by Shepard, McGreal and Hammer (1957), incidental to an investigation of new methods of analysing clinical material to isolate central factors. Forty somatic and behavioural measures were taken from 96 DS children, to produce 800 inter-correlation coefficients. Degree of DS was based on height percentile, cephalic index, hyperextensibility, hand involvement and eye involvement. A correlation coefficient between degree of DS and IQ percentile, in the order of +0.65, was found. Intelligence test scores appeared, however, to have been one of the criteria for determining degree of somatic expressions for DS. Gibson and Gibbins (1958) tested the proposed link for stigma frequency and Binet IQ using only the classical cardinal stigmata. Thirty-two cases (16 males and 16 females) were examined for presence of 14 traditional diagnostic signs. These signs were selected for degree of pathogonomy, ease of recognition and relative age stability. There was the expected tendency to decreasing IQ with increasing age but not significantly so. The mean CA of the sample was 9.4 years. No case was less than 4 years CA (below which the sharpest growth deceleration is known to occur) while the upper limit of CA 21 years was selected so as to avoid some of the intellectual decline associated with premature 'ageing'.

Statistical analysis of IQ, on number of stigmata, yielded a significant regression-based correlation coefficient of 0.422 (see addenda, Gibson, 1962). The purpose of the study was to support the argument that individual clinical patterns within the syndrome might be related to differential involvement of the major tissue systems in embryo (i.e., the skeletal and nervous systems reaching maximum general susceptibility to internally or externally initiated pathological influences at different periods of foetal development). Benda (1960 a, b) was of the opinion that the clinical stereotype for DS was fundamentally an expression of skeletal system arrest. Arey (1954) stated that at between 10 and 12 foetal weeks, ossification is spreading and that by 16 weeks some bones are distinctly indicated. With respect to the nervous system, however, not until between 20 and 40 weeks do cerebral fissures and convolutions appear and myelinization of the brain begins. The cerebral cortex is layered typically during this period. Baumeister and Williams (1967) have similarly proposed the matching of pathological effects with the maturational timing of the various body systems in embryo, and these, in turn, with subtype of cytogenetic anomaly.

The initial statistical studies of the correlation of physical and psychological artifacts for DS were unreliable with respect to methodology and to assumptions made. It will help to review the difficulties, by class, before beginning to consider recent evidence.

(1) First, it would be essential to establish and adequately compensate for the age variability of the physical stigmata of DS. Both IQ and stigma occurrence (along with stigma severity and sampling frequency) are thought to change with age (Gibson and Frank, 1961). If the physical anomalies of DS tend to recede with age, and if amentia level quite independently deepens with age, then an entirely fortuitous but statistically significant relation could be shown between the two sets of observations.

(2) Criteria for selection of stigma are of importance insofar as relatively few of the several hundred physical anomalies of DS can be viewed as especially pathognomonic. A pathognomonic or cardinal diagnostic sign of DS (i) must occur with a high frequency in DS and a low frequency in other forms of mental retardation, and in the normal population, (ii) must be ethnologically independent in any major sense, (iii) should have a suitable degree of assessment reliability, (iv) must be substantially independent of the occurrence of most other pathognomic signs and (v) should be age stable or at least age accountable. Some questions have been raised about each of these conditions in relation to previous studies (Gibson, Pozsonyi and Zarfas, 1964; Gibson and Frank, 1961; Baumeister and Williams, 1967).

(3) A corollary to the foregoing, involves the extent to which the stigmata of DS can be mathematically manipulated so as to permit the establishment of comparative frequencies of pooled diagnostic signs. Some rationalization would be needed so that individual cardinal signs would be of equal diagnostic weight. Otherwise, indicators A and B might have more diagnostic influence than signs C through G, thereby making arithmetical nonsense of summed stigma frequency comparisons. Differential weighting of the cardinal indices of DS was attempted by Gibson (1966) on the basis of the occurrence of each across a number of independent samples.

(4) Instrumentation for the measurement of intelligence for the syndrome has descended largely from usage and convenience. Most previous studies have employed some form of the Binet scales or item-related infant schedules, e.g., the Kuhlmann. These instruments have been useful with normal populations but generate perplexing questions about relevance, reliability and prediction when used with DS. A variety of other devices have been tried (e.g., Porteus Mazes, Columbia mental maturity scale) but are unsuitable because of the narrow skill base they represent. The effective testing of somatic–behavioural specificity hypotheses would require the use of a multidimensional psychometric battery combined with life performance indices.

(5) The assumption of a linear distribution for any proposed amentia–stigma interaction has been applied to most statistical treatments of such connections; despite the Penrose (1949) caution that 'biological–psychological phenomena are typically arranged in non-linear fashion'. Gibson (1966) attempted a curvilinear solution of the regression of amentia level on weighted physical stigmata, with encouraging results.

(6) Since many of the physical stigmata included in the traditional diagnostic battery occur at very low frequencies, any evident IQ-stigma connection might be unreliable when samples are small; as has been usually the case. Sampling is further biased (i) by the high early mortality rate for DS which operates to leave a clinically atypical residue for later study, and (ii) by the frequent use of institutional populations. The distribution of IQ tends to be attenuated within custodial programmes. On the other hand, IQ distributions of community samples can be distorted by intensive rote training of DS children for test-related skills. The effect is either to obscure or magnify IQ-stigma frequency relationships.

Gibson (1966) and Baumeister and Williams (1967) have summarized the foregoing methodological difficulties, along with a number of additional problems. Among these is the possibility that the stigma–intelligence association might be genuine only for certain abilities and/or confined to particular subgroups of physical stigmata. Also mentioned is the possibility that the traditional (pre-cytogenetic) diagnostic approach might have required the brighter DS individual to demonstrate more convincing clinical evidence, than would a less intelligent member. The effect would be for a positive correlation in the direction of higher IQ with greater stigma frequency. There is the final point that children with low IQ *and* many typical stigmata are probably institutionalized earlier thus creating institutional samples which favour significant stigma–IQ concordance.

Evaluating the evidence

The retest of Gibson and Gibbins (1958) original hypothesis for a positive correlation between cardinal stigma frequency and IQ began with the work of Johnson and Barnett (1961). They engaged 88 institutionalized DS patients. The CA range was 6 years 6 months to 45 years with a mean of 21 years. The Stanford–Binet findings spanned 24 months to 72 months MA with a mean of 43 months. Twenty-three physical signs of DS were evaluated. Age stability ranges, for individual stigmata, were established against the Oster (1953) criteria. They found no significant statistical connection between test intelligence and stigma frequency. The Johnson and Barnett study had incorporated suitable controls for some of the problems already cited. However, their study used many stigmata not especially cardinal or pathognomonic for the syndrome. Numerous specific physical anomalies, seen equally in DS and other forms of mental retardation, were employed. Oster (1953) has identified some of these 'universal' anomalies of mental retardation (p. 44). Furthermore, selection of a sample having a mean CA of 21 years invites a type II statistical error; a product of the effects of ageing on intelligence as well as the tendency for adult DS to be suppressed for range, variety and power of intellectual expression following a number of years of routine custodial care. Johnson and Barnett (1961) indicate an IQ range of 14 to 40 points for their patients (mean = 26 points) but offered no standard deviations on which to assess the appropriateness of Pearson product–moment correlational analysis. Non-linearity of regression was noted but not incorporated in the statistical analysis.

Kaariainen and Dingman (1961) examined several aspects of performance for DS against a variety of clinical and case history variables. These authors identified a major sampling difficulty to be the more frequent and earlier institutionalization of the less clinically typical. They proposed too, that older DS subjects are a somatically distorted residue of the population because of the influence of high early mortality. Gibson, Pozsonyi and Zarfas (1964) demonstrated the probability that there are differences in the clinical stereotype among surviving DS, i.e., between those with congenital heart disorder (CHD), a major cause of early death in DS, and those without. The 22% of their series having congenital heart defect produced a mean stigma frequency of 6.82, while those cases with no evidence for CHD had a mean stigma frequency of 5.75. The study was based on 100 cases and indicated that the less clinically typical cases of DS tend to survive longer. There is the further possibility that sex plays some role in spurious correlations insofar as the female of the syndrome is said to expire earlier than the male and, at the same time, is more clinically typical. The problem is elaborated in the chapter to follow.

The stigma–IQ link is distorted by the change, in time, of the clinical expression of individual stigmata. The tendency is for cephalic indices to approach normal criteria with advancing age, for fissuring of the tongue to increase with time, for nostril direction to be less typically 'mongoloid' as age advances, and for recession of the epicanthic fold as adulthood approaches. These microsymptoms are especially important in contributing to the visual stereotype of DS and have acquired diagnostic importance beyond their empirical value (Gibson and Frank, 1961). Especially noticeable is a tendency for the presumably age stable dermal stigmata to vary with age;

indicating the effects of differential mortality and/or of differential institutional intake trends with advancing age. Cross-sectional sampling of institutionalized DS might, accordingly, reveal fewer stigmata and declining intelligence with advancing CA, both as independent events.

The approach of Kaariainen and Dingman (1961) illustrates some of the foregoing difficulties. Forty subjects were examined at a Finnish institution. Ten diagnostic signs, postulated by Oster as cardinal, comprised the definition of 'degree' of DS. A number of these signs are, however, age variable according to the findings of Gibson and Frank (1961). Secondly, since range and standard deviations for CA are not offered by Kaariainen and Dingman, it is impossible to estimate how representative their sample was clinically. Adult populations, institutionalized for many years have often deteriorated intellectually and display recession of microsymptoms such that no reliable conclusions for biological–behavioural specificity are possible.

The Kaariainen and Dingman correlation between subject age and degree of mongolism (frequency of selected microsymptoms) was not significant; indicating that their sample was older and clinically stable. Measures of intelligence included a pegboard, formboard, picture–vocabulary test, colour tests, and 'degree of subnormality'. There is no indication of how the latter was computed or of the source, validity or reliability of the specific skill and aptitude tests mentioned. None of the usual standardized measures of intelligence had apparently been used in this study. The unreliability of specialized performance items, when used with DS for the assessment of intelligence, has been discussed. Nevertheless, they find some interesting links between 'degree' of DS and pegboard, formboard, and picture–vocabulary test scores. Subsequent factor analysis led provisionally to the conclusion that the lower the pegboard score, the greater the degree of DS, clinically. Evaluation is difficult without details of the methods employed.

Domino and Newman (1965) examined 128 institutional DS for 82 physical characteristics. Many of these signs were 'not necessarily pathognomonic of mongolism', and therefore not cardinal in the sense of generally accepted diagnostic criteria. Six signs involved some sort of quantification, whereas the 76 other stigmata were evaluated only qualitatively. The Stanford–Binet and the Cattell scales were used throughout. No correlations were computed between CA and test intelligence. The stigmata were weighted according to frequency of occurrence, deduced from the average of a number of independent samples, in order to award appropriate diagnostic emphasis to the most common stigmata. No adjustments were made for the uniqueness of a given symptom to the syndrome, or for symptom independence. These difficulties of stigma-based diagnosis are mentioned by Oster (1953), Penrose

(1949) and Gibson and Frank (1961). Domino and Newman found five of the commonly accepted signs of DS to be significantly correlated with IQ. These are IQ and protrusion of the tongue (-0.28), furrowed tongue (-0.22), wide toe space (-0.10), irregular dentition (-0.19) and dry skin (-0.19). All five significant coefficients are in a direction opposite to that usually postulated. These particular indices are also significantly variable with age. Since no control of the age factor was undertaken for the individual signs, the few positive findings of Domino and Newman are suspect.

An expectation has been that if the individual stigmata of DS are not correlated with test intelligence then no stigma frequency–IQ relationship could exist. The Gibson and Gibbins data showed that none of 13 individual cardinal signs of DS were significantly related to IQ level. The frequency occurrence of these same signs did nevertheless vary with intelligence level. Possibly, the diagnostic signs for DS relate to intellectual potential on a configural rather than on an additive basis. Or else, no single diagnostic indicator accounts for sufficient variance to be manifest statistically. In any event, Domino and Newman concluded that there was no functional relation between the psychological and physiological particulars of the syndrome.

Newman (1960) likewise reported no connection between IQ and single stigma occurrence. His major concern was to identify the relation of stigma frequency to test intelligence. He employed 40 cases having ages ranging from seven to 28 years, with a median CA of 15 years. The IQ range was from seven to 28 points on the Binet scale. Fifteen stigmata were identified as meeting the various selection criteria for cardinal signs. Chronological age and test intelligence were not significantly correlated. Preliminary analysis showed a simple product–moment correlation coefficient, between IQ and stigma frequency, in the order of 0.46 for the males and 0.28 for the females (0.05 level of significance for both). Semi-log and log-log adjustments of the IQ–stigma frequency correlations yielded 0.44 (raised from a total sample correlation coefficient of 0.31) and 0.59 respectively. Some other interesting phenomena isolated by Newman are the marked sex differences in intelligence level, the relentless deterioration of IQ with advancing age, and the considerable interdependence of the individual cardinal diagnostic signs of DS. The heterogeneity of the features of DS suggested to him that the syndrome might encompass a number of related but overlapping subgroups, both clinically and causally. It was Newman's contention that stratification for additional variables, such as aberrant cytogenetic subtype, might expose other and even stronger somatic–behavioural interactions for DS.

Single stigma studies abound. Engler (1949) suggested that 'the more pronounced the degree of mongolism in a case, the greater the likelihood of epicanthus being present' (p. 21). Dunsdon, Carter, and Huntley (1960) tested one clinical sign of DS, the palmar axial triradius (ATD) angle against test intelligence for a community sample. Their tables revealed no connection between magnitude of ATD angle and 'bright' (IQ 45+) or 'not bright' (undefined) patients matched for sex and age. Range and standard deviation of the sum of the ATD angles, for the two groups, are quite divergent and in the direction of greater homogeneity for the 'bright' group ($N = 10$). The futility of testing the relation of single stigmata, to other artifacts of DS is well documented. Pozsonyi, Gibson and Zarfas (1964) found a correlation of -0.41 for IQ and bone age. First-order partial correlation, accounting for the effect of the IQ–CA and the CA–bone age relation, produced a final IQ–bone age correlation of -0.08.

Evidently, actuarial studies of the interaction of structure and function in DS are little more certain than was the naturalistic evidence. Perhaps the major virtue of the statistical approach has been to identify the variables which mask exposure of these interactions. The central problems, for the statistical analysis of clinical-behavioural phenomena for DS have been (i) a neglect of age effects, (ii) the tendency of most investigators to treat the physical concomitants of DS as of equal pathognomonic stature, and (iii) a failure to adjust statistical treatments to the observed non-linearity of the regressions of intellectual indices and cardinal sign frequencies in full age-range samples. A study by Gibson (1966) attempted to meet these limitations.

Gibson (1966) selected 100 diagnostically confirmed cases of DS from an age range (5 to 19 years) where least variability of cardinal physical stigmata is thought to occur. Age variability, for each physical sign, was nevertheless calculated and controlled by computation. The physical stigmata were then assigned a weight proportional to their individual frequency occurrences in the sample. The frequency occurrence of the cardinal diagnostic signs was consistent with those presented by Gibson *et al.* (1964) and by Domino and Newman (1965). Two problems were examined. First, the diagnostic potency of the cardinal physical stigmata was tested ranking each by magnitude of relation to test intelligence. The simple frequency occurrence of individual physical signs was then ranked so as to calculate a rho coefficient for the two continua. A correlation coefficient of 0.61 resulted, indicating some validity for the belief that the various traditional cardinal diagnostic criteria of DS have unequal pathognomonic importance. A second analysis tested the relation of the resulting weighted frequency of physical stigmata and IQ level. The product–moment correlation coefficient, between these 13 weighted cardinal signs and IQ levels, was 0.12 (not statistically significant).

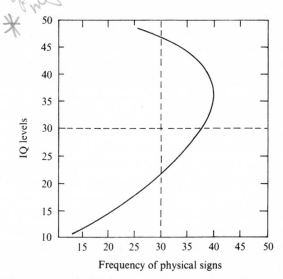

Fig. 3. Distribution of weighted frequency of 13 physical signs of Down's syndrome with IQ. (From D. Gibson (1966). *American Journal of Mental Deficiency*, **71**, 433–6.)

Fig. 3 traces the nature of the distribution of frequency of physical signs, with IQ level. The linear assumption is clearly inappropriate. The IQ-stigma frequency regressions were then computed using correlation ratios (eta). Analysis of variance results, for predicting frequency (weighted) of physical indices from IQ, was not significant. However, the analysis of variance for predicting the IQ of DS from frequency (weighted) of physical stigmata, was statistically significant. These findings indicate a reasonably consistent connection between the somatic and performance dimensions of the syndrome and the possibility (though presently remote) of forecasting performance levels on the basis of somatic status.

Morphology and intelligence in Down's syndrome

A quite different approach to understanding the reciprocity of the physiological and psychological dimensions of DS was initiated by Crookshank (1925). His book, *The mongol in our midst*, detailed a conspiratorial fantasy concerning the origins of the syndrome, along with supporting anecdotal evidence. His thesis was that DS is atavistic or racially regressive in origin and that only the more 'advanced' peoples suffer these genetic throw-backs. Racially Mongolian peoples do not produce clinical 'mongolism', he claimed, although evidence appearing since has identified DS across all racial and ethnic groups. Only some 'mongoloids' moreover are retarded. The others are intellectually normal and said to be among us. They are cast as less noble than is the birthright for European peoples and are said to be easily recognized by their mongol-like physical appearance. These 'normal' mongoloids (DS) lack creativity but possess dangerous cunning and often rise to important positions in society. The significance of Crookshank's work has been discussed previously, in an historical context.

Notwithstanding the Darwinian distortions of Crookshank, a number of workers in the field of morphological enquiry have been impressed by the dwarfism and generally consistent rotund appearance of DS, while being perplexed by the frequent exceptions to the rule, such as a taller, slimmer variety. It was an easy next step to polarize DS by body type, searching for distinctive behavioural outcomes. Some of these writers have preferred the term 'congenital acromicria' (shortening of the distal bones) to describe morphologically typical DS (Schuller, 1907; Clift, 1922; Benda, 1949). The clinical evidence is scanty. The developmental morphology of DS was explored by Scano (1958) who catalogued the body build of 65 DS children during their first 2 years of life. He reported that, as early as six months, they are different in body build from normal infants, and presumably owe these differences to inherent aberration of growth. Goldstein (1956a, b) searched for behavioural variables associated with body build in DS. He identified two groups, using criteria of morphology and behaviour; (i) the thyroid deficient was marked by dwarfism, atonia, wide facial features, pudgy hands and feet, docile personality, and relatively high IQ and (ii) the pituitary deficient who seemed taller and slimmer, was of lower IQ and displayed the incurved fifth palmar digit more frequently than the first type. The second type of DS was also said to be more restless and to succumb to a greater frequency and depth of emotional disturbance. These findings have been reviewed by Hallenbeck (1960). She treated Goldstein's conclusions as speculative but anticipated that a proven link between morphological and behavioural potentials for DS would enhance the effectiveness of parent counselling.

The Goldstein hypothesis has been tested directly on two occasions, first by Mosier (1962) and again by Tang and Chagnon (1967). Mosier, using the Gray and Ayers growth norms for children, undertook a cross-sectional anthropometric comparison of hospitalized DS and non-DS patients. The finding were for a correlation of shorter stature with lower IQ. However, a similar trend was noted for other aetiological groups of retardates and in the normal population, suggesting a host of non-genetic, non-syndromic explanations. Tang and Chagnon tested the view that there is a systematic relation between intelligence and height/weight ratios, across a sample of

258 DS cases. The sample was stratified for age and split into two groups within each age level: those in the upper and those in the lower quartiles of the height/weight ratio. The upper height/weight ratio group (from 0.74 to 3.13) showed a mean IQ of 33.62 points. The lower height/weight ratio group (from 0.35 to 1.45) showed a mean IQ of 27.95 points. Chronological age was similar for the two groups. The mean IQ differences of almost 6 points was statistically significant. There is a tendency then for the shorter and heavier DS subject (the typical cases) to display higher IQs than the taller and slimmer 'type'. The relationship is not a strong one and is of questionable practical value. Tang and Chagnon tested the predictive power of the finding, using the chi-square method, and concluded (i) that in forecasting IQ from body build for the two extreme groups, 42% of the total sample would be incorrectly placed and (ii) that individual prognosis on these criteria alone is not yet possible. A replication of the study might attempt additional stratification for aberrant cytological subgroup, diagnostic particulars, nutritional and nurtural factors, and sex.

Karyotype and the IQ–stigma debate

Baumeister and Williams (1967) re-evaluated the IQ–stigma research using recent studies of the behavioural outcomes of variation of karyotype for DS. They proposed a connection between the concept of foetal timing of insult (different timetables of maximum susceptibility of distortion of tissue systems in embryo) and selective chromosome action. Their proposition is summarized as follows:

Gibson and Gibbins (1958) interpreted the results of a positive relationship between frequency of stigmata and intellectual functioning in terms of onset of the biochemical anomalies and their influence on embryonic development. Most of the common signs are directly or indirectly related to the skeletal system. The skeletal and nervous system commence their differentiation from cellular mass at different embryonic periods. Therefore, the two systems would reach different critical points in respect to their maximum susceptibility to pathology. Moreover, Gibson and Gibbins assume that there are differences among individuals in the relative susceptibility of the two systems to the cause or causes of Down's syndrome. (p. 590)

Baumeister and Williams identified the weakness of the argument as a failure to account for 'individual variability with respect to timing of the onset of the condition in embryo' but offered that:

In view of recent cytological discoveries showing that mongolism can be associated with a number of chromosome disorders, it is possible that the different genetic errors involved would differentially affect skeletal and nervous development. An explanation such as that proposed by Gibson may have some merit in this context. (p. 590)

The identification of genotypic variables allied with the biological and behavioural features of DS is more promising than debating such surface phenomena as IQ–stigma frequency correlations. Considering the extensive biochemical and metabolic consequences of the chromosome anomaly it would be surprising to find no somatic or behavioural concomitants attributable to variations of karyotype within the syndrome. For example, low abnormal cell frequency (mosaicism) DS, having both atypical or minimal clinical features and high intelligence, has been reported (Rosecrans, 1968) but not subsequently supported. Other cytological–somatic comparisons have been drawn between classical trisomy and translocation DS. Gibson and Pozsonyi (1965) examined the frequency of cardinal stigmata for a group of 20 age-matched translocated and standard trisomy cases. Stigma frequency differences, while in the direction of a more stereotyped clinical configuration and higher IQs for the translocation DS, were not large. An additional impression was of a more obvious dwarfism in the standard trisomy (80%) than in the translocation series. Dermatoglyphic patterns differed; (i) there being higher average palmar axial triradii for the trisomy group and (ii) the translocation dermatoglyphic indices (Walker method) tending, comparatively, to fall in the diagnostically equivocal range. Palmar differences, representing position of the ATD angle and presence or absence of the simian crease, are related apparently to skeletal distortions (Gibson and Frank, 1961). The more pronounced acromicria of standard trisomy DS, and thus the more obviously squared hand, might enhance fuller expression of the classical dermatoglyphic picture. These findings are in dispute (Soltan, 1965; Gibson, 1965; Ong et al., 1967). It is not intended here to review the dermatoglyphics of DS but merely to focus the debate on a possible relation of karyotype to somatic–behavioural expression across the syndrome.

On the other hand, Ong et al. (1967) found no height/weight differences between translocation and trisomy DS. Clinical distinctions included evidence for congenital heart disorder in five translocations ($N = 12$) and in only one trisomy control case. The implication of the finding is that differential mortality rates might be governed by karyotype. Other clinical distinctions noted included poorer muscle tone, a greater frequency of simian crease, high arched palate, flat nasal bridge, and other deviant skeletal characteristics, all for the standard trisomy sample. These data reinforce the view that translocation DS cases possess less of the classical symptoms than do the standard trisomy variety. Given also the eight point IQ difference, favouring the translocation series, the findings of Ong et al. might support a relation between the physical and intellectual particulars of DS, at least inferentially, based on genotypic variation within the syndrome.

Johnson and Abelson (1969 a, b) examined stigma differences (type and frequency) for translocation, standard trisomy and mosaicism DS. The trisomy group displayed a lower IQ than the translocation and, at the same time, a higher stigma frequency. The latter finding was not statistically significant. The 14 diagnostic signs employed included such ethereal items as rosy cheeks, impressions about toe length, hand length, space between the big toe and second toe and so on. Many of these clinical minutiae are not pathognomonic for the condition and are highly impressionistic, sex variable and age variable.

Shipe, Reisman, Chung, Chin-Young, Darnell and Kelly (1968) attempted to discover stigma–IQ correlations *within* discrete aberrant cytological subgroups. Twenty-five were trisomic, three were D/G translocations and three were mosaic for DS. All children had been seen in a community clinic over a 5 year period. They concluded, 'It does appear evident, however, that mosaic individuals scored above the trisomic children in addition to showing fewer physical evidences of Down's syndrome.' (p. 790). Polani (1963) had similarly claimed that an observed discrepancy for stigma count and IQ in DS might provide an index of potential mosaicism. No such findings were obtained exclusively for the trisomy group. Of the 19 individual stigmata studied, only the occurrence of dry skin and slanting eyes were associated significantly with lower IQ levels. The mosaicism subgroup was too small to support further analyses. In any event, the frequency mosaicism–IQ relationship is in doubt (Gibson, 1973; Fishler, 1975). Fishler does confirm that mosaics are brighter than age and sex matched trisomy-21 (mean IQ 67 versus 53 points) individuals.

Somatic or behavioural uniqueness, as a product of karyotype variation in DS, has been briefly reviewed here to account possibly for some of the discord in the stigma frequency–IQ literature. A more critical examination is made in the chapter to follow.

Predicting psychological events on the basis of the clinical and somatic configuration of DS is promising but still inconclusive overall. The methodological and sampling complexities are partly to blame. To return to Fig. 3, it is clear that if a wide ranging IQ (and therefore age) sample is drawn, the curvilinear expression of the IQ–Stigma relation would work against significant linear correlations. On accelerating portions of this curve, a more severely retarded sample might manifest a positive correlation between frequency of physical markers and intellectual level. A thoroughly institutionalized group of older DS patients, where there has been suppression of individuality or intellectual deterioration, would support no significant IQ–stigma frequency correlation. The other possibility, that of a negative relation between degree of defect and physical stigmatization, might be understood in terms of subtype of chromosome anomaly, if at all. Robinson and Robinson in their 1976 edition of *The mentally retarded child* dismiss the problem with one study (Domino & Newman, 1965). The lay literature also tends to reject the hypothesis (Brinkworth & Collins, 1969), perhaps because it is distasteful to think that biological or cytogenetic status in infancy could indicate future behavioural outcomes for DS or any other human condition. Conceivably, a more refined index of somatic events could facilitate prediction of typical versus atypical intellectual growth rates and mental status at maturity for individual cases of DS. One such approach would be to develop a clinical forecast instrument considering the cardinal stigmata and morphological data together with the intellectual growth formulae proposed by Zeaman and House (1962) and Gibson (1966). Known sources of IQ–stigma variance associated with cytogenetic subclass, secondary pathology and sex could be incorporated. The device would be at least of research value.

Evaluation

Investigations of the structure of intelligence in DS have been largely descriptive and without regard for the likely antecedents. The neglect is understandable. The syndrome was thought to be non-genetic, unicausal, and more or less, clinically uniform. Prior to the finding of manifold cytogenetic causes, with their patterned but overlapping biological and psychological consequences physical and behavioural differences, when acknowledged, were attributed to the caprice of this or that causal condition. Our understanding of the dimensions of intelligence for the syndrome is therefore in flux.

Studies of central tendency for intelligence in DS were undertaken to show up the falsity of the pre-1900 clinical dogma that the syndrome was invariably of custodial (idiot) quality. Later psychodiagnostic testing placed most in the trainable (imbecile) category, at least during childhood. The psychometric stereotype of the post-clinical era became increasingly ambiguous, however, as further advances in mental testing showed DS infants to be close to normal and some younger children to achieve educable (moron) levels. Many older institutionalized patients regressed to custodial status while other DS adults exceeded expectation by carrying a stable trainable level of intelligence into adulthood to perform moderately well in protected community settings. So it was that purely environmental explanations of these differences become popular, biological accounts being dismissed as uncertain and deterministic. The study of syndromic events, in relation to behavioural expectations, is too recent to counterbalance the long-standing nurtural constructs.

Whatever the motivation, the search for parameters of intelligence in DS has disclosed a greater than expected range and diversity of behavioural potential and has generated a concern for (i) the efficacy of various care systems, (ii) the vagaries and roots of intellectual 'deterioration', with increasing age, (iii) a unique intellectual status for the syndrome, and (iv) whether or not DS is more or less retarded, as a group, now than in previous years. The resolution of these issues will enhance management effectiveness; but only if future study abandons cross-sectional sampling (where the consequences of differential mortality rate are difficult to assess) and is more sensitive to the biological and maturational factors.

The influence of selective mortality, on the mapping of the dimensions of intelligence for DS, deserves a special word. Warner (1935) reported that half of her sample had died during the course of study, at an average age of 12.6 months. Berg and Stern (1963) discovered that of 141 DS autopsies, 79 included lesions of the cardiovascular system. Tennies (1943) claimed that most of the early deaths were cases of idiot calibre, the older survivors being predominantly imbecile. One effect, in the short-run, would be the impression of increased intelligence for the syndrome. For the longer term, Tennies predicted that improving medical and other care standards would ensure the increasing survival of custodial level DS, thereby securing a decrease of mean IQ. Thus, there can be no simple or unyielding composite picture of intellectual modes, limits and patterning for DS. Perhaps it hardly matters insofar as the principal applied research goal is for the improvement of environmental and biological intervention techniques for individual DS children. Until the sources of the variablity of intelligence for DS can be determined, questions about majority mental age, the nature of the deceleration of intellectual growth rates of ageing, upper IQ limits, and the qualitative dimensions of intelligence, will remain unanswered.

4

The foundations of intelligence

Mapping the dimensions of intelligence for DS has not been a remarkable success, either clinically or statistically. The reasons have more to do with assumptions than with the nature of the data. One problem is that the physical configuration of the syndrome is so compelling that we expect attenuated ranges of psychological deficits and reliable modal characteristics. Instead, the literature shows considerable variability between cases and across age groups. A companion problem is our inclination to explain individual differences in environmental terms only. It is customary of late to regard DS children who flourish as the product of superior care and those who languish, as victims of mismanagement. What we know or suspect now is that (i) neuro-maturational status differs between cases from birth, (ii) the sources of developmental variability are concomitant with abnormal structural, neurophysiological and metabolic processes, in some cases exacerbated by nurtural conditions, and (iii) bio-behavioural similarities and differences are more or less programmed by the aberrant karyotype. It is unreasonable, therefore, to impose the same expectations on all DS individuals or to dismiss the syndromic modalities in programme planning for the disorder as a whole. The purpose of the present chapter is to examine the correlates of intelligence, for the syndrome, in terms of what these tell us about the origins of the behavioural stereotype. Deduction of a management policy is not a difficult final step.

Intelligence and karyotype

Connecting karyotype, through its variations, with physical or psychological outcomes, is a first stage in understanding mediational processes and in promoting behavioural prediction and intervention.

Hypotheses about the psychological outcomes of karyotype date from Clarke, Edward and Smallpiece (1961) who described trisomy mosaicism in

78

an intelligent girl having some features of the syndrome. Other clinical reports explored frequency of aberrant cells and level of intelligence, but with little agreement. Valencia *et al.* (1963) described a case having 62% and 70% abnormal cells on blood and marrow analysis and an IQ of 75 points. Lindstein *et al.* (1962) claimed normal intelligence for a DS individual having 61% trisomic cells. Chaudhuri and Chaudhuri (1965) guessed that their patient was seriously retarded, having 59% trisomic cells. Some of the dissonance might be attributable to the use of incompatible diagnostic standards (clinically) and to the age differences across cases (see Hayashi *et al.*, 1962; Weinstein and Warkany, 1963; Verresen *et al.*, 1964; Finley *et al.*, 1965; Hamerton *et al.*, 1965). Later studies compared samples of trisomy mosaicism with translocation and standard trisomy DS. Overall findings suggest that (i) mosaics are less severely retarded than translocations or standard trisomy DS, (ii) translocation DS displays less intellectual deficit than does standard trisomy DS, and (iii) some somatic and personality traits are distributed according to subclass of karyotype. The extent of agreement is by no means perfect and methodological faults abound, as will be evident in the two following passages.

Mosaicism studies

The most insidious of the methodological problems surrounding correlations of frequency of affected cells and intelligence for DS is the CA/IQ interaction. A finding of significant intellectual variation with percentage mosaicism, was first offered by Zellweger and Abbo (1963). They assembled seven clinical reports, concluding that severe mental handicap was most apparent where over half of the cells cultured were abnormal for karyotype. Near-normal intelligence was evident where the majority of cultured cells were unaffected. Their hope was that behavioural outcomes, and appropriate management decisions, might be anticipated from a knowledge of karyotype deviation. The thesis was advanced by Shipe *et al.* (1968) who added three cases to a collection of previously published case reports of trisomy DS to find that when over 50% normal cells are evident, intelligence level is mildly retarded or better. Where there is less than 50%, the mid-trainable range of mental defect is more common. While no check for age effect was conducted, it is prophetic that a correlation of −0.31 occurred between CA and IQ for the non-mosaicism control sample. Johnson and Abelson (1969 *a*) compared 18 mosaicism DS with 238 standard trisomy DS. Their mosaicism cases displayed a mean IQ of 28.94 and the non-mosaic trisomies, 31.11 points. No CA data were reported. Rosecrans (1968) examined 20 cases of mosaicism

DS, finding a mean IQ of 66 points and correlation coefficients of −0.89 (skin analysis), and −0.31 (blood analysis) between IQ and frequency of abnormal cells. These findings attribute almost 30% of the variance associated with retardation levels for DS to a single within-syndrome karyotypic index. Kohn et al. (1970) questioned the appropriateness of including the IQs of phenotypically normal adults in the computations.

Rosecrans' sample included 16 DS subjects. Of these, IQ and karyotype data (based on blood samples) were available for eight. It was thus possible to recalculate his correlations making the necessary corrections for sample composition and CA effects. Adjusted correlation coefficients for the refined sample were −0.50 (0.05 level) for IQ and abnormal cell frequency (skin tissue analysis), and −0.14 for IQ and the blood cell data. The combination for tissue sources proved non-significant. Age effects were then assessed using first-order partial correlation technique. A coefficient of −0.41 emerged between Rosecrans' CA and IQ scores for the clinically confirmed subjects suggesting that the older suffer progressively declining IQ scores. The age adjusted correlation coefficient, for degree of mosaicism with IQ, proved to be 0.06. There is, then, no support for the Rosecrans conclusion. In any case, age confounding of mosaicism–IQ studies has been evident since the original observation by Clarke et al. (1961) of high IQ for a low frequency mosaic DS child; their 1963 follow-up report indicating significant intellectual decline even during that brief period.

Kohn et al. (1970) published data on five children and three adults who were mosaic for DS. All exhibited the usual physical signs of the syndrome but no 'apparent correlation' between percentage of trisomic cells and IQ, although correlation coefficients were not reported. The Kohn et al. paper is of particular interest because it exposes some additional methodological problems; including the employment of a pot-pourri of non-comparable behavioural measures. Curiously, many of the studies examined here have suffered from poorly rationalized behavioural assessment procedures, against which to compare presumably more precise laboratory findings. Another problem is that Kohn et al. contrasted their mean IQ of 37 points (for 15 adult mosaicism subjects) with Sternlich and Wanderer's (1962) institutional DS adults having a mean IQ of 23 points. Had the adult mosaics been compared with Kuenzel's (1929) young adults (median IQ 31 points) or with Wallin's (1944) sample (mean IQ of 46 points) their inference for less retardation in mosaicism DS would collapse.

More general biases encompass the almost certain effects on sampling of selective institutionalization, mortality rates related to sample age and different nurtural conditions across care systems. These difficulties are evident throughout the literature. It is known that institutional and community Down's individuals deviate significantly for early IQ and for rate of IQ decline throughout their lifespan. The unfolding of neuropathological processes, in DS, has long been associated with progressive IQ erosion (Benda, 1960a, b; Carr, 1960; Cowie, 1970), with the early appearance of pre-senile dementia (Jervis, 1970a, b; Owens et al., 1971) and with behaviour disorders associated with 'chronic brain syndrome' (Menolascino, 1967). Behavioural decline continues throughout adolescence and adulthood and requires that age-related pathological changes continue to be acknowledged when attempting to match karyotypic events with phenotypic outcomes.

Still another age-related methodological puzzle is the difference in proliferation rates between normal and abnormal cells. Richards (1969) observed that

if trisomic cells proliferate more slowly, then this differential proliferation rate will be most effective in reducing the proportion of trisomic cells in rapidly dividing tissue, such as blood. Such an effect should be age related, the proportion of trisomic cells falling with increasing age of the mongol, the difference between the proportion of trisomic cells in blood and in skin increasing with age likewise. (p. 75)

Richards' cross-sectional data indicates a fall in the proportion of trisomic cells, principally during the first year. A longitudinal study by Taylor (1968) showed a progressive decrease in trisomic cells for five children, an increase for two, and no change for the three adults examined. Richards observed that (i) subjects with 50% trisomic cells will seldom be missed or misdiagnosed, (ii) errors of diagnosis, for less than 10% trisomic mosaicism, will usually be of clinical rather than of cytogenetic origin (especially for babies displaying only slight somatic evidence), and (iii) a general tendency to count too few cells might mean that mosaicism 'arising at a fourth cleavage would often be missed, and that the sixth cleavage, usually' (p. 81). Thus past studies have mainly included 'cytogenetically detectable mosaicism in clinically recognizable mongols...' who might be a small and unrepresentative proportion of a much larger mosaicism population.

What we do know is that some or many of the least retarded cases of Down's syndrome are mosaic (Hamerton, Gianelli & Polani, 1965), and that a relatively good IQ, coupled with discrepancies in the traditional clinical picture, might indicate potential mosaicism (Polani, 1963). On the whole, mosaicism DS appears to be less retarded than standard trisomy DS. Fishler (1975) compared 15 mosaics against age and sex matched standard trisomy cases. The mosaics ranged in IQ from 43 to 89 points with a mean of 67. No conclusions were drawn on the relation of percentage of normal cells, IQ and age. However, if frequency of normal cells in the Fishler sample is broken at plus and minus 55%, a non-significant difference of three IQ points is evident favouring the lower frequencies. Mean age is approximately 10 years for both groups.

Trisomy–translocation comparisons

Gibson and Pozsonyi (1965) Pozsonyi and Gibson (1965), Ong *et al.* (1967), Shipe *et al.* (1968) and Johnson and Abelson (1969) have proposed behavioural differences between standard trisomy and translocation DS. Among the differences is an IQ advantage of between 4 and 8 points favouring the translocations. Because the samples are small, the reliability of the IQ spread is uncertain (Belmont 1971); although the differences from pooled data exceed chance expectation. Other difficulties include the effects of diagnostic practices and differential mortality across variations of karyotype. Biased sampling can be associated with timing of original diagnosis and whether or not cell analysis was requested or required. There is evidence that translocation DS is less classically stigmatized than standard trisomy, the equivocal cases attracting a request for karyotyping more frequently and earlier. Support for this view has been offered by Johnson and Abelson (1969) reporting from a regional census of 2606 institutional DS patients. They found a mean IQ of 28.61 points for the total sample and 32.33 points for the karyotyped subjects. Although Johnson and Abelson claimed the foregoing IQ difference to be 'relatively slight', a spread of close to 4 IQ points for a quite large sample, having a severely attenuated IQ range, cannot be dismissed. It is probable that the non-karyotyped members included, disproportionately, the older institutional patients who would exhibit terminal (deteriorated) IQs and who would not have access to continuing diagnostic services. The clinically doubtful would attract karyotyping more certainly and at younger ages than would the more classically stereotyped, the older, and the very severely retarded. The translocations might, therefore, be younger and brighter than the standard trisomies for these reasons only. Too few of the published trisomy–translocation comparisons offer CA data or sampling parameters against which to check selection bias.

A second major sampling distortion has to do with variety of karyotype and life expectancy. Ong *et al.* (1967) recorded congenital heart disorder (CHD) for five of twelve translocation and for only one of the trisomy control series. They also contended that the translocations are less classical for physical symptoms than standard trisomy DS. A similar observation was made by Gibson and Pozsonyi (1965), Shipe *et al.* (1968) and Johnson and Abelson (1969 *a*, *b*). Fabia and Drolette (1970) complicated the problem by showing the extent of high infant mortality for DS and its major cause; CHD. If the earlier deaths over-represent the clinically less typical (e.g. Gibson, Pozsonyi and Zarfas, 1964), the translocation samples reviewed here would comprise a survival group which might not provide a suitable base for the discovery of phenotypic outcomes attributable to karyotype deviation within the syndrome.

The relation of variation of abnormal karyotype to other psychological dimensions of DS, has been studied by Gibson and Pozsonyi (1965) and by Johnson and Abelson (1969 a, b). The former argued that translocation DS is more adequately socialized, more passive and less aggressive than is the trisomy variety. Psychopathology took the form of withdrawal and autism for the translocations. Habit disorder and hostility marked the trisomy condition. Differences were modest and samples small. Understandably, Johnson and Abelson could as easily claim that translocation DS scores higher in aggression and activity ratings than does trisomy DS. They compared a set of 'problem behaviours' (samples matched for CA) noting that the high scores (negative) were all from the translocation group. These subjects were from 8 to 25 years CA and had a mean IQ of 36.20 points. Reservations about age and 'deterioration' influences seem to have been satisfied. Belmont (1971) challenged both investigations finding them overgeneralized and contradictory. One problem lies in attempting to project the essentially unvalidated behavioural stereotype rather than starting with objective measures which owe nothing to expectation.

Shaky procedures and conflicting conclusions have not inhibited speculation about mediation. Slater and Cowie (1971) summed up a prevailing opinion that 'an admixture of normal cells with trisomy-21 may ameliorate the mental defect in mongolism to some extent'. Rosecrans (1971) spoke of 'amount' of surplus genetic material and its 'chromosomal location' as being critical to physical and behavioural outcomes. Finley et al. (1965) referred to amount of extra chromosomal material as being related to magnitude of IQ deficit. The translocation–trisomy studies show no evidence for positioning effect (G/G versus D/G) and the matter has not been pursued. Mention has been made, too, of the potentially different clinical effects of fused versus detached chromosome fragments. There is no statistical support for the idea. Embryological mediation has been discussed by Baumeister and Williams (1967). Building on speculation by Gibson and Gibbins (1958), they proposed that subtype of chromosome anomaly might be critical with respect to embryological time-tabling. The hypothesis implied would be difficult to test, i.e., that 'it is possible that the different genetic errors involved would differentially affect skeletal and nervous development' (p. 590).

The research to date has identified no certain biological or psychological differences among mosaicism, translocation and standard trisomy DS, with the possible exception of a higher mean IQ for the translocation over the standard trisomy condition, and for the mosaics over both. It is likely that any departure from the majority karyotype would contribute to increased somatic and psychological variability (Gibson & Pozsony, 1965; Reisman, Shipe & Williams, 1966) and that non-authentic directional differences among the cytogenetic subclasses might therefore emerge, especially if samples are small or otherwise unsuitable.

Familial residuals and intelligence

Stickland (1954) described two DS individuals of relatively mild deficit who were members of families exhibiting superior intelligence. He proposed that aberrant cytogenetic action might not entirely mask the transmission of normal familial characteristics, e.g., intellect and temperament. 'Each seems to have a good hereditary endowment apart from any genetical factors which may have influenced the condition, and each has received intensive education'. (p. 82). It has been the impression of some workers (Brinkworth & Collins, 1969; Pitt, 1974) that familial resemblances, physically and behaviourally, can be identified when the DS child is seen together with the family. Benda (1946), however, observed no particular association of intelligence level for DS with that of other members of the family and there are no formal investigations of physical resemblances other than for stigmatization. The problem would be the proper separation of nurtural and genetic influences. Because experimental manipulation of the relevant variables is not practical, and statistical control difficult, some rather circuitous tests of the familial residuals hypothesis for DS have been attempted. The objectives have been to determine the pervasiveness of the effects of the supernumerary chromosome and to support an hereditability hypothesis for the origins of intelligence in general.

The simplest approach to the problem was taken by Kostrzewski (1965) who investigated the connection between level of parental education and intellectual status in the DS offspring. He divided his parent group into four units; those having university training, those having secondary schooling, those with completed primary school, and a fourth unit with less than full primary school education. The first group was too small for analysis. The parents having secondary schooling counted 18 DS children among them. These achieved a mean IQ of 41.6 points. The DS offspring of parents with only primary schooling showed a mean IQ of 35.6 points while the educationally most disadvantaged parent group had DS children with a mean IQ of 32.2 points. These IQ differences by educational level were statistically significant. Kostrzewski favoured an environmental interpretation over the possibility of familial residuals. It was his contention that an intellectually stimulating environment, along with an *early* concern for the cognitive development of the DS child, would have a significant impact in the order of about 10 IQ points. The conclusion is attractive, from a pedogogical standpoint, but is otherwise empty in view of Kostrzewski's failure to test the relation of CA to IQ scores for his 155 cases. Much of the testing was probably conducted during childhood when IQ for the syndrome is highest and most unstable. Moreover, DS children are first seen in clinics or institutions at ages which vary according to parental socio-economic class and rural–urban origins. The educationally superior and the urban dwelling parent might seek a first psychometric and paediatric examination quite early in the life of the child and when test intelligence is appreciably higher than it will be in subsequent months. An IQ decline of even 50% is not uncommon for DS children during the pre-school years (Gibson, 1966).

Subsequent explorations of the relation of intelligence for DS to that of the parents (Gibson, 1967), and with normal siblings (Rimland, Stone & Dameron, 1969), have attempted statistical division of natural and nurtural backgrounds. Gibson selected three groups of DS children separated from the home environment at different ages ($N = 141$). Parental intelligence was inferred from educational and occupational history using the Haggerty and Nash (1924) and the Harrell and Harrell (1945) procedures. Paternal intelligence was evaluated because male occupational and educational status is more likely to reflect 'natural' ability (than for the mother) and because the father is often more remote from the subtleties of child nurture. The relation of paternal school leaving level and IQ, for the DS offspring, proved to be non-linear. The data were thus treated using eta coefficients. The regression of DS with parent intelligence is curvilinear, possibly because of the influence of secondary neuropathological factors at lower IQ levels and neuro-maturational end-effect at the upper range of the IQ continuum. Karyotype variation (within-syndrome) could also operate to distort the distribution insofar as parental age and cytological subgroup are interdependent. The first 39 cases examined (mean CA of 18 months at time of separation from the family) produced a mean developmental quotient of 45 points. The 77 DS subjects past 11 years of home nurture had a mean IQ of 26 points. The final sample was similar for initial age except that these 25 subjects had been examined 5 years after institutionalization (mean CA of 16 years and a mean IQ of 22 points). Fig. 4 depicts the visual fit for the distribution of IQ and

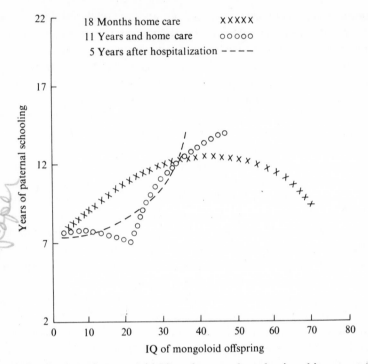

Fig. 4. Distribution of mongoloid IQ and paternal academic achievement ($N = 141$). (From D. Gibson (1967). *American Journal of Mental Deficiency*, **71**, 1014–16.)

paternal academic achievement across the three segments. The eta coefficients represent the regression of IQ on paternal educational standard. There was no significant eta coefficient between inferred paternal IQ and the developmental quotient of the DS offspring following an average of 18 months of home nurture. Eleven years of home care supported an eta coefficient of 0.75 (significant at the 0.01 level). The paternal–DS child IQ correlation, 5 years after separation, was statistically significant. It would appear that test intelligence for the young DS child (from 6 to 24 months of CA) is substantially under the control of aberrant genotypic forces, there being no evidence favouring the transmission of either familial genetic residuals or nurtural effects in respect to intelligence for DS at particularly young ages. At later stages of growth, there is a reliable connection between intelligence for parent and DS offspring and one which survives subsequent separation. Altogether, the findings favour the influence of nurture past infancy and also the tenacity of these gains following separation from the home. A more convincing test would employ DS subjects hospitalized shortly after birth and would select from among those who are comparatively free of secondary handicaps and of relatively good initial developmental status.

Another examination of the familial residuals hypothesis was undertaken by Rimland, Stone and Dameron (1969). They considered the normal siblings of DS children. Rimland *et al.* speculated that since an IQ correlation of about 0.50 exists between siblings, whether raised together or not, a 'constant subtraction' hypothesis for the origins of intelligence for DS could be tested by comparing DS performance measures with those of normal siblings. The resulting correlation coefficient was −0.064. The 36 DS subjects were of institutional origin having been admitted to hospital between CA 56 months and about 11 years. Duration of previous exposure to family environment or quality of home situation is not provided. More telling evidence is offered by Carr (1975). She finds a developmental spread for normal infants, as between manual and non-manual families, as early as 10 weeks of life. A similar separation, is not observed for the DS infants.

The step from familial to ethnological residuals is a large one. Caccamo and Yater (1972) build on the assumption that auditory memory is superior to other abilities for normal negro children and superior to the norms for caucasian children (Kirk and Kirk, 1971). The difference does not survive for negro and white children classified as Down's syndrome.

It is reasonable to conclude that intelligence for DS is not dependent, even in part, on hereditable competency in the parents. Whether the IQ advantage of the DS offspring of better educated parents is a nurtural bonus, or a result of different diagnostic and placement practices across socio-economic levels, is not clear.

Environmental correlates of intelligence

Care regimes compared

Many parents and professionals have been driven to expose institutional care as damaging and to lobby for increasing government and private support of family-centred facilities. The claims, whatever their respective merits, have generated a good deal of data about the role of the environment in the development of the DS individual.

The comparison of management regimes for DS dates from Pototzky and Grigg (1942). They challenged the established growth norms and projections for DS infants and children derived from institutional data. The increasing trend towards home care was by them, providing an alternative source of growth data. The norms for psychological and physical status, between institutional and community DS children, favoured the home samples; an important finding because Quaytman (1953) estimated that only between 10 and 20% of all DS cases are resident in institutions. He screened forty home-based DS children having a mean CA of 7 years 7 months. The average mental age was 3 years, representing a mean IQ of 44 points – 10 to 15 IQ points higher than the level characteristic of institutional samples at that time. However, hospital samples tend to be older so an IQ spread of 15 points, between CA 7 years and 20 or more years, might indicate merely the effects of IQ erosion with age. A second limiting factor is that most care comparison studies have used the Binet scales to assess intellectual performance, despite the tendency of this and other tests to favour the family-reared child.

Centerwall and Centerwall (1960) evaluated the physical and mental growth of two groups of DS children ($N = 64$). One half of the total were institutionalized at the start of the study and the other half after a lapse of 30 months or more. The authors reported that the home-reared group (deferred institutionalization) showed significantly superior intellectual, social and motor development over the institutional group. These differences persisted following hospitalization of the delayed placement group. The difference was attributed to the effects of superior family nurture. It would be necessary, of course, to match or otherwise control members of each treatment class for age and IQ (or DQ) at the start of any such study. Overburdened institutions tend to admit the more serious cases and to defer the less urgent. Low priority DS children are usually those enjoying stable and able home circumstances, those displaying less pronounced retardation, and those who are relatively free of secondary handicap requiring specialized attention.

McNeill (1955) stressed the dangers of ascribing growth differences, between home and hospital DS children, solely to the management locale. He compared mental age, IQ, social quotient, vocabulary quotient and eye–hand coordination for incidental samples of home-based and hospitalized DS children. Intelligence ratings were 19.23 points for the hospitalized group and 33.04 points for the home group. Social Quotients were 23.45 points and 41.79 points, verbal quotients 23.74 and 36.00 points and eye–hand coordination 27.10 points and 34.92 points for the institution- and home-reared groups respectively. Some interesting qualitative differences between care groups were extracted by arranging areas of greatest development to areas of least development within samples. For the hospital group, eye–hand coordination was stronger and social and vocabulary ratings weaker than for the home sample. The order of strengths could represent (i) a tendency for different environments to extract different behavioural priorities to suit specialized survival requirements or (ii) the habit of institutionalizing DS children who are less socially and verbally able. A later study by Kugel and Reque (1961), employing 8-year-olds who had remained at home and 9-year-olds who had been institutionalized at 1 year of age, showed the latter group to be inferior in all areas of growth including both verbal and motor attainment. Stedman and Eichorn (1964) could find no difference in motor development between home-reared and hospitalized groups of DS. Performance heirarchies for DS are still uncertain, possibly because gross cagetories of nurture tell us little about the type and quality of care within each or about the interaction of care regime and maturational staging.

Shotwell and Shipe (1964) undertook a longitudinal examination of the effect of type of out-of-home care on the intellectual and social development of DS children. Some were placed in private facilities at birth while others were institutionalized directly from the parent's home after 2 years of age (25 and 17 cases for each condition). Differences were identified initially between the two groups in respect to ethnic, socio-economic and educational factors in the families. There was a tendency for middle-class families to seek out-of-home care for the DS child at or shortly after birth. Kuhlmann, Binet and Vineland testing was done prior to admission, on admission to institution, and 18 months after institutionalization had occurred. No distinctions for overall medical history were detected between the two groups. The results indicate significant mental age and social age (CA controlled) advantages for the home-reared children. Shotwell and Shipe appear to support earlier cross-sectional finding for the superiority of home care. Their 1964 investigation, however, makes the assumption that the DS children placed in private institutions, close to birth, did not differ in developmental potential from those retained at home. Otherwise, a proper conclusion might be that home nurture is usually adequate and that some or many private nursing homes are grossly inadequate. The first nursing homes, for the very young retarded, were quickly organized to take advantage of the lengthening waiting lists for public institutions and were strongly profit motivated. They offered only routine cot care, there being little or no programmed sensory stimulation and minimal handling. While we can assume 'that the superiority of the home-reared children in both intellectual and social skills is to be attributed to their own home environment' (p. 696), the comparison is conceivably between something and nothing. Shotwell and Shipe had certain reservations. Among these is that since all cases were eventually institutionalized they might have differed from a third group, i.e., DS individuals who are not institutionalized and who do not appear on any pre-admission clinic file or hospital waiting list. Moreover, 44% of the home-reared group and 35% of the hospitalized group received alternate forms of care during the course of the study, i.e., were rotated between 'family care' situations and other forms of care.

In a second study, Shipe and Shotwell (1965) explored the long-term stability of nurtural gains to find that deterioration of IQ for the home-reared is more rapid than for the hospital-reared, once the former had been hospitalized. Both samples of DS children were followed through 3 or more years of institutional experience. The difference in IQ between the two groups, following the period of shared environment, was 6 points whereas the IQ difference at the time of institutionalization (for the home-reared) had been almost double that figure. Presumably, 5 or even 10 years of a common environment (institution or whatever) might yield no IQ disparity between DS patients having had different early care experiences. Shipe and Shotwell appealed to the unpublished study of Richards and Sands. These workers compared two groups of DS subjects between CA 8 and 9 years. The home group achieved a mean IQ of 43.4 points and the institutional children a mean IQ of 19.7 points. So large a difference suggests that the two samples might have differed for clinical status at the outset. A supporting observation, made by Shotwell and Shipe, was the extent to which the children within care groups differed among themselves, some in the early hospitalization group doing poorly and others doing comparatively well. Yet the nurtural milieu was ostensibly the same.

Adequate identification and control of the retrospective variables relevant to the effects of home versus hospital regimes could prove impossible. Stedman and Eichorn (1964) choose to manipulate environments experimentally. At the outset, they followed the usual tactic of comparing hospitalized with at-home DS infants. Results are as expected, with IQs of 37 and 52 points, social quotients (SQs) of 24 and 29 points and motor performance scores of 45 and 48 points each favouring the home sample. The results again permit no cause–effect inference. A second phase of the study involved an experimental care unit housed in the research wing of a hospital and redecorated as a nursery. The staff-to-child ratio was never less than one to five and personalized care and handling were the rule. Further details of the sample are contained in Dameron (1963). The DS children were from 17 to 37 months of CA at the time of assessment. A home-reared control series was matched with the laboratory series for age, sex and health status. The Bayley infant scale and the Vineland social maturity scale were used to assess mental, social, and motor growth. These findings are depicted in tabular form (see Table 6). Outcomes favoured the home-reared sample for the social and intellectual indices but not for the motor development scores. The overall

Table 6. *Mean motor, mental and social maturity scales*

	Hospital	Home	t	p (two-tail)
Mental				
Point score	90.6	108.4	4.02	0.01
Intelligence quotient	37.3	52.1	3.76	0.01
Standard score	−6.31	−4.41	3.85	0.01
Social				
Point score	24.0	29.0	3.27	0.01
Social quotient	61.8	75.0	3.20	0.02
Motor				
Point score	45.0	47.8	1.48	
Motor quotient	45.8	51.6	1.34	
Standard score	−4.44	−3.80	1.36	

After Stedman and Eichorn (1964).

tendency was for most growth to occur for social performance, followed by intellectual and motor functioning.

The value of Stedman and Eichorn's work, for present purposes, is in the item analysis. Table 7 shows only those differences which statistically separate the two samples. The important distinctions involve mainly the use or understanding of speech and the ability to manipulate small items and creative materials (crayons). The authors observed that 'the interpretation of the inferior performances of institutional infants in terms of deficiency of experience rather than lack of basic skills is strengthened by contrasts within the mental tests' (p. 396). However, while the groups were generally similar there was a tendency for the home-based sample to be physically larger. Other studies have recorded differences in initial physical status between home-based and institutionalized DS children, the disparity being assigned usually to the superior nutrition and physical care obtained at home. The physical size disimilarity, between the home and hospital nurtured, was attributed to leg length and linked to age at onset of walking. It is presumed that the home-reared are encouraged to walk earlier than those in group custody.

Leaving aside the matching problems, Stedman and Eichorn suggest that institutional care programmes can simulate many of the opportunities of a good home regime while retaining the advantages of the former. Carr (1970) initiated a longitudinal examination of motor and mental growth for 54 DS

Table 7. *Item analysis – mental and social scales*

Scale	Item	*p* (one-tail)
Mental		
82	Attempts to secure 3 cubes	0.005
84	Listens selectively to familiar words	0.005
87	Adjusts to words	0.005
92	Inhibits on command	0.005
92	Attempts to imitate scribble	0.005
101	Uses expressive jargon	0.005
107	Turns pages of book	0.005
111	One round block in Bayley board	0.005
85	Says da-da or equivalent	0.01
88	Fingers holes in pegboard	0.01
97	Holds crayon adaptively	0.01
89	Puts cube in cup on command	0.05
91	Looks for contents of box	0.05
105	Places 1 peg repeatedly	0.05
113	Removes pellet from bottle	0.05
Social		
17	Follows simple instructions	0.05
31	Uses names of familiar objects	0.05

After Stedman and Eichorn (1964).

babies raised at home, in foster-homes and in institutions. Her study was an advance over previous work because the matching was carefully executed and the subjects quite young. Normal infants were used as controls. Developmental tests include the Bayley infant scales and the California scale of motor development, given at intervals from 6 weeks onwards. Mothers were given questionnaires requiring a nurtural history of the infant. The DS sample was further divided for social class (manual and non-manual family groups), the at-home DS babies being matched with normal children for social stratum, age and sex. Carr's findings include: (i) depressed DIQ scores (Bayley mental scale quotients) for the boarded-out children versus the home-reared children, and (ii) a growing divergence, developmentally, for home-reared DS children depending on whether or not the families were rated as manual or non-manual. The normal control series exhibited a clear initial and later DIQ advantage favouring the non-manual families.

A key finding of the Carr investigation is that home-reared DS children regress from a mean DIQ of 80.96 (at 6 months of age) to 34.72 points by 2 years of age, whereas boarded-out DS infants drop from a mean DIQ of 77.28 points (at 6 months) to 15.84 points by 2 years of age. Since there was no intentional selection bias between the two samples, family environments appear pre-eminent. One must account, however, for the fact that developmental motor age (DMA) scores for the home-reared and boarded out DS infants were different at the outset. Neuromotor indices for DS infants, while surely subject to some environmental influence, have been viewed by past workers as strong correlates of early neuropathological status. Furthermore, score fluctuation was marked, some children showing rapid drops in DIQ while others retained gains or resisted losses, regardless of type of care regime. It would be useful in future to identify the somatic, maturational and cytogenetic characteristics of DS children who exhibit early and rapid developmental decline from those who hold gains; environmental factors controlled.

Fields and Gibson (1971) pursued a factor analytic solution for apportioning the effects of physiological and environmental influences on intellectual maturity levels. Ages of walking, talking, toileting and teething were determined for all DS adult residents in a culturally similar and relatively isolated community. The statistical outcome indicated that some early growth markers for DS were more environmentally susceptible than others and that a secure relation exists between early developmental indices and maturity level MA for the syndrome. The translation from physiological to behavioural maturation for DS is possibly more direct than is usually supposed, a result of the failure of DS children to move ahead to abstract levels of intelligence where there is greater opportunity for environmental impact. The early growth markers which proved to be most predictive of later mental age were of a simple motor and sensory nature.

Conclusions and problems

The home versus hospital studies have been motivated to justify the beliefs that intelligence for DS is quite plastic and that family care is superior to group care. At present no conclusions are warranted from the data presented because of the following methodological flaws:

(i) Various investigators have compared home-reared DS children with those exposed to boarding homes, private custodial and nursing homes, experimental community residences, residential nursery schools and modified hospital situations. A wide range of large custodial (public) institutions serving diverse populations and regions and having different budgets, staffing and goals, have also been engaged. These regimes all fall under the rubric 'institutional' for sampling purposes. Findings, favouring the benefits of family care, have almost always involved control samples from large and poorly staffed public institutions. By comparison, the style and quality of home-care regimes has varied little from study to study. Most investigators have sampled concerned middle-class families working closely with clinic research centres; hardly a typical combination. We need to test home-care programmes, graded for general adequacy, while isolating the positive and negative components within each. A substantial number of home-care situations might well prove to be inferior to many group facilities.

(2) The failure of the literature to establish initial comparability of samples is almost universal. Community and hospital groups have not been equated at the outset for neuro-maturation, extent of secondary handicap, or adequacy of neonatal care. Wolfensberger and Halliday (1970) reviewed the clinical and family care–decision literature on DS. They implied that (i) the institutional over home care decision is not a random process and (ii) there is little likelihood that samples from the two decision groups are similar for the important somatic or behavioural dimension.

The reasons parents choose early institutionalization over long-term community care are complex, but not accidental with regard to the clinical and psychological status of the handicapped offspring (Saenger, 1960). A re-analysis of the Centerwall and Centerwall (1960) data by Stedman and Eichorn (1964) is instructive. They demonstrated that if only those children (in both home and hospital samples) who walked by CA 5½ years are compared, the IQ and SQ differences, across care regimes, disappear. Birch and Belmont (1961) noted that IQ deterioration was more precipitous for those institutionalized later than earlier. This fact, coupled with the different timing of early developmental landmarks for the two samples, led them to suspect that the home and hospital groups were not maturationally or pathologically equivalent at the start of the study.

(3) Interpretative limitations are imposed by the criterion measures used. Instrumentation has included all forms and revisions of the Binet scales and the popular infant growth scales (the Kuhlmann, Cattell, Gesell and Bayley). These devices were designed to monitor the interaction of maturation and family environments for the normal infant and child. High calibre institutional programmes can and do have salutary outcomes which are not fully measurable using scales standardized on behaviours appropriate to functioning in a nuclear family unit.

(4) Intellectual and social growth, across care systems, is usually reported without any indication for the tenacity or quality of the gains. Birch and

Belmont (1961) remarked on the rapid loss of IQ points, for home-reared DS subjects, after institutionalization. They question whether home training produces much more than a social and academic veneer which is subsequently maintained in delicately balanced environments and at great cost. Extensive social and academic training for DS should serve more than a family and community need for 'appearances'.

(5) In general, support for the superiority of home care over institutional care has failed to consider outcome goals. No one has seriously articulated the possible and probable lifestyles open to the DS adult, or reflected on the community status of DS individuals following the demise of parents and the scattering of normal siblings. It should be determined how each nurtural option shapes competence and masks incompetence in relation to realistic adult survival options. The highly protected and intimate home care programme need not provide the most adequate or humane preparation for later adult life in community or institution. Although the trainable MR adult is finding a role in community life settings and in industrial and agricultural villages, these are essentially group facilities.

Physical correlates of intelligence
Neuropathology and intelligence

The behavioural phenotype for Down's is a product both of nurtural and syndromic events. With respect to the latter, performance profiles are influenced across the lifespan of the syndrome by circulatory, sensory, neurological and structural limitations. McIntire, Menolascino and Wiley (1965) found double the accepted rate for prematurity, and about 50% pregnancy, labour and delivery complications. They observed that 7% of cases were breech deliveries, and found relatively high frequencies of generalized hypotonia, hearing loss, abnormal EEG and later psychiatric complication. Cassel (1953) traced the extent of secondary organic factors for 21 DS males and 15 DS females between 7 years 9 months and 50 years of age. He demonstrated that 86% of the males and 60% of the females suffered organic defects of the kind which would limit behavioural competence. Therefore, while DS is a *primary* mental deficiency it is also important as a *secondary* disorder. Both sets of conditions determine intellectual limits and qualities; for the individual and for the syndrome as a whole.

The assertion that the 'potential mental development (of DS) depends on the degree of biological maturity which was present at birth and the amount of training and therapy given during infancy and childhood' (Benda, 1960a,

p. 66) is tidy but incomplete. Benda himself has detailed many of the complex secondary and progressive circulatory, sensory and neurological system defects which would alter the competency status of the syndrome over time and contribute to growing variation between cases. Penrose and Smith (1966) have also remarked on the disparity of developmental events for DS, by age and between individuals, i.e., that progressive circulatory, central and peripheral nervous system pathology contributes to increasing behavioural variability within the condition. There is ample evidence for example, of widespread vascular system defect in DS. Benda (1960 a) noted hypoplasia of the vascular system, the narrow and thin quality of the arteries, and the more sparse branching of the vascular tree, as compared with normal controls. These limitations are most conspicuous in the brain where the capillaries appear increasingly congested and enlarged. He said, 'in mongoloids beyond 25 years of age atheromatosis of the arteries is common' (1960 a, p. 148). Progressive cardiovascular limitations are prevalent throughout the nervous and endocrine systems probably contributing to declining behavioural capacities over time. Tennies (1943) claimed that, 'deterioration is constantly present at all age levels, involving atrophy of the cortex and small hemorrhages into the brain and cord'. Masland, Sarason and Gladwin (1958) referred to trophic inadequacies leading to ongoing damage of the nervous system in DS.

Benda (1960 a) has provided other evidence of the primary neuropathology of DS. He catalogued developmental anomalies of the cerebellum, reduced weight and size of the pons and medulla, thinner cerebral vessels than in normal brains, and in particular delayed myelinization. There was less than usual white matter, lack of cytoplasm in the nerve cells and a lower brain weight than comparable normals. Reduced development of the frontal lobes was evident when compared with normal children of similar ages and growth stages. Poor differentiation of the cerebral cortex, reduction in the number of cells in the nucleus supraopticus of the hypothalamus, and fusion of the cerebral fissures accompanied these difficulties. Little study has been undertaken of the range and type of neuro-morphological differences among DS newborn or of the relation of such differences to subsequent psychological development. Nor is much known about the ongoing degenerative changes in brain metabolism or of the corruption of neuro-maturation in terms of timing of onset or sources. Owens et al. (1971) described 'changes in the brain consisting of shortened anteroposterior diameter, exposed insula, irregular gyral sulcal pattern, small cerebellum and occipital lobes, and narrow superior temporal gyrus. On section, the cortex is said to be thickened and the white matter reduced. Microscopically, the cortical laminations are indistinct and neurons are clustered in groups separated by acellular areas. Abnormalities of the brain may be due in part to slowed growth of the skull.' (p. 606.)

Much of the neuropathological progress is accompanied by eroding behavioural potentials. Demyelinization advances with CA. Progressive cerebral necrosis, presumably related to a decreasing circulatory system capability has been noted. Benda (1960 a) observed 'continuous edematous submerging of nerve tissue in which cell after cell meets death by suffocation' (p. 108). Benda was also impressed by the growing disorder of the cerebral fissures, the atrophy of the cortex with gliosis, the ever-present pachymeningeal fibrosis and the ongoing evidence for coagulation necrosis. These activities were not observed to the same extent in all DS cases thus providing a physiological rationale for understanding its behavioural variability. With respect to the venous system, the vascular walls show degeneration and signs of perivascular calcification. While the mechanisms are poorly understood, it appears that degenerative alterations begin early, are progressive and display considerable individual variation. Owens et al. (1971) were able to identify the early onset and progression of pre-senile Alzheimer's disease using an object identification task. Dalton, Crapper and Schlotterer (1974) found progressive short-term memory defect to be associated with ageing and the onset of Alzheimer's disease.

Specific neuropathological–behavioural links for DS have been exposed by Loesch-Mdzewska (1968), Cowie (1970), and Crome et al. (1966). The Cowie findings for early behavioural-motor interaction have been reviewed. Loesch-Mdzewska noted many of the deficiencies summarized by Benda – including hypotonia, absence of Moro reflex, prolongation over time of the infantile reflexes, reduced sensory functioning and a variety of EEG changes with age. He examined 123 DS patients from ages 3 to 62 years. Karyotype was established for 117 DS subjects including 107 trisomics, 1 mosaic and 9 D/G translocations. For most subjects, including the youngest, some abnormal neurological signs were present and increased with age. Hypotonia decreased in frequency with age. Owens et al. (1971) described hypotonia as present only in DS under 20 years of CA. Neuropathological signs were most common for the more severely retarded. The highest occurrence of paralysis and epilepsy were also in the groups of low IQ and high neuropathology. Since these were the oldest, re-analysis was conducted by stratifying the sample for CA. An increasing connection between IQ erosion and neurological deterioration over time, was evident. Loesch-Mdzewska concluded that:

slight but definite neurological abnormalities, non-specific, not confined to one system (although frequently involving the pyramidal system) can be observed in the majority of patients with Down's syndrome...The relationship of most symptoms to age, showing an increase both in frequency of occurrence and in intensity with increasing age of the subject, suggests that the neuropathological changes in Down's syndrome are not only developmental...but that progressive degenerative changes also occur. (pp. 240–1)

Crome, Cowie and Slater (1966) compared the brain, the cerebellum, and brain stem weight for DS and normal subjects, and found lower weights for each for Down's. They supposed that the smallness of brain stem and cerebellum could be associated with low muscle tone. Hypotonia of the muscles was said to be a major factor in the early psychomotor development of the syndrome, an opinion later corroborated by Cowie (1970). The Chrome et al. findings are consistent with those of Jebsen et al. (1961) and Loesch-Mdzewska (1968) who classified infantile muscular hypotonia as originating in the central nervous system.

A number of post-mortem studies have been conducted using mainly older deteriorated cases. Solitare and Lamarche (1966) found in favour of the early occurrence of senile deterioration or Alzheimer's disease. Senile changes were not evident in the brains of cases of other forms of mental deficiency at similar ages, an observation which tends to support the hypothesis of premature neurological ageing specific to DS. Solitare and Lamarche were not so certain, however, that the associated behavioural picture is that of typical senile dementia. They also questioned whether a DS brain, especially of an older patient, could be reliably identified as such by virtue of any specific structural characteristics. In a later study, these same authors (1967) reported brain weights for DS (from 20–67 years of age) to be less than for either normals or mental defectives in general. Parenthetically, Alzheimer's disease in DS is described morphologically as including granulovascular cytoplasmic changes, senile plaques, and neuro-fibrillary changes in abundance. Solitare and Lamarche recommenced that the histochemical and morphological features of ageing, and their behavioural correlates, be studied in younger subjects to determine the relation of performance potential to the unique growth and decline of the nervous system of DS. Electron microscopic studies of the brain in DS have expanded the picture. O'Hara (1972) sectioned the cerebral cortex of five DS cases to find plaques (cores of hollow fibres surrounded by various cell processes) and neuro-fibrillary tangles (bundles of twisted tubules) like those detected in Alzheimer's disease. Synapses without vesicles or with increased numbers of complex vesicles were also recorded.

Additional evidence of the neuropathological base of behavioural potential in DS can be found in the epilepsy and EEG studies. The coverage in this and the foregoing sections is less than exhaustive, being intended only to demonstrate the chaining of progressive organic and psychological events for the condition.

EEG and intelligence

Prior to Kirman's (1951) account, it was widely held that convulsive disorders were rare or absent for the syndrome. The pioneering evidence of Brousseau and Brainerd (1928) for a 2.6% occurrence of epilepsy and of Engler (1949) for an 8.8% frequency of epilepsy in DS, had not been influential. As recently as 1960, Mayer-Gross, Slater and Roth, in their textbook *Clinical psychiatry*, state that neither epileptic seizures nor other manifestations of epilepsy are to be found in DS.

A number of statistical surveys followed Kirman's clinical report. Walter, Yeager and Rubin (1955) examined 200 cases claiming a 2% frequency of episodes of 'spontaneous' grand mal seizures. Another 2% of the histories recorded episodes of a convulsive nature. These workers compared DS with undifferentiated mentally retarded (and against norms for the general population) for epilepsy potential employing EEG tracings, photic stimulation and metrazol monitoring. It could not be shown, for the two 'treatments', that DS exhibits a lower convulsive threshold than normals. Others have claimed frequencies of epileptic-like behaviour in DS ranging as high as 12% and as low as 1 or 2%. Comparability among studies is poor, because (i) variables relevant to epilepsy such as age level and amentia level had not been considered, (ii) differential mortality in DS is influenced by CHD which is, in turn, related to epilepsy (Seppalainen & Kivalo, 1967) and (iii) seizures in DS are infrequent and mild and can be easily overlooked clinically or epidemiologically (MacGillivray, 1967). Veall (1974) found an overall prevalence of epilepsy at 5.8%. With respect to age distribution however, the distribution was dimodal with age, the peaks occurring between CA 16–23 years and 45–54 years. It is suggested that both epilepsy and Alzheimer's disease are related to progressive neurophysiological changes but are otherwise independent events.

EEG phenomena for DS have also been studied as correlates of various behavioural manifestations. The latter investigations fall into two categories; those concerned with electrophysiological predictors of general behaviour and those which seek psychophysiological correlates of convulsive thresholds.

Investigations of epileptiform EEG activity have reported a higher convulsive threshold for the syndrome than for other classes of mental retardation (Walter *et al.*, 1955). Levinson, Friedman and Stamps (1955) recorded spike discharges for 16% of their series of 50 cases. Gibbs, Gibbs and Hirsch (1964) identified a 20% incidence of epileptiformic activity for DS subjects having no indicators of clinical epilepsy. Seppalainen and Kivalo (1967) examined EEG tracings for 92 DS patients. Almost 9% had a history of epileptic seizures and 2.2% of 'probable' epileptic seizures. Another 3.3% presented evidence of febrile convulsions. EEG examination produced mostly abnormal records, including a diffuse irregularity for 82%, episodic subcortical disturbance for 16% and paroxysmal activity for 20% of the series. The EEG irregularity was described as 'of more than slight severity' for 72% of the sample. These findings are very much higher than those of previous reports and might indicate sampling distortion. LaVeck and de la Cruz (1963) uncovered 60% abnormal EEGs for their 20 cases. However, since 25% suffered from clinical epilepsy, the sample cannot be considered representative of the syndrome. The clinical epileptics, most studied, are usually more severely retarded mentally than the majority of DS.

Age differences, allied with clinically positive EEG findings, have been mentioned by many recent workers and with good agreement that the incidence of EEG abnormality in DS increases up to about 11 years CA, decreasing subsequently into adulthood. These cross-sectional results do not account for sampling bias related to differential mortality effects. Ellingson, Menolascino and Eison (1970) concluded that 'abnormal EEGs in these patients tend to become normal with time' (p. 649). Their later work supported this (Ellingson, Eisen & Ottersberg, 1973). EEG abnormalities were studied for 202 DS subjects confirmed for karyotype and ranging from 1 month to 63 years of age. Up to 25% exhibited abnormalities, the highest rate being prior to the age of 14. The rate for young adults was the same as for the general population, increasing again in the fifth decade of life. Incidental findings were of no difference in percentage EEG abnormality across trisomy, translocation and mosaicism samples and of no obvious connections between EEG status and specific clinical or behavioural conditions.

Extended longitudinal investigation of electrocortical irregularity in DS would be useful. To this point, the clinical EEG literature supports the presence of early-appearing and progressive neuropathology associated with degree of mental retardation. It is not certain (i) if the changing frequency of EEG abnormality with age is sampling error only, or (ii) whether or not the electrocortical phenomena associated with the syndrome represent ongoing genotypic processes, or result from the secondary afflictions detailed by McIntyre, Menolascino and Wiley (1965).

A second body of evidence attempts to relate alpha rhythm to developmental and intellectual status. Kreezer (1939) was the first to find a significant positive correlation between (occipital) alpha index and mental age (Binet) for DS. The enterprise was extended by Gunnarson (1945) who demonstrated slower frequencies of alpha rhythm for a series of eleven cases, as against a control series of non-DS mentally retarded. Godinova (1963) noted excessively slow EEG activity for 50% of his sample of 66 DS cases (ages 4 to 17 years). Possibly, the generally lower frequency of alpha for the syndrome is an indication of slower neuro-maturational process. A predictable statistical effect might be a significant alpha–IQ correlation, although Ellingson and Lathrop (1973) failed to uncover any useful correlations between alpha frequency and Wechsler adult intelligence scale subtest scores for 39 DS subjects aged 13 to 42 years. In any event, the EEG artifacts of progressive neuropathology in DS could yield entirely spurious IQ–alpha correlations, i.e., that the 'damaged' brains in any random series of DS subjects, across age groups, would distort the data in favour of the hypothesis. A possible connection between degree of mental defect and extent of the clinical–EEG evidence was shown previously to be a result of CNS damage rather than of primary maturational events.

Alpha studies, designed to test purely developmental hypotheses, have not controlled neuropathological variability and cannot, therefore, insist that extent of neuro-maturation is related to magnitude of MA or IQ. Studies of sleep reactivity contradict the belief that slow maturation of the brain is an adequate explanation for variability of alpha rhythm in DS. Borselli and Sferlazzo (1963) reported that 66% of their sample displayed asymmetrical cortical reactivity, disturbance of the left hemisphere, and so on, indicating a greater variety of subtle clinical CNS manifestations than is usually acknowledged for the syndrome. Goldie et al. (1968) examined sleep patterns in DS, including the newborn (five cases). They found that periods of non-rapid eye movement sleep were longer for the newborn and that for DS, in general, there was less clearly demarcated episodic sleep activity. Hirai and Izawa (1964) examined 40 cases having no history of seizures. They conceded the diffuse neural immaturity documented by other workers but stressed that the presence of more than usual fast activity in their records, displaying no 'seizure discharges', points to neuropathological change which is evident very early and accelerates into adulthood.

On balance, the EEG literature lends considerably less support for a neuro-maturational than a neuropathological hypothesis for the nature of intelligence in DS. A fresh approach to charting the neuro-maturational aspects of mental growth for DS could be based on the work of Ertl and Schafer (1969) and Vogel and Broverman (1964) where the measures are more sensitive than the rudimentary alpha indices or 'clinical correlates' approaches.

Biochemical–metabolic correlates of intelligence

There is considerable biochemical research which focuses on questions of metabolic functioning within karyotypic subclasses of DS and between DS and other forms of mental retardation. A few of these studies have searched for behavioural correlates. Selected studies are mentioned here only to illustrate the approach.

Masland, Sarason and Gladwin (1958) were disappointed by the minor pathological changes accompanying the more or less severe intellectual limitations of DS. The disparity suggests that the few demonstrated cerebral limitations must be highly critical, or that 'we are dealing here with some more generalized toxic or metabolic disorder which leads to impairment not only through anatomical lack but also through interference with physiological activity' (pp. 91–2). Conel's (1939) work is cited as the normative authority. The biochemical and metabolic concomitants of behaviour for DS are less appreciated than are the structural factors perhaps because as Penrose (1963 b) observed 'functional biochemical tests have not yielded very characteristic results' (p. 206). Findings of the period involved low basal metabolism rate, decreased quantities of blood calcium, decreased urinary excretions of tryptophane metabolites, a diminution of cerebral metabolism (based on measures of oxygen use), and irregularity of Vitamin A absorption, among others. The confirmation of distinctive metabolic and biochemical process, having more or less direct consequences, could result in techniques for chemical intervention. Bazelson and Paine (1967), in this regard, have experimented with 5-hydroxytryptophan for reversal of hypotonia in DS infants.

It has been generally held that hypothyroidism and pituitary gland malfunction in DS is of aetiological importance (Benda, 1960 a, b). Myers (1938 a, b), using an epidemiological control group method, tested the relation between thyroid disorders in mothers of DS children and the regional distribution of the syndrome. The mothers displayed a greater frequency of thyroid disorder and 'nervous excitement'. Laboratory studies have not supported easy generalization (Lilenfeld & Benesch, 1969; Uchida, 1970) and, specifically, are uncertain about any genuine bond between thyroid disease and DS (Mellon, Pay & Green, 1963). More relevant to our purposes was the Mellon *et al.* finding that of seven DS subjects, with thyroid autoantibodies, only three were the common trisomy-21 type. Other students of the chemical characteristics of DS (serum esterose, fasting blood sugar, steroids, etc.) are concerned with behavioural correlates. Klebba's (1973) bio-clinical comparisons are typical. He collected blood, urine, IQ test and perceptual-motor test evidence on DS. A number of chemical indices (e.g., albumin to globulin ratio, calcium, phosphorus and alkaline phosphatase) correlated positively with intelligence. Negatively correlated with test intelligence were measures for gamma globulin, uric acid, blood lipid fatty acids 20:0 and 15:0, total bilirubin, phosphohexose isomerase, micro-haematocrit and haemoglobin.

The research into blood sugar levels in DS might be of particular importance behaviourally; although Dutton (1961) rejected the earlier findings of Runge (1959) which placed fasting blood sugar levels in the hypoglycaemic range. Later work by Pozsonyi and Gibson (1965) established no difference in blood sugar level between trisomy and translocation DS, despite apparent behavioural differences. Further search disclosed no significant biochemical trends, as between trisomics and translocations, for haemoglobin, leucocytes, serum cholesterol, ALK phosphatase, protein, amino acids, 17-ketosteroids, and skeletal age. One exception, was an indication of euthyroidism. There was a significant increase in protein bound iodine no change in butanol extractable iodine and radio-active ^{131}I intake for the translocation group, but the opposite results for the trisomy sample after stimulation (Thytopar-Armour). The evidence here for a chaining of subtype of chromosome aberration, biochemical change, and behavioural status, is not encouraging. Keegan, Pettigrew and Parker (1974) had better results using behavioural extremes (two psychotic DS females). There were signs of hypothyroidism and diminished T_4 level suggesting a disturbance of serotonin activity. Serotonin deficiency is associated, in turn, with hypotonia and hyperkinesis. Progressive disorders of cerebral metabolism have been traced to cytogenetic factors of Rosner *et al.* (1965 *a*, *b*). Michejda and Menolascino (1975) in their review of skull base abnormalities in DS proposed an interaction of structural disorder (Roche *et al.*, 1972), enzyme activity and the supernumerary chromosome (Nadler *et al.*, 1967; Hall and Dohlgvist, 1969) but considered that the specific biochemical pathways are not yet known. Advances in the area might clarify the biological foundations of behaviour for the syndrome and permit chemical remediation.

Sex and intelligence

Sex ratios

To what extent DS occurs more often in males than females and whether or not the sexes expire unequally, over time, is a crucial issue when charting the behavioural dimensions of the syndrome. The present section looks at the sex-specific characteristics of growth, neuropathology, karyotype, morphology and behaviour. A practical concern will be to implicate sex differences for management purposes.

Conventional opinion is that DS occurs in a ratio of about 60 males to 40 females. Malzberg (1953) found an institutional admission rate of 151 males per 100 females for DS. Penrose (1963 b) assigned the imbalance to the bias of institutionalization, although Wunsch (1957) reported a similarly disproportionate sex ratio for clinic-evaluated DS. Sex-ratio imbalance decreased as the age of admission increased, according to Malzberg. He argued that a true sex difference probably exists because 'selective mortality operates during the years following birth so as to decrease the number of surviving males' (p. 304). While Carter and Maley (1958) indicated that 53% of DS cases are dead by 1 year of age, Fabia and Drolette (1970) added that females expire disproportionately during the early period of high mortality; congenital heart disorder being identified as the most important cause of death. Data has been presented to show that DS, with CHD, might differ for other somatic features as well. A tentative conclusion is that sex-related psychological and biological traits could be artifacts of differential mortality and institutional placement practices. Whatever the source, there will be sampling distortion where psychological variables are being studied.

Returning to the issue of sex ratios at birth, quite complete natality statistics for DS have been offered by Oster (1953). Of all DS births in a regional hospital, between 1923 and 1948 inclusive, 54.79% were boys. During the same period 51.15% of all children born were boys. No data were offered for frequency of miscarriages, abortions and stillbirths for DS as compared with normals, or by sex. Subsequent sex-ratio comparisons, across types of care regime, showed 133 males to 102 females in institutions and 136 males to 155 females residing at home. The facts would seem to indicate that natal sex ratios for DS are almost the same as for the general population, that there is a greater tendency to institutionalize males (and earlier), that females expire more frequently in infancy, and that the most retarded expire first. One consequence is that older DS females would be less retarded than males of the same age. Differential survival rates by sex might, therefore, pervert our impressions about temperament, health status, intelligence and

Table 8. *Percentage occurrence by sex for thirteen cardinal indices of mongolism*

Stigmata	Male percentage	Female percentage	Direction and percentage of bias
Cephalic index	36	50	14 (F)*
Nostril direction	55	48	7 (M)
Toe spacing	52	33	19 (M)*
Short 5th digit	33	52	19 (F)*
Curved 5th digit	54	57	3 (F)
Square hand	69	62	7 (M)
Epicanthus	55	81	26 (F)*
Fissured tongue	86	76	10 (M)*
Simian crease	57	60	3 (F)
Single 5th flexion	19	14	5 (M)
Abnormal ear	30	31	1 (F)
Adherent lobule	41	60	19 (F)*
Abnormal heart	22	21	1 (M)

After Gibson, Pozsonyi and Zarfas (1964).
* 0.05 level of confidence or better.

the clinical features of the syndrome. The latter probability has been studied most extensively.

Somatic differences by sex

Gibson, Pozsonyi and Zarfas (1964) have depicted the distribution by sex of 13 cardinal stigmata of DS (Table 8). The cardinal signs are viewed as the most representative of the syndrome, for purposes of clinical diagnosis. Sample ages ranged from 5 to 20 years CA. Differences supported the view that females are most physically typical, 67% of the cardinal signs being identified as female-specific and 33% as male-specific. Possibly a disproportionate number of clinically atypical females had expired prior to 5 years CA, the survivors being more classic for the syndrome. Evidence for a connection between cardiac defect, the occurrence of specific somatic anomalies and sex has been offered by Gibson *et al.* (1964) and by Fabia and Drolette (1970). These affinities would tend to distort stigma frequency comparisons, by sex, progressively with advancing age. Nevertheless, some workers have proposed that the trisomy is somehow sex-related thereby accounting for sex differences in cellular terms (Levinson and Bigler, 1960).

Demidov (1972) observed skeletal-motor anomalies, evident at birth and shortly after, more commonly in males.

Other sex-specific somatic differences have been reported by Roche (1965) who uncovered a significant male–female difference for mean standard deviation of stature. His samples were comprised of otherwise comparable male and female DS patients. There was a tendency for expanding growth variability to occur about 2 years earlier in the females than in the males, i.e., for the onset of wider fluctuation of mean stature with CA. Increases in stature ceased for males at CA 15.5 years and for females at CA 14.3 years. Finally, Fabia and Drolette (1970) noted an excess of females over males among cases of autosomal trisomy. They speculated that one reason for a high infant mortality in DS females (attributable to CHD) might be that trisomy-G is more lethal in females, or else that females suffer different types of cardiac defects than do males.

Whether somatic and behavioural differences by sex are cytologically determined or are merely a deception of sex-specific survival rates, is unclear. The search for distinctive bio-behavioural patterning by sex for DS is further complicated by child-rearing traditions which differ for boys and girls. A number of these concerns are explored now.

Behavioural differences by sex

Both institutions and community schools for the retarded cling to the belief that DS females are inherently more alert, more tractable and more intelligent than are DS males. There are honourable clinical origins. Engler (1949) claimed that 'in the upper (intellectual) group the female patients predominate and in the lower the male' (p. 88). He summarized thus: 'that girls are generally more vivacious and more impulsive and that they possess willpower and initiative' (p. 88). He continued: 'They are more interested in their surroundings, in dancing, and in playing, and it is easier to keep them engaged in conversation than male patients'. (p. 88). A separation of modal intelligence between the sexes can be explained in terms of (i) dissimilar care quality in sex-segregated institutions, (ii) differential mortality by sex, (iii) cytogenetically programmed differences evident from birth and (iv) a tendency for DS males to be less tolerated in the family and community (than females of a similar biological status) so that they are institutionalized more commonly and earlier in life. Which of these factors predominate is a matter of conjecture.

Magnitude of IQ differences, between DS males and females, has varied across reports. Estimates are not especially reliable because there is seldom adequate control for CA, environments or survivor effects. For example, Sternlicht and Wanderer, (1962) found a significant sex–IQ difference for an institutional sample. The males showed a mean IQ of 22.8 points against 29.1 points for the females, but the females were significantly younger than the males. Nakamura (1961) had previously documented a minor sex–IQ difference in favour of DS females. Gibson's (Gibson and Frank, 1961; Gibson, Pozsonyi and Zarfas, 1964) studies of long-term institutional cases have failed to expose any significant sex–IQ differences, although direction of differences consistently favoured the female. Initial differences might not survive prolonged custody. Demidov (1972) compared level of retardation for 312 boys and 225 girls from birth to 3 years of age. Of the girls, 16% were mildly retarded and 2% profoundly so. The boys were 3.61% mildly retarded and 11.91% profoundly retarded. His explanation is that the male foetus has greater sensitivity to all intra-uterine abnormalities and that the new-born male is subject more often to infectious diseases and other vigour reducing health problems. It has been claimed, however, that most DS infants expire before age 1 or 2 years and that these are disproportionately female. The surviving female, even in in infancy, might thus be less retarded than the males (Carter, 1958; Fabia & Drolette, 1970; Carr, 1975).

Other comments have concerned variability of performance by sex. Brousseau and Brainerd (1927), while claiming that modal IQ was about the same for both sexes, established greatest variability of IQ distribution for the female sample; even by 6 weeks of age. Carr's (1970) developmental quotients (DQs) for DS infants showed a range from 96 to 65 points for boys and from 111 to 71 points for girls. Differences in dispersion of scores were observed across five age levels up to 2 years CA. Moreover, while DQ scores decreased with age, for both male and female infants, the variability of scores up the age ladder continued to increase for the females. The tendency was not observed for normal infant controls. Motor development scores supported no significant differences for either central tendency or dispersion indices according to sex. The infant research has served, therefore, to identify sex differences which seem programmed but has not dealt satisfactorily with the environmental variables.

Differential age stability of IQ for DS males and females has been the subject of several studies. Newman (1960) reported a correlation between IQ and CA of −0.273 for DS males (having a CA range of 7–28 years with a median of 15 years for the combined sample), but of only −0.083 for the females. Evidently, DS females 'hold' for learning and general performance longer than do males: progressive intellectual deterioration with age being more marked for the males. Clements, Bates and Hafer (1976) found males to decline from 55 to 38 IQ points and females from 62 to 43 IQ points (over an age span of 36 to 155 months). All subjects were resident in the community and diagnosed as trisomy-21. These two studies suggest that females are more intact intellectually at all age levels but are otherwise in disagreement. Further, the Binet age levels sampled are essentially non-verbal and should have favoured the boys. Clements *et al.* offered the interesting suggestion that the female sex-chromosome may tend to reduce the severity of retardation, although differential survival rate is mentioned as a potential source of IQ differences by sex.

Although sex-specific mortality effects on sampling provide the soundest present explanation, the possibility of karyotypic influence, by sex, cannot be discounted. Fabia and Drolette (1970) reported an excess of females over males for cases of autosomal trisomy. Gibson and Pozsonyi (1965), comparing a series of translocation DS and standard trisomy controls, contended that the males fell disproportionately within the translocation group. Differences in IQ were also observed between these cytogenetic subgroups in a direction consistent with past trends. Rosecrans (1968), assembling studies of mosaicism DS up to 1966, revealed that of 14 verified DS mosaics all IQ levels of 50 points or less occurred in the males (seven cases) while all but one instance of IQ scores of plus 50 points occurred in the females. One could argue that sex status is not randomly distributed across cytogenetic categories or that phenotypes are modified biologically and psychologically according to sex status.

Distinctive clinical and psychological manifestations for male and female DS might be genuine. The sex-specific disparities, declared to date, have included a more typical picture of physical stigmatization and greater variability of stature for females. Sex differences have been mentioned for bone growth, intelligence level and personality status, all favouring the DS female. The reasons can only be guessed. In summary, they include a greater frequency of CHD in DS females and thus a higher and earlier mortality. The female survivor group, substantially established by the second year of life, might exhibit median somatic and psychological features slightly in advance of males as a group. The second hypothesis, of sex differences in developmental patterning from birth, has been introduced by Carr (1970, 1975) but requires further work.

Future investigation will need to pursue the foregoing issues and, as well, (i) trace the suspected behavioural differences for DS males and females through the various chromosomal subtypes, and (ii) determine whether sex-specific patterns of nurture, in both family and institutional settings, are sufficient explanation. As improving paediatric regimes redress the mortality imbalance, the distribution of psychological profiles, by sex, will also change. Meanwhile, it is operationally sound to consider sex status among the percursors of intellectual potential (or performance) and to plan accordingly.

Evaluation

The foundations of intelligence for Down's syndrome are likely to be inter-dependent and of greater complexity than we know. Some workers are convinced that karyotype is critical for determining the limits and quality of intellectual potential. Many of these investigators have proposed that translocation DS is an average of 6 IQ points ahead of standard trisomy DS and mosaicism DS superior to both. Others have argued, unsuccessfully, that the mosaicisms vary by intellectual level according to the percentage of aberrant cells. Still to be determined is the amount of IQ variance which can be assigned to subclass of chromosome anomaly and if development forecasting and management can be based, in part, on cytogenetic data. The search for familial residuals of intelligence in DS is so far a failure. A secondary result of the research is that the character of the parent–child bond might be different for the DS offspring than for their normal siblings. The usual family nurtural process is socio-cultural in nature and is on a base of shared genetics. Reliable parent–child IQ correlations are therefore to be expected. The presence of a significant IQ link between DS offspring and their parents and the absence of such correlations for DS children and their normal siblings might indicate that (i) the normal genetic links are totally masked by the aberrant karyotype, (ii) the shaping of the DS child in the home is more an affectional than intellectual enterprise and (iii) DS children have a developmental plasticity which exceeds that of other varieties of severely to moderately retarded children. Nurture of DS children by well-motivated parents can result in a 10 point or more IQ advantage, an impressive increment in view of the modest IQ limits of the disorder.

Adventures into the psychological outcomes of family versus institutional care have methodological difficulties. The general impression is that different care regimes elicit different kinds or levels of social, psychomotor, cognitive and affective skills but that (i) psychometric studies select and sample these skills to the advantage of home care and (ii) DS children are hospitalized, or not, depending on degree of handicap and the coping skills of the home. In any event, the wide range of individual behavioural differences, evident within any single care regime, point to more than environmental forces at work. A kindred problem is the permanence of IQ gains achieved in a given 'good' environment. Hospitalization, subsequent to home care, has been accompanied by precipitous declines in test intelligence. These losses could attest to the effects of over-training, to the impotency of institutions as care agents, to the superficiality of environmental absorption for DS, or to the strong community bias in IQ test standardization. The issue is complicated by the practice of institutionalizing DS children at ages (6 and 11 years CA being the most common) which correspond with the first behaviourally visible effects of neurophysiological corrosion. Cowie (1970) offers the strongest demonstration of the parallels between neurological and behavioural development and as early as 6 months of life.

The matching of essentially global environments with psychological outcomes has therefore been unsuccessful. A better approach would be to identify the range of communication, psychomotor, cognitive, self-help, and affectional potentials and deficiencies for DS, as these co-vary with the stimulus properties of the environment and with shifting somatic events. Some sensitivity to the rates and timing of developmental trends would be necessary, especially as these are affected by environmental and biological forces. Future care options are surely richer than merely a choice of traditional family versus classical institutional care and the admonition to 'love' the child.

Arguments have been advanced for a sex-specific biological susceptibility to the effects of chromosome anomaly. According to others, clinical and psychological differences between DS males and females are a consequence of differential mortality rates, care practices within institutions and placement practices. The four sets of considerations are not necessarily exclusive. It is sufficient for now, to demonstrate that sex status for DS can be considered an important correlate of intellectual status. The hypotheses that the phenotype is variably expressed by sex or that DS females enjoy greater resistance to deteriorative processes, need additional study. Sex-biased mortality rates over time and the greater susceptibility of males to secondary damage are at present the most plausible explanations.

A final impression about the foundations of intellectual growth and decline is the pre-eminence of biological forces and our failure to understand these as relevant to management planning, both for the syndrome and its individual members. Evidence shows that the dynamics of genotype are also influential, favouring an early plasticity of behavioural potential for DS and some characteristic ability–disability profiles as age advances. A need for early and intensive remediation, built around the maturational and pathological sequencing of the disorder, is indicated.

5

Personality: normal and abnormal

Down's syndrome is one of those conditions about which professionals and laymen speak with confidence. The DS child or adult is widely described as affable, mischievous, docile, aggressive, affectionate, stubborn, pleasing and self-willed. These traits of personality and temperament are said to be characteristic of the syndrome and in some way innate. They are also contradictory. The pioneer studies were naturalistic, followed by efforts to catalogue DS personality by types and to identify the varieties of psychopathology associated with the syndrome. The recent research is actuarial and experimental in method. It attempts to trace the interaction of intelligence levels, sex, extent of secondary organic factors, communication and arousal potentials, and the conditions of nurture with personality status across ages and karyotypes. The movement has, therefore, been away from unproductive debate about the structure of the stereotype and toward the discovery of the origins and distribution of personality characteristics relevant to management.

The stereotype

Naturalistic observations

The personality stereotype, including its surety and internal inconsistencies, can be traced to Down (1866). As 'instances of degeneracy' they were presumed by him to display the more rudimentary, simplistic and child-like personality patterns of modern (European) man's remote racial ancestors. Penrose and Smith (1966), quoting from an 1887 report by Down concerning the proposed talent for mimicry, claimed that 'several patients who have been under my care had been wont to convert their pillowslips into surplices and to imitate, in tone and gesture, the clergyman or chaplain they have recently heard.' A second supposedly unique feature was also identified by Down, i.e., 'They have a strong sense of the ridiculous; this is indicated by their humorous remarks and the laughter with which they hail accidental falls, even of those to whom they are most attached.' A third major feature of the DS personality was said by Down to be obstinacy: 'No amount of coercion will induce them to do that which they have made up their minds not to do. Sometimes they initiate a struggle for mastery, and the day previous will determine what they will or will not do on the next day. Often they will talk to themselves and they may be heard rehearsing the disputes which they think will be the feature of the following day.' And finally: 'They are always amiable both to their companions and to animals. They are not passionate nor strongly affectionate.' (Down as quoted in Penrose and Smith, 1966, pp. 54–5.) Down's prescription for management reflects his belief about the constancy of these personality features, e.g., 'Whether it be the question of going to church, to school, or for a walk, discretion will often be the better part of valour, by not giving orders which will run counter to the intended disobedience and thus maintaining the appearance of authority while being virtually beaten.' (Down, 1866.)

These descriptions of the typical personality of DS are anthropomorphic, optimistic and over-generalized, as later evidence will show. Implied throughout was a degree of cunning, foresight, resourcefulness, recall ability and capacity for interpersonal collaboration which is not consistent with what is now known of the behavioural (especially the intellectual) potentials of the typical DS child or adult. The times were partly culpable. During the nineteenth century, psychological propensities of all kinds were thought to be instinctual in origin, not necessarily tied to general intelligence, and discretely evolved as biological adaptations to meet finite environments. In retrospect, the chief value of Down's characterization was to draw attention to the existence of the syndrome and its special management needs.

Later comment generally adhered to Down's opinion except for a few near contemporaries who made parenthetic note of 'atypical' cases where restlessness, poor control and either aggressiveness or marked withdrawal predominated. Barr (1904) questioned the 'mongolian type' as a behaviourally bounded class of mental retardation. He described five institutional cases as representative. One case (aged 15 years) answered the classical description, the man having a good nature, some obstinacy, a keen sense of the ridiculous, a facility for imitation and an excellent memory. A female aged 23 years was described as disobedient but affectionate; a male (18 years) as semi-mute and classifiable as an 'apathetic idiot'; and finally, a 24-year-old male who was an idiot–imbecile epileptic. Notwithstanding Barr's singular diagnostic practice, his evidence does not support the classical personality picture as described by Down. Since Barr's sample appears severely retarded, under terminal custodial care and somewhat older, it is perhaps not representative of those first cases described by Down. Sherlock and Donkin (1911) recognized that the severity of retardation would qualify his otherwise kindly account of DS individuals as good-tempered and submissive to authority, i.e., that they should be 'sufficiently intelligent to be capable of such manifestations'. Yet as late as 1924, Brushfield was describing DS as 'always cheerful, lively, restless and very happy'.

With the exception of Barr, the clinical impression of a consistent and uniform personality for DS remained unchallenged until 1928 when Brousseau and Brainerd traced the development of personality in DS. They claimed that 'emotionality' is lacking in the DS infant, 'expressive movements showing emotional states' (p. 120) being evident in only one infant examined by them. The sudden smiles, seen only on occasion, are attributed to momentary external stimulus conditions which are able to elicit a reflexive facial response much like a grimace or a gas smile. The general placidity of DS infants, compared with normal infants or with other moderately retarded, is taken as evidence of quite depressed sensory thresholds. The sudden and late appearance of more age-appropriate affective responses would be proof that the DS child has finally matured the minimal sensory apparatus necessary to support reliable stimulus–response circuiting. Otherwise, volitional reactions are dismissed as 'largely instinctive' and dependent upon the impulse of the moment. These opinions were impressionistic and based on small samples of mostly quite young cases. It was not until 1953 (Oster) that a large sample study, representative demographically and by age, was available. Oster was impressed by the dispersion of personality reaction corresponding to age class. He claimed that while young DS patients are usually good-natured, ongoing constraint and 'failing understanding' with age contributed to a growing restlessness, aggressiveness and obstinacy. The hypothesis is for progressive personality change as a function of an early and progressive erosion of intellectual status, coupled possibly with restrictive care practices. Temperament was said to be good in 273 cases (71%), fluctuating in 32, neutral in 15, and poor in three cases only. Stubbornness and aggressiveness were claimed to be the most common and consistent personality characteristics. Marked aggressiveness was especially evident for older DS individuals. Stubbornness occurred at all age levels, and about equally for the sexes. The inference is that some aspects of DS temperament are constitutional in nature while other features are dependent upon the vagaries of secondary handicap and environment.

Benda (1956) initially suggested a situational understanding of personality. He viewed DS as temperamentally placid or neutral; positive or negative responses being elicited by the nature and quality of the surroundings. His later explanations (Benda, 1960 *a*) depended less on environmental factors, moving instead to 'a very characteristic behaviour pattern of mongoloid patients: their stubbornness' (p. 67). He acknowledged the difficulty of establishing suitable psychiatric or behavioural definitions for stubbornness and settled finally for 'inflexibility of intentions' which is innate and the basis of a good deal of their interpersonal style. For example,

Stubbornness can be observed in very young mongoloids and seems to depend upon their inability to shift quickly from one object to another and to react to new situations. With great patience, the stubbornness may be overcome in a certain test condition, but it remains a fundamental tendency of the patient in all new situations. Contrasted with the lack of attention and the distractibility common to many subnormal patients, I venture to suggest that the stubbornness of mongoloids is a psychological manifestation of the peculiar discrepancy in the development of the nervous system, in which the central subcortical areas serving emotional responses are fairly well developed while the 'long-circuiting' system of the cortex, serving the evaluation of sensory stimuli and responses, and therefore, intelligent interaction with the environment, remains immature and undeveloped. (Benda, 1960 *a*, p. 68)

Benda thus supports Oster's view of stubbornness as a focus for understanding personality in DS but goes on to propose neuro-maturational mechanisms underlying the predisposition.

At the outset, single case observations favoured a benign and trouble-free personality picture which was more or less uniform and predictable from one DS child to another. Subsequent observation contributed a growing number of exceptions to the rule. These have been explained, with little real evidence, as the effects of environmental corruption, advancing age, or the result of innate stubbornness. Others have identified the alleged stubbornness as a product of a too high intellectual expectation stimulated by the pleasing temperament of many young DS children. Another explanation is that sensory and motor immaturity, peculiar to DS children, frustrates a relatively more intact intellectual potential and contributes to a general recalcitrance. Evaluation of these early impressions requires examination of the trait classification and actuarial literature, followed by a consideration of the varieties of psychopathology for Down's syndrome and the interaction of personality with age, cognition, sex, karyotype, constitution and nurtural conditions.

Temperament and personality typing

Contradictory naturalistic evidence is often reconciled by claiming exceptions to a rule or by promoting 'types' within a system. Wallin (1949) proposed two major personality variants for DS; a lively, good-natured, affectionate, amiable, docile and cheerful type, and a shy, reticent, apathetic, destructive, noisy and negativistic type. He was inclined to accept the positive personality stereotype as primary, attributing the large group of exceptions to emotional and CNS process aberration presumably acquired or expressed later in life. Rollin (1946) had earlier offered a similar view but within the framework of a behavioural typology. His intent was to differentiate two distinct emotional types, the introverted and extroverted. It was his belief that the more attractive psychological artifacts of DS might be natural to the syndrome and that progressive neuropathology or environmental spoiling shaped the less attractive personality configuration.

Engler's (1949) notions about DS temperament closely follow those of Wallin and Rollin. The first type delineated by him included the happy, gentle and good-natured members of the syndrome. Engler was more enthusiastic than objective. For example: 'Their innate need for affection and tenderness quickly forms a bridge between them and those around them. Their gay and pleasing mood is not easily changed. When annoyed, in any way, a few words or a caress are sufficient to restore their happiness. One rarely sees or hears them crying, and then only when they are in real pain or get the worse of an argument which is always started by somebody else' (p. 94). A second personality group included the dull, listless and unresponsive. A final personality type was characterized as being aggressive, destructive, incompetent, uncontrollable and in every respect the opposite of the first. These personality divisions shift and erode with age, according to Engler, and 'Those among them who pass a certain precarious age gradually become duller and relatively early lose all the characteristics which made them so delightful in youth. They become listless, and uninterested, sit silently in a corner, and scarcely reply to any questions. Meals constitute the only happy break in their monotonous existence.' (p. 95). Perhaps the most parsimonious conclusion is that the first personality type is a romanticized view of the classical stereotype, the second (the severely and profoundly retarded DS) having little or no intellectual potential on which to build contact patterns and the third the older deteriorated cases. The effects of prolonged custodial care and advancing age could be the primary sources of Engler's typology.

Only Rollin (1946) attempted to bring theoretical respectability to the personality typologies then postulated for DS. He proposed an introvert–

extrovert dichotomy for DS and distinguished them thus: 'Environmental stimuli, biologically, can produce two fundamental modes of reaction. Firstly, the organism may seek to re-establish equilibrium by bringing about alterations in the environment itself. Secondly, the organism may passively accept the environmental alterations and bring about changes within itself to suit the new conditions. The essential difference between the two types of reaction is one of motor discharge.' (p. 225). Rollin applied the terms hyperkinetic and hypokinetic to mark motor outcomes for the two personality classes. He believed that a polarization of personality is more evident in DS than for normals because these 'primitive modes of reaction' are somehow less blunted by the forces of environment and learning. What stands out for the syndrome is pure, simple and unimpaired affect, negative or positive, the expression of which is all the more direct and uncomplicated as a consequence of poor capacity for cognitive mediation and modification. Others who are moderately retarded do not exhibit this characteristic because their neuropathology is often more capricious, or centered at more primitive neurological layers such as to corrupt affect more severely. 'It is, therefore, not surprising that amongst them the primitive instinctual–affective patterns approach a high degree of purity, rendering the division of the two groups much easier than in normal individuals who, as is well known, tend to cluster about the average in any personality scale.' (p. 225). Rollin conceived, also, a third or 'mixed' type of DS personality, as is usual when a host of exceptions are to be dealt with.

Rollin's supporting data were both descriptive and experimental. Of 73 cases studied, 50 were male and 23 female with ages ranging from 8 to 48 years. Most of these were in the 10- to 20-year age group, followed by the 20- and 30-year age category. Thirty-two DS cases (43.8%) were described as extroverted, conforming to the positive personality stereotype as described by Engler. Notwithstanding, of 44 who displayed behaviour disorders, 11 were classified as extroverts. The second largest group was comprised of the introverted personalities (42.4%). The mixed group made up the balance (13.7%). The relation of temperament to clinical status in DS was evaluated using various criteria: IQs below 29 points (criterion A), cephalic index (0.83 or higher) (B), epicanthic fold (C), fissured tongue (D), conjunctivitis (E), simian crease (F) and single crease on the fifth palmar digit (G). While the introverts placed more frequently in the low IQ pool, the extroverts exhibited a more classical expression for all somatic features. Tests of statistical significance were not offered, although scanning suggests the operation of non-chance factors for direction and magnitude of intelligence differences in respect to the six somatic characteristics. The extroverted, according to Rollin, total about half of all cases, are brighter, and appear more clinically stereotyped than the introverted members of the syndrome. Rollin next attempted to relate personality type to manipulated behaviour. All patients were assembled and seated in a recreation hall. Simple dance music was played and each patient was encouraged to respond. Only 24 attempted to dance, 16 of whom were extroverts. Four were introverts, and four others of the venturesome were of the mixed personality variety. Rollin added that the quality of performance was notably poor, whatever the personality class. The introverted cases remained largely unmoved by either the music or by the activity surrounding them. The experiment is hardly critical, there being no control group and no information about comparative ages or quality of institutional care. Nor is it clear how personality ratings were obtained.

A third arm of the study tested the connection between psychometric performance and personality type. The devices employed included the revised Stanford–Binet, the Goddard formboard, and a single Merrill–Palmer item (mare and foal). The IQ results indicated extroverts to be generally brighter than introverts, and apparently significantly so. Re-grouping of the IQ test content, into verbal or performance categories, is also of interest for the elaboration of the personality dichotomy. The extroverts' verbal responses during testing were self-assured and superficially impressive, with easy answers and random guesses predominating. Test performance of a non-verbal nature was impulsive, rushed and confident, but generally of poor quality. Performance approach, Rollin said, was largely trial and error with little evidence of what he called 'Gestalt' or conceptualization ability. Introverts, by comparison, were shy and reticent on both verbal and performance tests and, without suitable encouragement, did poorly. Rollin offered that perhaps the introverted merely appear to be of lower average IQ, both as a result of their reticence and its magnification in the form of inhibitory schizoid reaction. The thesis evidently is that, for the introverted, intellectual prowess is masked by psychosis (for 22 of his sample). Otherwise, the introvert was (given adequate examiner patience and affection) able to make finer motor coordinations and to display a rudimentary conceptual ability superior to that reported for the extroverted sample. Length of home care versus institutional care and age are, however, not controlled and would be critical to any interpretation relevant to differential management.

The Wunsch (1957) typological ratings for 'manifest' behaviour are important principally because non-institutional DS is engaged and because the potential influence of age and sex are remembered in the computations. DS was divided into docile-affective and aggressive-hostile types of personality.

Wunsch indicates that 51% of 77 DS children were docile-affective, 14.3% were aggressive-hostile, and the balance notably neither. Docile-affective ratings were about equal between the sexes but with a larger number of boys being aggressive-hostile. Wunsch noted that 'a greater proportion of those under 5 years and over 14 years of age were aggressive-hostile while the docile-affective type were concentrated in the 5 to 13 year age group'(p. 125). Some additional tests of the interaction of intelligence level with proposed personality type, sex and age would be of value in order to assign appropriate sources of variance. The gross findings are, in any case, similar to those of Rollin with the largest single group satisfying the favourable stereotype for DS and the positive proportion being greater (51% versus 43.8%) for the community over the institutionalized cases.

Hallenbeck (1960) carried Rollin's topographical hypothesis into the field of somatotyping, based on Goldstein's work. Goldstein (1956) had contended that DS was distributed behaviourally as two overlapping groups; the thyroid deficient exhibiting short stature, atonia, awkward gait and higher IQ, and a second group which displayed lower IQs, a greater degree of emotional lability, tall and thin stature, general restlessness and metabolic differences. Pursuing the division, Hallenbeck classed the ectomorphic variety of DS (tall, thin and introverted) as hostile-aggressive and the endomorphic (shorter, heavier and extroverted) as of superior disposition and intelligence. The ectomorphic were described as hyperactive and thus likely to be viewed, by parents and other care agents, as aggressive. Aggressive behaviours would, the argument goes, attract hostile responses to the child and thereby reinforce less agreeable behaviours. The more positively out-going or extroverted endomorph would attract more salutary opportunities for personal growth.

The Hallenbeck speculation is that (i) temperament for DS is founded on physiological predisposition expressed in classical somatotypic terms, and (ii) appropriate environments are important for guiding the behavioural unfolding of the somatotype. Simpler explanations come to mind based on the lack of an acceptable operational definition of 'personality' for DS and the absence of proper controls for the influence of CA, karyotype, quality of early care regimes, prominence of secondary handicap and amentia level. Moreover, studies founded on abstracted, unidimensional and often inconsistent theoretical dichotomies, such as extroversion–introversion, docile-affective, hostile-aggressive, etc., offer little opportunity for critical hypotheses testing. It is even premature to make the nurtural claim that 'the pattern of docility-affectiveness versus aggression-hostility (Wunsch terminology) apparently depends in large part on the child's affectional environment' (Forman, 1967, p. 9). The newer studies to be reviewed have demonstrated that about half of all DS children (in the favourable age range of approximately 5–14 years) display a more or less attractive temperamental status depending upon degree of intellectual and other handicap. Across all age categories, however, personality stereotypes have not proved to be reliable concepts for prediction or management purposes.

Empirical evidence

The only data-supported studies mentioned thus far, those by Rollin and by Wunsch, were designed to demonstrate a theoretical position. Using non-DS varieties of MR for comparison, most other empirical studies have tested the null-hypothesis in respect to (i) the validity of the personality stereotype for DS, and (ii) the range and type of psychopathology exhibited by the syndrome.

Some actuarial contradictions

The first attempts to quantify and sample specific psychological traits for DS (see Kuenzel, 1929) added little to the impressionistic evidence. Pototzky and Grigg (1942), for example, applied the Marston personality rating scale to an institutional sample of 19 cases of DS. The cutting score, between the two personality types (extroversion–introversion) was 60 points with a theoretical range of from 20 to 100 points. About 70% of the cases were in the extroverted range. The impact of this finding is greatly reduced insofar as the mean score of 65 points for the entire sample is close to the arithmetic border between the two personality 'types'. Further treatment of these data was possible, CA and IQ scores being available for 18 comparisons. Ranking CA and IQ with personality ratings (taking a Marston score of 71 as the midpoint) produced a mean IQ of 47.44 points for the upper half and 42.10 points for the lower half of the personality distribution. Upper scale personality ratings represented a mean CA of approximately 18 years and lower scale personality ratings, on the average, of 25 years CA. The high scorers are therefore both younger and less retarded. Given that IQ for DS is known to deteriorate with advancing CA and that institutional time would likely be greater for the older group than the younger group, there is no justification for the Pototzky and Grigg contention for a polarization of personality in DS. There is some suggestion, though, that sex may be an important variable in determining magnitude of personality score for DS, the female being both more 'extroverted' and at the same time more intelligent.

Blacketer-Simmonds (1953) did not build on the prior work of Pototzky and Grigg and thus invited many of the same methodological and theoretical problems. The study is important chiefly because of its use of environmental and aetiological controls. The Blacketer-Simmonds procedure was to assemble data, concerning temperament, both before and after institution-alization. Pre-admission behavioural information was scaled and compared with later hospital staff ratings for largely the same individuals. Non-DS controls (100) were selected so as to be compatible 'intellectually and physically' with the DS cases. The particular personality criteria considered included such adjectives as affectionate, cheerful, friendly, docile, imitative, solitary, destructive, mischievous and a number of others related more strictly to level of social performance. Percentage frequency of each adjec-tive was compared for the pre-admission status of DS subjects and controls. Of 15 psychological characteristics, only the qualities docile, solitary, and mischievous yielded significant chi-squares. The DS sample was apparently less docile and more mischievous than other retardates in the same intel-lectual range but otherwise were similar. Nor are three differences, from a series of 15 comparisons, statistically reliable. The conclusions did not favour a special pre-institutional personality status for the syndrome.

A second phase of the Blacketer-Simmonds study was undertaken within the institution using a questionnaire method and nursing staff evaluations. DS patients ($N = 60$) were randomly dispersed throughout a population of non-DS patients ($N = 300$) so as to obscure their group identity. Each patient was rated plus or minus for a given trait. The mute and non-ambulatory were excluded. No differences proved significant, indicating that the few suggestive trends of the first study were unreliable, or that community-originated behavioural differences are superficial and disappear following hospitalization. The overall tendency, unconfirmed statistically, was for the DS sample to be less good-tempered and more mischievous than other comparable MR and, at the same time, to be both more affectionate and more restless. Finally, a separate analysis of homogeneity of behavioural responses showed the DS group to be about as variable as other moderate MR. These findings, too, provide little closure on the question of unique personality patterning for DS. Testing the personality stereotype for just institutional patients or candidates, against the opinions of admitting physicians and nursing personnel, is bound to generate sampling bias and also subjective bias. A more useful strategy would be a comparison across institutional, pre-institutional (waiting list) and community established samples of DS.

Blessing (1959) selected 83 DS children resident in community special schools (and presumably not pressing for admission to institution) for behavioural scaling by their teachers. The test items and tabular results are examined more closely in the chapter on socialization. The conclusion reached was that most of the social performance characteristics of DS did not adequately differentiate the condition from other retarded children. It is of interest that the few significant differences related more closely to temperament than to the overt aspects of socialization. Teachers classed a variety of behaviours according to Goldberg's (1957) categories of 'satisfactions and problems', derived from his study of teacher attitudes towards DS children. Blessing lists the 'satisfactory' and the 'problem' traits according to whether they are seen more and less frequently. Most frequently occurring positive personality features included cheerfulness, good disposition, obedience and independence. Most frequently expressed problems included communication disorder, stubbornness, short attention span, attention seeking and easy fatigue. Overall, Blessing claimed that DS ranked first in ease of management, compared with other aetiological groups of mental retardation, but not first in ease of instruction or training. The Blessing sample was clearly a selected group insofar as these cases were sufficiently intact intellectually to attend school, of optimum age for favourable social and personality expression, community-based, comparatively free of secondary handicaps, and of good socio-economic background. Had these findings been reported against an appropriate control group, using a more closely rationalized or stratified sampling procedure, a case might have been made for a unique personality pattern for DS. As it is, the study provides a mixture of negative and positive psychological traits distributed more or less randomly across aetiological groups.

Silverstein's (1964) statistical test of the behavioural stereotype for Down's will be explored later in the context of social growth or 'general adjustment' (identified as factor I). A second important aspect of the paper is its investigation of personality (factor II) for DS and matched controls. The approach is more precise than in the Blacketer-Simmonds studies. DS subjects and controls were paired for age, sex, IQ and length of institutionalization. The mean age of Down's and controls was 12.1 years. Mean IQ was 25 and 26 points respectively. The duration of hospitalization was 5.1 and 5.0 years. The rating scale employed was derived from Peterson (1960) and designed to isolate introverted and extroverted personality styles. The ratings (on each subject pair) were completed by nurses and attendants and the scores analysed to determine factor loading. Analysis of variance tests were undertaken for those variables identified with the introversion–extroversion dimension for the DS cases ($N = 30$) and the controls ($N = 30$). Six significant behavioural differences emerged from the survey of 20 performance traits but only two related specifically to temperament. These were degree of cheerfulness and degree of gregariousness. The other significant differences were for behavioural characteristics of a social nature (manners, responsibility, etc.). Factor II results (introversion–extroversion) therefore supported no difference between Down's and non-Down's, even though factor I content (general adjustment) had been shown to be different in favour of superior social adjustment for the DS sample; a paradox insofar as social response capacity is usually a reflection of qualities of temperament and personality.

Additional sampling and methodological frustrations are evident in the study of Domino, Goldschmid and Kaplan (1964). Their sample was limited to DS females (mean IQ of 30 points) resident in a single ward containing 21 DS cases and 35 other retarded girls. The controls were described as uncomplicated 'cerebral dysgenesis' of unknown cause. Behavioural ratings were obtained mainly from 12 ward staff. The major instrument was a checklist of descriptive adjectives from case book and ward reports and standardized as the 'sonoma checklist'. The staff were instructed to select 40 adjectives which best described the patient. A second data gathering procedure was to require ward staff (i) to judge whether they would accept or reject a given patient, and (ii) to rate their degree of familiarity with a given patient along a 7-point scale. Thirty-five adjectives correlated significantly with the diagnosis of DS. These were, for the most part, related to patterns of temperament rather than to socialization. The results suggest a favourable and somewhat distinct personality configuration for DS. Even the mooted stubbornness was absent. Since a good effort had been made to control the bias of the staff and other bias, the major interpretive options would seem to be (i) that a special and positive personality stereotype is valid for DS females or (ii) that the aetiologically mixed controls were less able to benefit from an apparently good quality ward care regime.

A second project by Domino (1965) generalized his initial finding of a special constellation of DS personality traits to both males and females and tested the bias of the staff as a form of 'stereotypic projection'. Naive, non-staff judges were used. The 'sonoma checklist' was applied to 21 pairs of DS and non-DS retarded, appropriately matched. Each student (of 210 freshman college students) observed one pair of patients and rated each for 210 behavioural adjectives. Fifty-six items distinguished significantly between pairs. Consistent with the usual stereotype were such words as clownish, content, active, affectionate, calm, chatters, co-operative, friendly, good-natured, happy, lively, manageable, playful, pleasant, relaxed, show-off, sweet, tries to please and warm. At the same time, the DS cases were seen by naive observers as significantly hostile, indifferent, secretive, shy, sulky, greedy, messy, sloppy, unfriendly and unteachable. The mean frequency of still other adjectives was higher for the non-DS series. These included such positive qualities as being stable, outgoing, educable, controllable and meticulous. Interpretation of the Domino findings will depend on the readers' tolerance of the more subtle methodological difficulties.

Some methodological traps

The resolution of inconsistent findings about the personality stereotype for DS would require (i) a better understanding of the nature of the various control groups used, (ii) reliable data on sample differences between DS subjects and controls for gradients of CA and IQ, and (iii) sounder information concerning the quality and type of support and training regimes within the various institutions or schools sampled. In one study reviewed no controls were exercised. In another, both the DS sample and controls were well advanced for age, the controls appearing rather hyperkinetic and the care programme merely custodial. A number of studies examined test the personality characteristics of brain-injured imbeciles, of whatever type and origin, and compare these with Down's syndrome. A more fruitful strategy would involve longitudinal comparisons of young DS children with both normal children of equivalent MA and other causally specified retarded children. Such studies should clearly define the behavioural expectations and the environmental conditions. End-effect, too, is a problem. The Silverstein sample, in common with others, was not closely representative intellectually of DS, his 12-year-olds having a mean IQ of only 26 points. The conclusion 'that stability and consistency of the personality syndrome in mongolism may spring from...genetic bases' (p. 570) is not yet justified. Belmont (1971) questions the findings further on the grounds that the observations have been too brief and not ideally quantified.

The empirical research has provided no firm grounds either for accepting or rejecting the classical personality stereotype for DS. The problems are many. The use, from study to study, of non-comparable and sometimes rudimentary personality assessment methods inhibits generalization. Samples, across studies, vary for such vital dimensions as CA, IQ and nurtural origins. Moreover, a cohesive behavioural constellation could probably be extracted for any subject group living together in a closely-managed institution; especially over a long period, and where care routines are prescribed, constant and reinforced by closed staff training programmes. Conditions of environment, as these impinge on the dimensions of personality for DS, have been neither manipulated experimentally nor acknowledged statistically. Personality trait differences, as between hospital and home resident DS, might flow entirely from the variety of subject conditions and family circumstances which lead to the placement of selected DS children in institutional settings. The various concepts of personality, translated for the study of DS, are inappropriate, as well. Some investigators have abstracted and rated along introversion–extroversion or affective–hostile continua. Others have defined personality, *ad hoc*, as ease of management or in terms of degree of social acceptability by either community or institution.

Whether an identifiable personality profile exists or not, for DS, can be explored on a broader base by considering (i) its extensions into psychopathology and (ii) the stability of its properties across developmental stages, degrees of intellectual deficit and conditions of nurture. With such information, a consideration of the issues will be possible.

Varieties of psychopathology
The structure of the evidence

Clear distinctions between normal and abnormal personality are always difficult, and even more so where the populations studied exhibit intellectual and neuromotor handicaps of developmental origin. Negative behaviours are not necessarily maladaptive, just as all apparently positive behaviours need not indicate a state of psychological well-being. The DS child responds to the conditions of his internal and external environment, like anyone else; only perhaps more so. The most adaptive response to a restrictive or negative environment might be stubbornness, aggressive acting-out, or retreat into docility and lethargy. Socially sanctioned responses might be symptomatic merely of poor internal and external conditions, e.g., habitually arid environments which invite intensive competition for attention at the expense of other psychological needs. Vigorous affection-seeking in poorly staffed group-care situations, while cute, is hardly indicative of emotional health and happiness. The much described imitative facility of the DS child further complicates the definition of his psychopathology if, for instance, he is easily able to model the deviant behaviour of those around him. The reliable mimicry of the peculiarities of 'significant others' may in truth be quite adaptive, especially if internal pressures are satisfied, e.g., outlets for impulsiveness.

Consideration of the psychopathology of DS will include the functional and organic psychotic states and the more severe anxiety-derived conditions which are ordinarily classified as symptom disorders. Habit disorders, comprised usually of magnifications of normal traits, have been covered in the consideration of the trait literature. Three general classes of psychiatric disorder, as distinct from behavioural idiosyncracy, are said to occur for the syndrome. These are the functional psychoses, a variety of neurotic symptom disorders and several major neuropsychological manifestations including convulsive disorders, pre-senile state and senile dementia. The neurotic states include chronic and disabling impulsiveness, distractability, recalcitrance, fearfulness, anxiety, poor self-control and general aggressiveness. Various writers have associated psychopathology in DS with (i) the lower levels of intelligence, (ii) the adult and prematurely aged, (iii) the male, (iv) patients displaying various secondary handicaps and obvious neuropathology, (v) karyotypic variation within the syndrome, (vi) poor care conditions and (vii) supposedly novel and genetically predisposed qualities of temperament. There is modest correlational and clinical evidence concerning these matters but limited experimental study. The literature can be assembled under two general headings; Maladaptive Behavioural States and Psychotic States.

Maladaptive behavioural states

The most striking feature of the psychopathology literature for DS is its contrariness. Unspecified behaviour disorders occurred in 25% of Oster's (1953) sample and about equally between the sexes. Fifty-seven of his cases were resident at home and 75 in institutions. Types of psychological 'disorder' most often cited included 'emotional instability, teasing, sulkiness and crossness, and anxiety states, a few with attending hallucinations. Others were destructive and self-mutilating; but only very few displayed violent behaviour to those of their own age or younger.' (p. 53). Menolascino (1965, 1967) elaborated the range and frequency of psychiatric manifestations in DS. His concern was whether or not behavioural deviation, of classical psychiatric proportions, existed for the syndrome and to what extent. Domino et al. (1964) and Silverstein (1964) concluded that DS is comparatively stable behaviourally. Webster (1963) claimed that his subjects were free from severe forms of emotional disturbance. Beley and Lecuyer (1960) had referred to a number of 'transitional' types of aberrant emotionality in DS but reported nothing of a serious psychiatric nature. Ellis and Beechley (1950) tested the frequency of emotional disturbance for 40 DS cases and a similar number of controls matched for IQ, sex and CA. Little or no emotional disturbance was found for 70% of the DS group and for 40% of the controls. An additional 20% of the DS group and 45% of the controls were placed in the moderately disturbed category.

Decker, Herberg, Haythornthwaite, Rupke and Smith (1968) studied the pattern of referral for specialty consultation, among institutional mentally retarded, as part of a general study of health care needs. DS was referred less often for psychiatric consultation than hydrocephalus, cerebral palsy or convulsive disorders. These statistically significant trends are deceptive. The authors freely acknowledged that frequency of referral for health impairment, and for severity of intellectual deficit, are closely related and that psychiatric referrals predominated for those resident for shorter periods, aetiology notwithstanding. Connor and Goldberg (1960) collected teacher ratings from educational settings for the trainable mentally retarded. Adjectives to be rated were classed either as teacher 'satisfactions' or 'problems', e.g., moody, fearful, obstinate, etc. Of the 350 children identified as DS, 54% exhibited problems contributing to difficulty of classroom management. Comparisons with other aetiological groups were not made. Blessing (1959), using a similar teacher rating method, had previously found DS to rank relatively high for ease of classroom management when compared with trainable level brain-injured, epileptic and cerebral palsied children. A less favourable account of the extent of emotional abnormality, for DS, can be found in a study by Rollin (1946). He reported a 60% occurrence of substantial psychiatric involvement among DS subjects. A high incidence of psychosis was first recorded by Earl (1934) and again by Bourne (1955), although in the latter case the diagnosis of 'protophrenia' has little descriptive or prognostic value for Down's syndrome.

Menalascino (1965) was among the first to give serious attention to psychopathology for DS within the framework of psychiatric practice. All children coming to a state clinic were psychiatrically screened. Eighty-six clients proved to be DS and of these eleven were classified in the range of clinical psychopathology. There were four females and seven males in the series. The sample is appreciably younger than former studies which have reported much higher frequencies of behavioural anomaly in DS. Data relating to intelligence rating, socio-economic background, potential institutional status, extent of secondary handicap and cytogenetic analysis were available for most of the children. Menolascino found severe amentia for four cases, moderate for five, and mild for two. Hearing problems were diagnosed for two and abnormal electroencephalographic findings were evident for five of the ten cases available for examination. Family psychopathology was absent in only three of the 11 families studied. Psychiatric diagnosis of the 11 behaviourally disturbed DS patients included chronic brain syndrome with behavioural reaction (seven), chronic brain syndrome with adjustment reaction (three), and chronic brain syndrome with psychiatric reaction (one). Family psychopathology was classified as reactive or structured, the former referring to families unable to adjust to the needs of their DS child and the latter to family units where one or both parents exhibited 'prominent and severe' personality disorder. Reactive psychopathology occurred in two of eight families and structured psychopathology in six of the eight atypical families.

Menolascino's three detailed histories of DS children showing abnormal personality are especially instructive. In each instance there emerged a pattern of 'disorganized' behaviour attributable to chronic brain syndrome and/or to severe mental retardation. Some secondary 'causal' factors were associated with environmental disruption (birth of another child, moving, etc.), or with disruption of a well-established interpersonal relationship. The single case of psychosis was said to be of the catatonic variety and occurred in a family where the father had also experienced a schizophrenic reaction. The DS child responded readily to treatment, leading Menolascino to the conclusion that the child 'had been literally nurtured on structured family psychopathology' (p. 657). These results indicate that serious psychopathology is common enough in DS and can be a product of neurological process or of either acute transitional or more insidious but chronic psychological influences. Down's syndrome, in a family context, is said to develop exaggerated affectional dependencies. Given its reputed suggestibility, the syndrome might indeed exhibit unusually strong reaction to environmental disruption; a *folie a deux* phenomenon in cases where the care agents themselves are psychiatrically afflicted. While 13% of Menolascino's cases displayed emotional instability to a serious degree the full sample of 616 MR children of all types showed a 30% incidence of psychiatric disturbance. Menolascino's reported frequency of serious behaviour disorders for DS is, furthermore, not much greater than that often quoted for normal children under 8 years of age.

Considering the massive biological disruption associated with DS, these estimates of relative psychiatric incidence are suspiciously modest. Perhaps DS children are more resistive to the forces shaping aberrant emotionality than are other mentally retarded children, except of course where more serious neuropathology is involved. Owens, Dawson and Losin (1971) made precisely this proposal in an attempt to explain the absence of behavioural sequelae for Alzheimer's disease in DS. Menolascino, too, urged caution in relating neuropathological findings, and particularly atypical EEG findings, to specific psychiatric outcomes for the syndrome. Regardless, emotionally disturbed DS children displayed a 50% frequency of abnormal EEG records, whereas the non-disturbed DS showed a 13.4% incidence of cerebral dysrhythmia. Surely, any serious somatic irregularity will predispose to a greater risk of psychiatric morbidity.

The clinical-psychiatric findings, for a randomly selected sample of 95 institutionalized DS patients, were more closely described by Menolascino (1967) in a second study. His concerns were, (i) to compare an institutional DS sample with the earlier clinic sample for extent and nature of psychiatric handicap, and (ii) to identify case history factors which might match the occurrence of psychiatric disturbance. The sample was comparised of 54 male and 41 female Down's with a mean age of 13.2 years. Examinations included a neurological survey, stigma counting, dermatoglyphic analysis and cytogenetic assessment. Psychiatric diagnosis was established by personal interviews, talking with care staff, and reviewing clinic and hospital histories. Thirty-five of the 95 DS patients fell within the definition of psychiatric disorder (37%). A comparison of these findings, with those of other workers, would require consideration of sample differences for CA and IQ levels. Of the emotionally afflicted, chronic brain syndrome (CBS) with behavioural reaction was the most frequently reported. The CBS cases, taken together, comprised 60% of the psychiatrically aberrant. Such other categories as trait disturbance, psychoneurosis and 'adjustment reaction of childhood', have not been defined operationally and are difficult to compare across studies.

The large group identified as chronic brain syndrome are of special interest. The CBS cases were pictured psychologically as hyperactive, impulsive, poorly integrated and having a disturbed attention span. This behavioural sequence is consistent with Menolascino's data from pre-admission records where the justification for institutionalization, most commonly offered (34.7% of 33 patients), centred on psychological symptoms of the sort usually associated with chronic brain symdrome. The dominant symptoms included judgement deficit (lack of caution on the street, around farm animals, etc.), impulsivity, hyperactivity, 'driven behaviour' and unprovoked outbursts. A comparison of Menolascino's two studies supports the view that institutional and community resident DS are likely to differ psychologically and physically on a simple selection basis. Menolascino concluded, however, that psychopathology in DS need not be a direct and inevitable consequence of syndromic events. He viewed emotional aberration in DS as more or less acquired in the same manner as for the population at large, but with a higher risk dependent upon the extent of neuropathology. The further point was made that the classical physical stigmatization attracts adverse environments and specific loci of stress which can produce psychopathology quite independent of nervous or metabolic system limitation.

An alternative contention is that psychopathology in DS is inherent, being an inevitable outcome of genotype. There are strong indications for the systematic action of a variety of progressive neurological and metabolic degenerative processes; perhaps more so for some cases than for others. The unfolding or regressive nature of the phenotype for intelligence in DS, along with the interdependence of affective and cognitive potential, has been reasonably established (see Chapters 3 and 4). Masland, Sarason and Gladwin (1958) after studying the literature, claimed that there is a likelihood,

that there occurs a progressive retardation of the patient's development, even after birth. In most maldevelopments, growth proceeds in a linear fashion in its later stages, and the occurrence of deterioration is suggestive of some continuing deleterious factor. The suggestion has been made that the original maldevelopment results in hormonal or trophic inadequacies which in turn lead to a secondary deficiency. Another possibility is that mongolism is actually associated with some chemical or metabolic error which, in addition to leading to antenatal maldevelopment, may also predispose to continuing damage of the nervous system. (p. 90)

Individual differences with respect to extent, type, and frequency of psycho-pathology in DS might well be some function of original karyotypic programming, as differentially expressed with advancing age and care conditions, but otherwise specific to the syndrome. A test of the latter hypothesis would require suitable comparative data.

Examination of particular maladaptive behaviours for DS and for non-DS retardates of various aetiological groups was undertaken by Moore, Thuline and Capes (1968). The samples were large (536 DS and 536 controls) and drawn from several institutions. The relative frequencies of those traits symptomatic of drive and impulse control disorder, generally associated with brain-damaged children, is of special concern. While the controls displayed most of the hyperkinetic symptoms, their frequency for DS is impressive. About one third of the DS sample was judged to be hyperactive and close to one half, aggressive. Another 79 of the 536 Down's were described as aggressive to other patients; 82 of 536 as destroying clothing; and 65 as having a history of breaking windows. The mean CA of the DS sample was 21.3 years and mean length of institutional residence 12.3 years. Intelligence test scores were not reported. A mean social quotient of 27.6 points suggests that the mean IQ might have been lower than usual for the syndrome, hospitalized or not. The direct effects of advancing age on frequency of maladaptive behaviour for DS (as distinct from possible behavioural erosion seen after many years of institutional custody) cannot be assessed from the data of Moore *et al.* What is striking is the so-called 'organic' flavour of much of the behaviour recorded for both groups.

A contrary and distinctly environmentalist view of the origins of hyperactivity for the institutionalized DS patient, at least, is offered by Buddenhagen and Sicker (1969). They charted relevant behaviours over a 48-hour period, recording the associated events which 'evoke and sustain such behaviours'. The background conditions examined were said to be characteristic of institutional care programmes. What transpired was a series of annoying, aggressive and destructive behaviours by a DS girl resulting in immediate control measures by ward staff. These controls, exercised in an otherwise attentionless setting, assumed a strong reinforcement quality. Her negative behaviours were thereby intensified, eliciting additional personal attention from the ward staff followed by still further behavioural deterioration. The authors recommended that ward staff give personal attention only when a patient displays desirable behaviours. As it happens, the aetiology of hyperactivity in mental retardation is in question on a broad front. The behaviour modification literature has demonstrated that, at best, some undesirable behaviours can be usefully modified for some cases of DS but that duration and general nature of gains are still in question. Environmental explanations are necessary but hardly sufficient because neurologically correlated drive and attention disorder is present in a sizable minority of DS children and in an even greater number of the older and severely retarded cases.

Studies of the more subtle psychological deficits of DS children, especially those related to attention and drive disorder, are useful for distinguishing organic from environmental precursors. Fisher (1970) surveyed attention and concentration deficits in brain-injured children including DS. The DS series consisted of 31 children with IQ less than 50 points. A battery of attention tests was administered to DS, brain-damaged and normal comparison groups. The psychometric instrumentation included (i) an impulse control test for which the child was required to draw a line between two points as slowly as possible, while being recorded for time elapsed, (ii) an incidental learning test in which the child concentrated on one visual feature and was later asked to identify some other peripheral feature, (iii) a 'dog and bone' test gauging ability to change set, (iv) an imbedded figure test to determine ability to 'resist contextual clues and to isolate the relevant aspects of the stimulus complex', (v) a 'matching familiar figures' test, requiring a good level of visual concentration, (vi) a card test to measure visual vigilance and (vii) an up–down test to measure auditory vigilance in terms of response to a time and tone mixed series of auditory cues. Fisher concluded that the DS and non-DS patients belong together as a brain-damaged group insofar as they display similar patterns of attention deficit. Extent of attention disorder was found to be a function of IQ level, the deficit increasing as intelligence level decreased.

Tentative conclusions are that maladaptive behaviours in DS are not much different in kind, though somewhat less in frequency, from those 'observed for non-DS subjects of similar age and IQ level. Also, more severe forms of psychopathology appear to be heralded by integrative and impulse control difficulties, compounded both of initial and progressive neuropathology, and modified to a lesser extent by environmental pressures.

Psychoses in DS

Kraepelin (1919) believed that the repetitious and sometimes bizarre mannerisms and movements of moderately to severely retarded individuals indicated the presence of larval, incomplete, or rudimentary forms of dementia praecox. Others interpreted the rocking, head banging and general self-abuse of the 'idiot' as purposeful, satisfying some primitive erotic need. These phenomena, evident especially in older custodial MR, are now believed to have origins in disturbances of the CNS and metabolism, and to be aggravated by poor conditions of physical and psychological care.

The first reliable epidemiological report of the frequency of psychoses in DS is that of Moore, Thuline and Capes (1968). They exploited a number of US hospital data sources, comparing DS with other forms of mental retardation. For all regional samples, 'manifest psychotic behaviour' was recorded for 56 of 536 cases of DS and for 105 of 536 non-DS mentally retarded controls. These controls consisted largely of neurologically handicapped individuals. Regional differences, as between DS and non-DS patients, were not significant. The samples examined had been in hospital an average of 12.3 years and had a mean chronological age of 21.3 years. Assuming that the term 'manifest psychotic reaction' has some operational importance, psychosis can be said to occur in 10% of young adult DS and in 20% or more of other forms of mental retardation; under similar life conditions and equated for age and degree of mental retardation. No data were gathered for non-institutionalized Down's of similar ages, although such figures might be difficult to interpret in view of the evidence that a major criterion for the institutionalization of any mental retardate is the presence of psycho-social disorder (Saenger, 1960).

The most commonly cited psychotic formation for DS has been catatonia. 'Apparent' psychosis of the catatonic type was initially identified among DS adults by Brousseau and Brainerd (1928). Evidence of catalepsy was the only clinical support offered. Earl (1934) culled two cases of 'primitive catatonic psychosis of idiocy' from a group of DS and identified them as the reactive type. Both subjects were the cataleptic variety, that is, displaying little or no motor initiative. An absence of motor initiative is common among older institutionalized DS, especially those who have no supervised exercise and whose main preoccupation is with their starchy diet, sleep and visceral processes.

   Actuarial support for catatonic psychosis as a common disorder of DS was first offered by Rollin (1946). He attributed the condition to an exaggeration of the personality configuration of the introverted DS patient. Of 57 DS patients, having accessible family history records, 16 were described as psychotic and 41 as non-psychotic. For the psychotic group, evidence of neuropsychiatric disorder in the family was found in six cases (epilepsy, imbecility, insanity and alcoholism). For the non-psychotic DS cases, there was a suggestion of 'tainted family histories' in nine. Psychosis in DS is evidently more common for families having a history of neuropsychiatric aberration. No tests of statistical significance and no rationalization of sampling practices were offered, hence, no reliable generalizations can be attempted. Rollin subsequently searched the personal history of the psychotic Down's for clues to the developmental origins of the psychiatric disorder. He found that psychotic process onset was often sudden and occurred particularly between 11 and 14 years CA. The behaviour change, he said, is marked by a swing from docility to manic-like restlessness, incessant talking, noisiness, and aggressiveness. More advanced stages displayed rapid behavioural deterioration, having a regressive quality. Personal habits were lost and articulate speech disappeared. Withdrawal and apathy became the rule, except where punctuated by brief periods of excitement. The terminal picture is for a total loss of volition, manifest in the usual automatic motor and speech suggestibility of classical catatonia. Earl's (1934) term 'primitive catatonic psychosis' of DS was preferred by Rollin so as to acknowledge the lack of hallucinations and delusions, claimed to be absent because the syndrome is too low intellectually to generate these ideational flights. Neville (1959), however, had described a DS patient with classical paranoid schizophrenia. Rollin remarked on how frequently stereotypy, repetitious movements, emotional dissociation and catalepsy are observed among the DS population, whatever the official psychiatric status.

   Prognosis, while generally poor, was best when onset of psychosis had been late in life. Concerning causes, Rollin conceded that 'it must be accepted that all mongols are defective usually grossly, and therefore the major factor in any gross alteration in behaviour and personality must be deterioration' (p. 229). Menolascino (1965, 1967) identified a similar mix of psychiatric problems for DS finding situational factors to be of some importance. Of Menolascino's 35 instances of general psychiatric disturbance in DS, two are described as props-schizophrenia, i.e., as a schizophrenic reaction engrafted upon primary mental retardation. Four other cases were classed as chronic brain syndrome with psychotic reaction and were said to 'display periods of rather complete uncontrollability', or else contact withdrawal. The two instances of props-schizophrenia were cast clinically as catatonia having 'bizarre language manifestations'. They had been hospitalized at 4 and 5 years of age. Early history was marked by fearfulness and introversion. Menolascino (1965) had previously identified a patient for whom the onset of catatonic posturing and bizarre speech occurred when the father experienced an acute schizophrenic reaction. As the father improved, and as the father and son were reunited, the child's psychosis dissipated. Thus, the behavioural reaction of the DS offspring may have been either imitative in nature or a separation reaction marked by profound withdrawal. The environmental evidence does not, however, exclude the role of neuropathological events or other predisposing factors.

Also mentioned in the psychiatric literature is Bourne's (1955) protophrenia, a sort of mental dwarfism in children attributable to perverted child-rearing practices. Bourne studied 154 children with IQ less than 50 points, including those with DS. He contended that some or all of the manifest mental defect could be consigned to psychic aberration of early and dramatic psychodynamic origin. The chief psychological characteristics are marked withdrawal from interpersonal contact and complete reliance on object contact. Still another form of psychosis, depression, was described by Roith (1961) in a 35-year-old 'pyknic mongoloid' (IQ 45 points). Depression followed a bout of influenza, prior to which the patient was characterized as cheerful, affectionate and good-tempered. The symptoms included food refusal, crying, agitation and fantasies about being bombed by Russians and Germans and a belief that mother had died. Treatment, specific to psychotic depression, was undertaken with good results. Roith was impressed with the high incidence of catatonia associated with introverted personality traits (for Rollin's sample) and, at the same time, the lack of psychosis among the extroverted DS population. Roith's expectation was for some evidence of manic-depressive psychosis among the extroverted members of the syndrome. The psychodynamic causal position for Down's has attracted little research support. More impressive is the quite common occurrence of psychotic-like symptoms in a wide range of confirmed brain-damaged, senile and organically deteriorated mentally retarded, including Down's syndrome at more advanced ages.

Clinical and statistical reports of the high frequency of early senile dementia, related to progressive neurological degenerative changes, comprises the bulk of the literature. Some of these studies were evaluated in a discussion of the origins of intelligence in DS. Evidence was cited which supported an approximation among the psychological indices of premature ageing, declining intelligence and personality change. The reliability and functional importance of these correlations, while not well established, are worth pursuing. Jervis (1948) described a series of instances of early senile dementia with psychiatric complication, offering both behavioural and postmortem evidence in support. One such case was a female Down's of IQ 40 points who had enjoyed good personal habits, was cheerful, able to read and write a little, and able to do routine housework. At the age of 38 years she suddenly became moody, seclusive, and destructive. Speech deteriorated, periods of noisy excitability increased, and indiscriminate eating became a problem. Hallucinations were judged to be present on the basis of her screamed, incomprehensible verbalizations. Structural and histological changes, associated with senile dementia, were subsequently found. Another case exhibited depression, loss of speech, and personal habits, and was in a continuous state of semi-torpor. She had formerly been a cheerful and helpful patient with an IQ estimated at between 40 and 50 points. Autopsy examination uncovered evidence of senile dementia. Later remarks by Jervis (1970) proposed that biological 'ageing' in DS might begin at the cellular level before birth and could be well advanced by late childhood. He also speculated on the direct influence of the aberrant karyotype in setting maturational time-tables for the syndrome.

Loesch-Mdzewska (1968) concluded that ongoing neurological abnormalities can be detected in the majority of the syndrome, appear quite early, and grow more severe into adulthood. Cassel (1953) claimed that evidence of unfolding or progressive neurological defect was often present in DS children as young as 7 years of age. Also involved were 86% of the male, and 60% of the female sample (of all ages). The neurological and histological alterations were usually those associated with pre-natal and early post-natal nervous system damage. Presumably, the neuropathological status of many cases of DS is similar to that of other severe forms of MR and would be accompanied by similar behavioural control problems. These behaviours are known to range from extreme hyperactivity and impulse disorder, to autism and mutism. Solitaire and Lamarche (1966), on post-mortem examination, documented the extent of neurological change in younger instances of DS.

Supporting investigations of the prevalence of dysrhythmia, and of the greater than expected frequency of convulsive disorders in DS, have been examined in previous chapters.

Just about the full range of psychotic disorders have been mentioned for DS (chiefly catatonic and paranoid schizophrenia and the depressions). Suggested causes are dependent on psychodynamic, genetic and injury concepts with little attention being given to interactive or eclectic positions. An ingenious approach to the resolution of differences is offered by Keegan, Pettigrew and Parker (1974). They attempted chemotherapy for two apparently catatonic DS girls (age 23 and 25 years) using agents known to be specific for either the cognitive or affective psychoses (e.g. Trifluoperazine Chlorpromazine, Haloperidol and Amitriptyline). Amitriptyline was alone satisfactory. The results led them 'to wonder whether our cases were affective (depression) in origin, possibly due to some organic biochemical disturbance in these mongoloid patients' (p. 382). In one girl there has been possible signs of hypothyroidism and diminished level of T_4. They hypothesize that their two cases 'may be progressive disturbances of serotonin deficiency further accentuating the serotonic deficit found in patients with trisomic Down's syndrome' (p. 382). (See also Rosner, Paine and Mahanand on serotonin activity in trisomic and translocation DS.) The mild hypothyroidism is linked insofar as there is 'an increased monamine oxidase activity which could further deplete serotonin...' (p. 382). They comment further on the diagnostic difficulty. On the one hand the condition could be a variant of classical affective disorder; on the other hand the hyperkinesis and impulse disorder of many DS 'psychotics' reminded them of hyperactive children. In an attempt to associate these they point out that hyperkinetic children do exhibit diminished levels of serum serotonin and that serotonin deficiency is associated with hypotonia in DS. The picture, if confirmed, serves to link behavioural symptoms and progressive disorders of cerebral metabolism which can be traced provisionally to cytogenetic events.

A second treatment-derived causal position is exclusively psychodynamic. Szurek and Philips (1966) described the case history and psychotherapy programme of a DS child. At the outset he was anxious, tense, depressed and destructive. The father was depicted as having unrealistic expectations for the child. Following 57 playroom sessions over 20 months, and counselling sessions with the father, the signs of tension and anxiety decreased, speech quality improved and socialization increased. Intelligence rating, however, declined from 70 to 40 IQ points. The authors speculate that expectation pressure had contributed to an unnaturally high drive level which could only be sustained on a neurotic base. Intensive instruction had shaped a large rote vocabulary which elevated mental test scores beyond any predictive value. These environmental antecedents to psychopathology for DS are plausible given the affectional needs and suggestibility of DS children. Over-compensating behaviours and chronic tension would be required for the maintenance of such patterns.

Patterns and origins of psychopathology for DS are far from clear. The major positions are doctrinal and relate to how one thinks about causes. The evidence so far has implicated (i) pre-natal factors which unfold a behavioural sequence much like the impulse–attention difficulties seen in many 'exogenous' MR (Strauss and Kephart, 1955), (ii) a premature and accelerating ageing pattern with neuropathological and behavioural decline, (iii) environmental factors which corrupt personality at a level and rate depending on initial IQ, and (iv) karyotypic programming of deviant cerebral metabolism. A consideration of the correlates of personality (age, sex, intelligence, karyotype, constitution, secondary organicity and nurture) should be useful for assigning priorities to the various hypotheses concerning the causes of personality deviation for the syndrome.

The correlates of personality

Frequencies of deviant behaviours

It will be helpful in judging the origins and character of personality in DS first to review the actuarial findings. Frequency estimates of frankly deviant personality for Down's have ranged from 0% (Webster, 1963) to 60% (Rollin, 1946). Oster (1953) identified 25% of his community sample as psychologically aberrant. Menolascino (1965) reported 13% of a clinic sample and 37% of an institutional sample to be within the range of psychiatric disorder. Moore, Thurline and Capes (1968) observed 'manifest psychotic behaviour' in 10% of their cases. Approximately 30% were classed as hyperactive and 50% as aggressive. Rollin (1946) labelled 44% of his patients as extroverted personalities. Wunsch (1957) claimed 51% of his series to be docile-affective and 14.3% to be aggressive-hostile. Differences can be accounted for in terms of sampling practice. Subject populations have ranged widely for age, quality of institutional programme, length of time in institution, pre-institutional history, regional and socio-economic class, degree of defect, and general health and nurtural status. Some investigators have used control groups of non-DS retardates, others not. Control samples have varied from the quite retarded, and the so-called organic syndromes, to the use of sub-cultural and other educable-level MR. How one views the distribution and deviancy of the particulars of personality for DS would depend partly on the background effect imposed by the nature of the control samples.

There are other limitations. Students of behaviour differ considerably in the way they assess traits. For some, the process is impressionistic and clinical. Others have devised checklists, rating scales, and time-sampling procedures in contrived situations. Experimentists have been professional and lay, students and parents, ward staff and volunteers, each experimenter performing within a personal perceptual context. Psychiatric criteria are equally disparate and with a number of equivocal usages. Pre-, proto-, manifest, primitive, rudimentary, and psychotic-like states are regularly described; a search for the reassurance which comes of using established psychiatric analogies. Others have invented terminology, making their findings difficult to replicate or generalize. Calculations of the extent of various personality features for DS are further warped by the professional cloistering of most investigators. The various professional disciplines tend to be referred different types and severity conditions of behavioural deviation and to operate within distinctive theoretical frames. The neurological studies, for instance, have demonstrated an impressive amount of aberrant behaviour in DS as a correlate of neurophysiological damage or degeneracy. The samples are usually severely retarded and older. Psychiatric reports have highlighted the extent of reactive personality disorder and the temperamental predisposition of DS to catatonic states, with ingenious stretching of the classical psychiatric categories. Psychological laboratory studies of personality for DS are too often exploratory with a profusion of data and with enough client and situational characteristics sampled to support almost any argument. If various disciplines pooled their skills, blending theoretical suppositions, the uniqueness, nature and origins of the personality characteristics of DS might become clearer. In the final analysis, the chief difficulty is a failure to index personality variables (normal and abnormal) against relevant history, maturational, somatic and situational factors. Some of these are explored now.

Antecedents of the personality spectrum

Age as a personality correlate

Some of the contradictions in research surrounding personality in DS can be attributed to age differences between samples. Investigators of pre-adolescent DS (under relatively good conditions of care) contend that about half, more or less, meet the pleasantly extroverted personality stereotype usually projected for the syndrome. Studies of pre-school DS support a picture of general lethargy attributed variously to motor lag, to unspecified developmental retardation of sensory physiology, or to some antenatal central nervous system deficiency. While the very young DS child hardly fits the traditionally pleasing personality description, he is at least little trouble behaviourally. The favourable stereotype, when seen, is manifest typically at between 6 and 12 years of CA and is closely dependent upon magnitude of individual IQ. Personality parameters are evidently quite variable depending on the rate of increase of MA in relation to CA. The classical personality stereotype is most evident past 3 years MA, representing a 6-year spread of physical age. The markedly less attractive behaviours, reported for older samples, suggest the acceleration of neuropathological and other somatic processes. But not all DS, of whatever age, conform to these expectations. Some say that only a minority, across all age groups, fit the positive stereotype.

More to the point, aggressiveness, hostility, sullenness and withdrawal are clearly evident in the post 14-year age group, or in those younger cases where there is demonstrable cerebral dysfunction. Neurological disorders begin to be visible clinically at about 8 years CA and are common by the late teenage period. Behavioural difficulty is most obvious then and is coincidental with accelerating IQ decline. Corroborative evidence, of a sort, is offered by Francis (1970) who found low-grade DS children to substitute constructive object-oriented play behaviours with pointless self-orientating activities such as rocking and diffuse movements, as age advanced. These changes surfaced at between 4 and 13 years of age for most. She favoured an environmental interpretation, although her data are nicely consistent with the premature ageing and early progressive organic deterioration hypotheses for the syndrome. It is relevant that peak hospitalization times for DS are about 14 years of CA. However, age 14 is also correlated with the onset of puberty. Still another problem is that the DS child, exposed to intimate home care for a long period, might suffer more separation stress and more subsequent adjustment difficulty than those institutionalized at the age of 6 or so. Neurologically confirmed senile changes have been observed in young adult Down's, accompanied by catatonic-like psychosis in some instances. Where these processes have been described there is an emergent pattern of cyclic excitability, deterioration of personal habits, food refusal, retreat and loss of speech. The notion is that biological ageing is well advanced in even younger DS cases, compared with the normal. A good deal more needs to be learned about the telescoped growth and decline process in DS and about the value of maturational evidence for behavioural prediction and programme planning.

Sex as a personality correlate

The positive personality stereotype has been less challenged for the DS female than the male. Most of the research reviewed to date has used hospital samples where the male predominates and where the male is of lower IQ than the female, on the average. It is likely that a severely retarded or recalcitrant DS male would be more quickly hospitalized than a similarly afflicted female DS, especially in the middle years of childhood. Then too, higher mortality rates among young DS females than males might build an institutionalized residue of more behaviourally attractive girls. Other disparities are environmental in origin. For example, the DS female probably receives more sensitive ward care from female staff than do DS males from male institutional staff. Home care conditions might differ for DS males and females, the latter being more acceptable in the family for a variety of culturally-toned reasons. Central to these considerations are the age correlates of personality and the tendency for institutionalized DS females to be less retarded mentally, on the average, than the males. Up to now there is no corroborative evidence based on community samples. Future research would require longitudinal sampling and adequate controls for sex differences across care practice, timing of mortality, frequency of secondary handicap, extent and quality of intellectual status, and institutionalization priorities by sex.

Intelligence, language and personality

Many Down's individuals are so severely retarded that useful affective and social repertoires are practically nil. Others, at home or in hospital, show upper trainable levels of retardation accompanied by good self-care habits and a positive emotionality. Negative behavioural changes, detected as the child grows older, seem to coincide with two developmental events; a failure to bridge concrete to conceptual styles of intellectual expression, and an absence of language skills appropriate to the expectations of advancing age. Both the ability to abstract and relate interpersonal events, and a suitably matched advance of communication skills, are critical to positive personality growth and maintenance. Speech and conceptual lags in DS do relate to declining test intelligence and to eroding neurophysiological status. Meno-lascino (1965) found severe or moderate speech retardation at all IQ levels in DS having chronic brain syndrome associated with behavioural reaction, adjustment reaction, or psychotic reaction. Johnson and Abelson (1969a, b) contended that the ability to 'communicate to others understandably' was the most noted handicap of DS (2606 cases studied), over comparable non-DS retarded (20606 cases studied). Only 18.80% of the DS subjects could communicate usefully, compared with 35.24% of the non-DS custodial and moderately retarded samples. The mean age of the DS sample was 21.18 years. There seems little doubt that personality formation and corruption in DS is a function of both quality of intelligence and extent of communication skill. These, in turn, are reciprocal and are subject to the influences of ongoing neuropathological processes, the structural disorders which inhibit speech growth in DS and quality of care.

Karyotype and the origins of personality

A first study of aberrant chromosome subtype and behavioural outcomes for DS was undertaken by Gibson and Pozsonyi (1965). They offered that

psychiatric and psychological findings show the translocation series to be socialized adequately in eight of the ten cases, as compared with six for the trisomy controls: to exhibit autistic tendencies in five of the translocation cases, as compared with three of the trisomy controls; to be passive in temperament in eight of the translocation cases, as compared with six of the trisomy controls; and to display neurotic features (various tics and mannerisms) in three of the translocation series, as compared with four of the trisomy controls.

These results are neither dramatic nor very reliable, given the modest number of cases studied. There was, however, a tendency for the trisomy child to be aggressive and, when frustrated, to exhibit temper tantrums and negativism:

Sustained pressure was manifested as enuresis, facial tics, nail biting, and the like. Under favourable conditions of nurture, the trisomy child was disposed to enthusiasm and mimicry. By contrast, the typical translocation DS tended to be passive and cautious. Under prolonged stress the translocation child seemed more disposed to withdraw, eventually displaying various ritualisms, stereotyping of behaviour, and bizarreness; a picture superficially like that of the psychotic child. (pp. 803–4)

The aberrant chromosome, and its subtypes, might account for some of the variance associated with the range of personality expression in DS.

Baumeister and Williams (1967) thought that 'IQ . . . varies with the nature of chromosome involvement'. Since IQ level influences the expression of various behavioural traits in DS, then personality trait distribution could have some basis in subtype of abnormal karyotype. A further test of the 'intellectual, behavioural and physical characteristics associated with trisomy, translocation and mosaic types of Down's syndrome' was conducted by Johnson and Abelson (1969). By 1969 these investigators had acquired a sufficient sample of mosaicism DS to permit behavioural comparisons with standard trisomy and translocation DS. Of 296 cases, 254 were standard trisomy, 21 were translocations and 18 were mosaic. The balance showed multiple chromosomal anomalies. All were resident in institutions and had a mean IQ of 32.33 points. The overall behavioural census contained 22 items rated on a four-point scale. Fourteen items assayed general activity indices and aggressiveness (e.g., hyperactive, passive, destroys clothing, requires restraint), while another eight items were said to represent psychotic manifestation, regressive behaviours and sexual activity. Translocation DS rated significantly higher on 12 of the 14 general activity and aggression measures, except that they were significantly more passive as well. The translocation sample exceeded the mosaicism series on 10 of 13 general activity and aggression indices, but not significantly so. Trisomies and mosaics provided little evidence of trait separation, although the tendency was toward higher scores for activity and aggression for the trisomy cases (5 of 14 traits tested). The second group of measures (psychotic, regressive and sexual anomalies) did not differentiate among chromosome sub-classifications. The translocation and mosaicism samples were subsequently compared (on a four-point scale) with age-matched trisomies for frequency of problem behaviours. The only interesting finding here was that the five highest scores, for activity–aggression, favoured the translocation series. Johnson and Abelson concluded that the traditional stereotype of the happy, affectionate and passive DS patient involves mainly the trisomies, most mosaics and a few translocations. A relatively smaller second behavioural group, characterized as overtly active and aggressive, were largely the translocations. Belmont (1971) has disputed these findings on procedural grounds.

The Gibson and Pozsonyi, and the Johnson and Abelson findings are difficult to reconcile except for some agreement that translocation DS is generally less retarded than trisomy DS. Mosaicism studies are equally unpromising, there being no evidence of a connection between behavioural status and percentage mosaicism (Gibson, 1973). The only consistent indications are that any deviation from the standard 21-trisomy karyotype appears to be accompanied by increased behavioural and somatic variation and that IQ for the translocations is superior by more than five points, on the average, to trisomy IQ. The result should be a more classically homogeneous personality picture for trisomy DS and a greater range of personality features for the translocation variety. A large sample study would help establish both the biological reliability of the personality stereotype and the relation of behavioural potential to discrete chromosome events.

Constitution and personality

Some writers have argued for a typical extroverted, outgoing, agreeable variety of temperament for DS which, when extended into psychopathology, takes the form of impulse disorder, aggressiveness and excitable catatonia. Its rarer opposite is an introverted, withdrawn and fearful form of DS, the psychiatric projection being a stuporous catatonia. Others see a division into a docile-friendly introvert as distinct from an aggressive-hostile extrovert. The implication is that temperament for DS, and its extension into psychopathology, is somehow inherent and unique among the mental retardations.

Others contend that while the higher brain centres for DS are afflicted diffusely and progressively, the lower brain centres (associated with emotionality) are comparatively free of pathology. The product would be a relatively intact personality. Ellis and Beechley (1950) made this point when comparing the range of temperament for DS versus non-DS mentally retarded subjects of similar IQ levels. Benda (1960 a) supported a similar view especially for the childhood years. A popular speculation is that pure temperament is thereby 'uncovered' as an intact emotional responsiveness with limited cognitive mediation. The outcome is said to be a benign though unrefined extroversion. It would be difficult to test this essentially constitutional concept in the absence of better anatomical data. An alternative approach is to examine those traits claimed to be of constitutional origin.

Stubbornness is the most frequently studied particular of the personality stereotype. Oster (1953) proposed that 'stubbornness' was uniformly present at all ages in DS, occurred equally for the easily managed and the troublesome, and was quite likely of constitutional origin. Benda (1956) identified stubbornness as an inherent reactional inflexibility peculiar to the syndrome, i.e., insofar as DS might have unique cortical deficiencies preventing optimum evaluation of sensory inputs. Others consider stubbornness as a personality expression of supposedly immature sensory thresholds, cognitive facility notwithstanding. Furthermore, the well-integrated (though rudimentary) emotionality claimed for DS might produce a behavioural expectation at a higher level than is intellectually realistic for the condition. In any event, constitutional explanation for the exaggerated affective qualities of DS defies the fact that most don't easily fit the classical behavioural stereotype, whatever its particulars.

Another facet of the constitutionality–personality debate grows from the small literature on family psychopathology. The hypotheses are firstly that residual forms of familial mental illness have survived to account for occasional psychiatric disorder in the DS offspring, and secondly that standard trisomy DS is genetically linked with other forms of psychiatric disorder. Walker (1956) considered the latter position in her examination of double occurrences of DS in one sibship (three families). In two such families (comprised of five and nine children) an older male sibling was schizophrenic. She cited two other instances of DS children born to schizophrenic mothers. All DS cases showed dermatoglyphic indices (Walker, 1957) in the overlap area, i.e., being atypical or diagnostically equivocal for DS. A similarity of dermal configuration, for the related Down's and schizophrenics, was observed suggesting to Walker a possible similarity in disturbance of early foetal growth. One of the schizophrenics was undifferentiated and the other catatonic. She supposed that these links had been overlooked because DS children and their families are screened for institutional admission before other abnormal genotypes are expressed in the siblings. Future investigation of these highly tenuous ideas might focus on the relation of cytogenetic irregularity (in child and relatives) with variety of psychiatric disorders of familial origin. The family residuals hypothesis has been examined by Menolascino (1965). Family psychopathology was documented for eight of the 11 DS families studied. Two of these families displayed reactive (to the DS child) forms of disturbed family interaction. The other family units were described as having structured familial psychopathology, with one or both parents exhibiting 'prominent and severe' personality difficulty. No comparative figures were presented on the frequency and type of family psychopathology for the more numerous DS cases who were themselves free of psychiatric disorder.

Among the many approaches to understanding the emotionality of DS, assuming its distinctiveness from other forms of MR, the constitutional approach is the most cumbersome. Less glamorous explanations are available both in the injury and the nurtural literature.

Secondary organic factors and the origins of personality

Impulse disorder, ego-integration difficulty, aggressiveness, attention disorder, cognitive concreteness, language pathology, hyperactivity, perceptual-learning and sensory handicap are common enough in MR. They are associated usually with the exogenous aetiologies. These same traits, although less obviously expressed, have been observed at all ages and in the majority of DS cases at more advanced ages. Studies recounted earlier have offered evidence for neuropathological and other secondary degenerative process paralleling behavioural decline in DS. A few of these investigations relate particularly to personality.

The neurophysiological evidence highlighted a number of possible somatic–behavioural connections. Among these was a proposed correlation between the timing and expression of abnormal EEG tracings and the age of onset of behavioural difficulty. Gibbs, Gibbs and Hirsch (1964) observed that the rarity of 6 and 14 cps spiking, in DS, was related to an 'extremely placid and gentle' personality (p. 583). Other studies in older Down's subjects have linked neurological findings with psychotic-like reactions (Menolascino, 1967), with the early manifestations of senile processes (Jervis, 1970) and with a host of indicators of hyperkinesis, attention disorder, specific learning handicaps and psychometric patterning usually associated with the brain-damaged types of MR. The evidence for uniqueness in this regard is by no means conclusive. Fisher (1970) demonstrated the similarities of both psychometric patterning and extent of attention deficit for DS and non-DS retarded children of similar IQ levels. Wolf, Wenar and Ruttenberg (1972) found DS children to display less cognitive fragmentation and compartmentalization and more generalization, between key areas of function, than did early infantile autistics. The disagreement, once again, comes down to non-comparability of studies for age, care status, sex, nature of control group and degree of mental retardation.

The importance of the foregoing variables has been demonstrated by Owens, Dawson and Losin (1971) in their study of Alzheimer's disease in DS, as a function of age. Rosecrans (1971), too, has a word on the subject. He described a 'partial' DS who was able to maintain an average IQ of 85 points during childhood. Personality was marked by over-activity and negativism. The child was sufficiently intact, intellectually, to perform on a variety of psychodiagnostic tests. These revealed poor visual–perceptual organization, distortions, perseveration, directional difficulty and all the usual signs of the exogenous mental retardations. Rosecrans speculated that such difficulties are 'more frequently associated with the right hemisphere disturbance than left hemisphere, although a generalized cortical deficit is evidenced' (p. 293). The study indicates that the DS subject is usually too handicapped to exhibit the expected behavioural consequences of their neuropathology in measurable form.

Owens et al. (1971) made nearly the same point. They described the usual signs of pre-senile dementia (or Alzheimer's) as progressing from psycho-neurotic and involutional psychotic states, to amnesia and aphasia, terminating in Parkinsonism and seizures. These events can occur in normals at about 50 years, but much earlier for DS. Neuropathologists have found Alzheimer-like changes in the brains of all DS subjects over age 35 and in many much sooner. The failure to identify the concomitant behavioural changes in all cases has been puzzling. Owens and his colleagues say that 'because of the relatively low level of personality integration and the poorly developed state of ego functioning, combined with weak libidinal and aggressive strivings, the changes of Alzheimer's disease manifest themselves more subtly and cryptically in Down's syndrome patients than in non-retarded individuals' (p. 608). To test this view, Owens *et al.* devised a checklist of neurological and behavioural signs to be used with 30- to 50-year-old DS subjects. These adults were free of known secondary neurological disorders, e.g., birth trauma, and had an IQ of at least 25 points. A second sample was comprised of much younger (20–25 years CA) cases but with similar IQ levels. The older Down's subjects demonstrated a higher frequency of aphasia–agnosia indicators, of frontal lobe dysfunction and of 'diffuse cerebral dysfunction in general'. Several ideas were put forward to explain the absence of clear-cut dementia, or of any classical psychological correlates of these neurological alterations. Among them is the view that institutional DS faces few genuine crises or anxieties which would trigger the usual extensions from neuropathological states to behavioural states. Secondly, it was proposed that DS subjects, compared with other retarded, are able to resist personality changes because they have enjoyed a good primary personality status in the early years. If these explanations have merit then the older community-based Down's population should show more obvious dementia associated with pre-senile organic changes; an unknown statistic at this point. If proven, the variety of abnormal manifestations of personality might be expected to increase as community care becomes more common and as DS individuals live longer. Still unsettled, though, is the inevitability of progressive neuropathology in DS, the reliability of its expression psychologically and the role of nurture in either process.

Nurture and personality

In North America, at least, behavioural scientists and laymen appeal mainly to environmental constructs for the provision of explanations about behavioural competence and incompetence. There are numerous accounts of behavioural status for DS as some function of family, community, school or institutional milieu. There is correspondingly less solid information about (i) the potency of managed environments for the shaping of personality in DS and (ii) the potential for matching therapeutic environments with syndromic events, particularly those which might be peculiar to DS.

The flexible temperament and imitative quality, claimed for the DS child, suggests an easy susceptibility to psychological programming, although in this regard the imprinting and modelling constructs, to be reviewed later, will be found wanting. The importance of environmental forces in a triggering sense have also been argued, e.g., the endomorphic DS individual who is predisposed to more negative adjustment modes and who might attract hostile reaction which would heighten his difficulties. There is a third position which takes a more strictly maturational and neuropathological view of the negative features of personality for DS, admitting to little external influence. Research support is available for each of these positions.

Menolascino (1967) likened the behaviour of his hyperactive DS cases, having evidence of chronic brain syndrome, to the 'terrible two's' of normal growth. Many of his children responded to any stimulus source with 'behavioral overactivity often of an undirected nature' (p. 72). Menolascino thought also that the overactivity might be an adaptive response to a negative or barren institutional situation. He said, 'they are attempting to replenish their literally vacant interpersonal worlds by engaging anyone and everyone within their immediate physical setting' (p. 72), a kind of 'titrated over-affection' characteristic of symbiotic psychosis. The neuro-maturational prolongation of certain early developmental states, in combination with the effects of poor institutional programming, would need to be considered in relation to pre-hospital environment. Menolascino claimed that many of his sample had been institutionalized because of sibling or parent rejection, or because the families were not themselves psychologically capable of coping with the special problems of the child. The more damaged DS child would, however, attract a rejecting environment leading to institutionalization and continuing erosion of personality on purely organic grounds.

Lyle (1960) favours a predispositional view of personality for DS. He found that while 43% of his non-DS institutional MR subjects had a disturbed pre-admission history, only 13% of the DS records had similar evidence. Unless it can be assumed that the parents of DS children are more mature, hardy or understanding than the parents of other custodial to moderate MR, the blame for disturbed family–child bonding would fall on the side of the inherent performance deficits of DS. The superior early temperament is said to be innate and able to attract appropriate family reinforcement. The advantage of DS over non-DS retarded survives into subsequent institutional and adult life. Projective research adds some weight to this view. Brink and Grundlingh (1976) found hospitalized DS individuals to show significantly higher human movement determinants and better form response on the Rorschach than non-DS retarded subjects, appropriately matched. They concluded for superior self-concept and social awareness in the DS group, the advantage being relatively independent of environmental considerations.

Tarjan, Dingman, Eyman and Brown (1960) reported DS subjects to be the most attractive diagnostic group for purposes of family-care placement. Curiously, they also had the highest return rate in comparison with the familial MR and the various exogenous aetiologies. The often dramatic personality decline of many post-pubescent DS youth might explain the latter contradiction. Parents of DS children are dismayed by the sudden changes and are poorly prepared for them. Parents of post-traumatic, and other initially quite difficult mental retardations have, from the outset, accepted a more realistic view of the child, prognostically, and experience few further surprises. The interaction of care and training conditions with the behavioural 'givens' of DS is probably age-bound but has been poorly explored and has enjoyed little expression in care technology.

A number of purely environmental mini-models have been proposed to explain personality deterioration for DS. Francis (1970) found an increase in rocking movements, unusual posturing, diffuse motor activity, decreasing general interest, and an expansion of self-orientated behaviours among low-grade institutionalized Down's, as age increased. Erosion occurred most precipitously between 4 and 13 years of CA and again after 30 years of CA. Francis was inclined to attribute these changes to institutional effects, rather than to age-related biological changes. Lang (1974) related the conformity, clinging affection and stubbornness of 27 institutional DS children to fixations on oral modes of reacting. The conclusions were two: that personality for DS depends on the initial acceptance of parents and that personality differences will be as varied as are parent acceptance levels and modes. Buddenhagen and Sickler (1969) demonstrated how attention-seeking behaviours, in an institutional environment, are reinforced and magnified. Similar mechanisms operate to shape over-affection in DS, especially on 'demonstration' wards, routinely a part of visitors' tours or used for staff indoctrination. Future experiments should be designed so that duration of hospital care can be separated from CA and each, in turn, distinguished for nature and intensity of ongoing biological stresses. There is a need, too, for knowledge of the impact of various nurtural conditions, by age, across community and institutional populations. Some work has been done but with limited results.

Ellis and Beechley (1950) compared 40 community (out-patient) DS subjects with 40 matched controls. The mean age for the sample was approximately 7 years, with a mean IQ of 38 points. Results indicate the DS children to be more stable, to originate with smaller families, for the mothers of DS children to be older, for both parents to be more intelligent and to have enjoyed superior economic status in comparison with the control sample. The DS children came less often from broken homes. Despite these largely chance level trends, the authors debate two alternative views: that DS retains a healthier personality than MR controls because of certain environmental advantages, or else, that the comparative emotional stability of Down's syndrome is inherent. The data supports neither position.

Schipper (1959) evaluated the potency of environmental conditions through the eyes of the therapist. He described nine community DS cases referred to him on account of their disturbed behaviour. Six were considered to be reactive to negative parent attitudes and were managed by parent counselling. Three others had parents with long-standing problems of their own. An element of poor impulse integration was evident throughout the histories. Otherwise, Schipper found most community DS children to be happy but with minor adjustment problems in the nature of 'dynamic, interpersonal relationships rather than a factor of mongolism *per se*'. Selective institutionalization tends, however, to leave in the community the least damaged, best nurtured and younger DS individuals such that extrapolations about the relative importance of nurtural and predispositional variables are difficult to make.

A few additional situational correlates of affective styles for DS can be mentioned, although there is no direct evidence. One includes an easy fatigue and the susceptibility of Down's to various illnesses derived from chronic circulatory and respiratory difficulties. Resulting periods of lethargy or general discomfort could generate acquiescense, stubbornness or any other component of the personality stereotype. Finally, the positive personality picture for DS might be mainly in the eye of the beholder; a phenomenon called 'stereotypic projection'. Given that DS children have been thought to be more attractive than other seriously retarded children, then the hypothesis would be self-fulfilling.

Evaluation

Uncertainties aside, there are a few points of near consensus.

(1) There is a compelling impression of characteristic developmental staging for personality in the syndrome. In caricature, the placid, sensorially insufficient infant becomes an emotionally intact and outgoing child who turns subsequently into a sullen adolescent and finally faces premature ageing and marked behavioural deterioration in early adulthood. But not always and maybe not even in the majority of instances. Many DS individuals defy cataloguing, remaining alert and partially self-sufficient well into adulthood despite demonstrated intellectual decline. We need to know much more about

the predictive reliability of the proposed personality stereotype and the sensory, metabolic and nervous system changes which appear to accompany it.

(2) More serious forms of psychopathology in DS have attracted various estimates of frequency and source. Among the few supportable conclusions is that behavioural difficulties in younger DS samples is less common and less acute than for other young moderately to seriously mentally retarded. The relative frequencies of psychopathology, across aetiological groups, perhaps change as adulthood approaches. The particulars of milder behavioural deviation are not much different in the beginning from other imbecile groups, e.g., hyperactivity, impulse disorder, attention deficit, etc. The later primitive catatonic states, depression and senile dementia appear to be more distinguishing of DS, focussed apparently on the affective system and based on progressive neuropathology. The timing and ordering of these behavioural events, leading to affective psychoses and premature senility, appear to be characteristic of the syndrome but not inevitable.

(3) Several major correlates of personality style for DS appear to be age, intelligence levels, communication facility, variety of abnormal karyotype and sex. Constitutional variables were discussed around the concepts of stubbornness and imitative facility but too little is known about these properties and whether they are a reliable outcome of cytogenetic events. The causal debate turns ultimately to the operation of specific (to DS) neurophysiological and metabolic mechanisms, the distortion of developmental timing, and the incongruity of expectation between early emotional promise and later cognitive fact. Evidence for family residuals, as a source of normal or deviant personality parameters, was not thought promising. It follows then that good personality prognoses for DS would favour the relatively bright, those on a gentle curve of IQ erosion, the younger, the female and the well-tended from birth.

Exposure to sound management, especially during the critical early and middle childhood growth stage, seems critical; although the ingredients of good management are unclear. The extreme current views are that the personality configuration for DS is (i) significantly maleable (good affect and modelling capacity) and therefore mutable, (ii) more or less directly programmed karyotypically in the form of the constitutional givens or residuals, (iii) unstable with age depending upon the progression of secondary organic process and (iv) a product purely of environment. The considerable variability of normal and atypical personality within DS suggests that no one explanation is exclusive. Our understanding of the origins of personality for the syndrome will be advanced as the long-term results of early stimulation programmes and the improved medical control of circulatory and metabolic insufficiency are known. The affective development of DS children will continue to be a commonsense venture, differing across family traditions and socio-cultural strata. Meanwhile, the personality stereotype lives on because as Norris (1971) claims, persons with DS laugh more.

6

Socialization

Textbooks in print (e.g., Kanner, 1957) perpetuate the opinion that DS individuals are mostly placid and cheerful, characteristics which make them more socially attractive than other forms of mental retardation. The present chapter examines the nature, origin and universality of the social stereotype. The main research burdens are the proper assessment of social capacity and the achieving of representative samples. Both are difficult. Moreover, the considerable heterogeneity of social behaviours for the syndrome will need to be examined in relation to other dimensions of behaviour. These include level of intellectual capacity, sensory equipment, motor abilities, cognitive styles, direction of temperament and the effects of different nurtural conditions. The relative importance of these background factors change, of course, with advancing age. The reader will decide if there is sufficient evidence to justify the classical or some alternative stereotype and whether or not the socialization promise of the syndrome warrants special consideration for management purposes.

The stereotype
Historical origins of the social descriptors
Formal origins of the social stereotype stem from the observations of J. Langdon H. Down (1866) and are largely impressionistic. Later actuarial opinions generally supported Down's view. More recent laboratory findings belie much of the traditional literature.

The social descriptors, offered by Down, assumed a high degree of behavioural homogeneity within the syndrome. Down's motive was to justify his concept of a uniform clinical condition based on ethnic degeneracy, or on corrupt physical environments, e.g., tuberculosis. Speaking of the social facade, Down claimed that 'they are humorous, and a lively sense of the ridiculous often colours their mimicry' (p. 261). Concerning social prognosis, 'they have considerable power of imitation even bordering on being mimics. This facility of imitation may be cultivated to a very great extent, and a practical direction given to the results obtained' (p. 261), presumably in the direction of better social adjustments.

Ten years later, DS was rediscovered by Fraser (1876) with the help of Mitchell. They called it Kalmuc idiocy. Fraser said of his single case, 'she remembered the faces of those who were kind to her, and of those who annoyed her, and sought notice from the former and avoided the latter. Her chief characteristic was an affectionate disposition. This was evidenced by her kind, contented, and happy expression and by her grasping the hand of anyone who took notice of her, patting it, and putting it to her cheek' (p. 171). Another distinction was her love of decoration: 'Any bright article of dress she wore with jealous care and drew everyone's attention to it. If any other patient had anything gay on she always pointed to it. She is reported as being very fond of music. She continually sat in a corner of a bench next to the fire with her feet under it. She had no sense of modesty and her habits were dirty. She had a great hatred of water and her struggles against being bathed were strong and persistent. On admission, she was extremely dirty, etc.' (p. 171). It would be difficult to separate those social habits associated with institutional living from those somehow particular to the syndrome. What does emerge from this account is evidence of good memory and temperament, major ingredients of the socialization process. Mitchell was especially impressed with the extent to which DS children 'would also be found to resemble each other in character, in capacity, in liking and disliking, in habits, in defects, in aptitudes' (p. 177). Another paper of the same period (Fletcher-Beach, 1882) claimed that while these patients were generally cheerful, they could be destructive and restless. Beach provided, to that point, the single negative component of an otherwise unblemished social image.

Anatomy of the social stereotype

By the early 1900s there was a spreading concern for the ingredients, universality and importance of the socialization potential alleged for DS children. Fennell (1904) claimed 'the child is cheerful, affectionate, easily amused, and often a born mimic and these traits are apt to raise false hopes of educational promise' (p. 34). And again, 'it has been stated that the mongol is readily taught habits of cleanliness, but only one child of my cases was reliable in this respect, while three of the remainder were habitually wet and dirty after years of careful attention' (p. 35). Shuttleworth (1909) thought that

DS was physically (number of stigmata) and behaviourally graded. He claimed one exception, 'but in all these were certain common mental characteristics, such as general backwardness, want of originality but remarkable imitativeness, retarded speech, often a taste for musical rhythm and usually a placid disposition, though in some cases a species of obstinancy which only yields to tactful management' (p. 664). Differentiating the condition from cretinism, he catalogued DS as having 'expression more or less vivacious and mobile, observant and imitative,' and the cretin as having 'expression dull and immobile; unobservant and apathetic' (p. 664). Differences between syndromes and types of MR were beginning to be noticed and, perhaps, served to heighten surety about the authenticity of the social stereotype for Down's syndrome. As late as 1924, Brushfield was offering sweeping social–psychological generalizations including musical supersensitivity, cheerful disposition, lively interpersonal patterns, marked curiosity, absence of erotic tendencies and so on (for 177 DS children under the age of 14). Many workers were less certain.

Tredgold (1947), remarking on the quality of social responding for DS, found positive results for most but was puzzled by the exceptions. Areas of handicap included a failure of social alertness and an absence of any carry-over from the widely acclaimed habit of mimicry to social learning. He also expressed surprise at the contrast between the very young DS child's social inertness and general lethargy and the good social sense, observation skill and curiosity evident in many older DS children. Tennies (1943) had previously remarked that the supposed social imitative facility of DS might suggest high mental promise, where in fact there is little transfer. Shuttleworth (1900) had claimed that an imitative social capacity should be an encouraging indication of educability, especially in regard to easily modelled skills such as writing and drawing. Benda (1949) interpreted the mimicry as probably non-syndromic, merely an exaggeration or protraction of a developmental phase seen in normal pre-school children. The first plateau of intellectual development for DS, occurring at a mental age of about 2½ years (Gibson, 1966), might indeed tend to prolong a normal age-specific susceptibility to imitation. Penrose (1933) was inclined to subscribe to the social stereotype as typical for some DS individuals and age groups but not for others. Marthisen (1947), seen in Oster (1953), described 20% of his cases as essentially unsociable.

Despite disagreement, a sufficient number of themes have emerged from the older clinical descriptions to justify a social profile of sorts. There was initial accord that DS children are often docile and socially suggestible. The implication was that specific social behaviours for DS are inherent, having little to do with learning, affective or intellectual potential. The view is a tenacious one. Blacketer-Simmonds (1953) thought of social imitativeness for DS as mindless, unoriginal and rather like echopraxia, e.g., 'the holding of attention by musical sounds is (as with bright lights) purely a response to pleasurable sensation absolutely void of real aesthetic appreciation' (p. 707). Moreover, the fixed social stereotype was reinforced and had some continuity as a result of traditional institutional care practices. DS patients are usually mixed with other severe to moderate forms of mental retardation and especially with the brain damaged who display patterns of hyperactivity, irritability or withdrawal. The social promise of the DS child would appear outstanding in comparison with his more overtly damaged companions. The social prognosis for the syndrome, within the family and community, attracts less enthusiasm.

Reliability of the social image for DS, from study to study, apparently depends on the age and care history of the sample. Rollin (1946) suggested that institutionalized DS is under closer discipline than those in the community and that, in the less permissive hospital setting, the full range of their social expression (positive or negative) might not be elicited. Rollin's social-behavioural profile was founded on 73 DS cases, only 43.8% of whom conformed to the generally accepted stereotype. The age spread between 10 and 48 years could have biased the outcome insofar as degenerative changes are evident in the older. For instance, Brousseau and Brainerd (1928) were of the opinion that infant and quite young DS children have little or no social expression and offer no response to a social initiative except for a reflexive tendency to grimace. Both Siegert and Scharling, writing in 1910 (see Oster, 1953), observed that reactivity for DS was sharply age variable and did not exhibit the unfolding maturational quality seen with normal children. At early age levels (2–3 years CA), they alternated between 'Topor and erithism' (Oster, p. 51). Oster (1953) reported social fear and shyness to be present for 20% of his 5- to 9-year-olds but for fewer of the older cases. We are invited to believe that social alertness for DS emerges later in childhood and rather more abruptly than for other MR children.

The classical social expectation for DS is a product, possibly, of institutional samples taken in late childhood and at median IQ levels. The social effigy is less convincing for the very young, the adult, or for those reared under permissive family and community conditions. The DS individual, according to Rollin (1946), is just as often withdrawn, aggressive, hyperactive, careless, anxious, and depressed, whether at home or in the institution. Tredgold's optimistic description was rejected by Blacketer-Simmonds (1953) as unfounded. Engler (1949) agreed with everybody, classifying social behaviours on a three-part scale; including the positive social stereotype, the severely retarded who had little capacity for social response of any kind, and a third smaller group who were consistently difficult.

There are many attempts to explain the exceptions to the rule. Sternlicht (1966) (writing for parents) attributed social recalcitrance in DS to defence against pressure to perform, inherent cognitive inflexibility, an inability to change perceptual foci, or all of these. He observed, as well, that imitative behaviours in DS are usually rudimentary, made up mainly of discrete and simple physical gestures (such as hand waving, clapping, head shaking) and are uselessly repetitive. Forman (1967) (writing for teachers) elaborated on the proper social expectations for DS. She asserted that some of the positive social stereotype might be anticipational, founded on the compassion and interest which an easily recognized, clinically cohesive and less 'damaged' MR student might invite. DS individuals, she says, are often socially attractive when seen with normal adults and singly. In groups, especially when not the object of adult attention, they are rather bad-tempered or quarrelsome and 'many people find their hyperkinesis trying' (p. 9). There is the interesting implication in the Forman statement that drive disorder and attentional flights are prominent and akin to the behaviours exhibited by the brain-damaged child. Further, the claimed preference of DS individuals for solitary rather than peer group activity was attributed to slow motor reactivity and perceptual rigidity.

Modern observers contend, on the whole, that the positive social stereotype for DS is not particularly universal and that their social responses could be a product of stereotype projection, compensatory drives, particular neurological deficits, or contextual factors. The problem of origins, related to outcomes, is not so simple. Butterfield (1961) described a DS adult male with a Binet mental age of 5 years and an IQ score of 28 points who was socially quite responsive in the community. Butterfield concluded that motivational and situational variables have a good deal to do with the quality of socialization in DS and that a relatively low intelligence, or other handicap, need not preclude a simple social adequacy. The contradictions in the clinical literature concerning the quality, frequencies and origins of social behaviour for the syndrome are, therefore, manifold. Their resolution will require a critical inspection of the data-based socialization literature in order (i) to establish the reliability of criteria and measurement techniques, and (ii) to sort out the many proposed antecedents of socialization status for the syndrome.

Empirical test of the social stereotype

Blacketer-Simmonds (1953) provided the first balanced test of the general behavioural stereotype for DS; prior to and following institutionalization, and against non-DS subjects who were intellectually and physically comparable. Pre-institutional behaviour ratings were derived from a checklist completed by intake nurses. Pertinent adjectives included 'friendly, sociable, mimics, solitary and docile'. Percentage differences between the DS sample and controls were tested by chi-square technique. Only two categories differed significantly; the pre-institutional DS appearing to be less docile and more solitary than the non-DS controls. The post-institutional check-list was so arranged that controls and Down's subjects could not be separately identified by observers. Three hundred non-DS control cases, of similar physical and intellectual status to the DS subjects, were available. Of the DS group, 20% were described as sociable, 31.6% as docile, 10% as given to mimicry, 16.6% as solitary and poor mixers, and 43.3% as restless. The controls showed a 40% frequency of restlessness, 15% were described as solitary, 7% as mimics, and 23.6% as sociable. Overall, there was a more attractive social status for the non-DS retarded than for the DS sample. The comparatively unattractive socialization pattern of the DS patients was evident both on admission and later.

Interpretation is difficult. The Blacketer-Simmonds study did not specify the age ranges for the two samples, e.g., the percentage of older cases in each. Nor did it compare the health and psychiatric status of the Down's individuals, whose commitment was being sought, against community cases not in need of hospitalization. Further, the devices and procedures used for assessing various traits were rudimentary and open to non-random influences.

A more complete test of the social stereotype for DS is provided by Silverstein (1964). In his study, 30 pairs of Down's and ward-mate controls were matched for age, sex, IQ and length of institutional residence. Average CA was approximately 12 years and IQ level about 26 points. Of the 30 pairs, 22 were males. Behavioural ratings were taken from a factor-based schedule. The two major factors examined were 'general adjustment' and 'introversion-extroversion'. Since these factors correspond roughly to socialization and personality status, respectively, only the former is discussed here. The DS sample was rated higher for such characteristics as 'mannerly, responsible, cooperative and scrupulous'. They also scored higher than controls for the factor of general adjustment (socialization). Re-analysis of these findings, using Blacketer-Simmonds' chi-square method, produced no item-specific socialization differences between the DS subjects and controls. Silverstein speculated that the widely accepted social stereotype for DS might have influenced the behaviour of observers as a consequence of expectation and projection.

Domino, Goldschmid and Kaplan (1964) involved a component of observer reliability in their examination of the social features of institutionalized DS females. A hospital ward of 21 Down's and 35 other mentally retarded girls of undifferentiated aetiology was used. The DS girls had an IQ of 30 points, had been in hospital 54 months, were 135 months of CA, and had been hospitalized at CA 81 months, on the average. The non-DS patients showed mean values as follows; IQ 35 points, CA 125 months, hospitalization duration 35 months, and age at admission 88 months. An objective instrument called the Sonoma checklist was devised for the study. Staff ratings were used to derive a staff 'acceptance index' and a familiarity score was defined for each patient by each staff observer. Observers included professionals, comprised of the usual MR hospital disciplines, and ward personnel. Each of the behavioural variables was subsequently correlated with a diagnosis, or not, of DS. Descriptive social adjectives such as 'friendly, sociable and open' correlated significantly and positively with the diagnosis of DS. There was no evidence of the stubbornness found to be associated with DS in the data of Domino *et al.* or in the data of Silverstein mentioned previously. The proposed 'restlessness' of DS patients was not noted by Domino *et al.* and is in contrast with most previous reports. Domino and his colleagues concluded that the positive and relatively cohesive social stereotype for DS was essentially supportable and that observer bias had been effectively managed. An alternative conclusion might be that the traditional social stereotype is sex-specific or that institutionalized DS females receive different and superior care regimes to male DS patients in the same institutions. Perhaps the greater length of hospitalization for the DS sample (4½ years), over the comparison group (2 years 11 months), contributed to greater stability and homogeniety of behavioural characteristics for the former. Domino *et al.* thought that the favourable social stereotype might be evident only in contrast with the non-DS subjects who manifested a significant number of central nervous system anomalies expressed as irritability, shortened attention and drive disorder.

Two general questions raised by Domino *et al.* were the subject of a second paper (1965). These concerned the extent to which the first results can be applied to both the male and female and the possibility that a positive and distinctive social stereotype, at least for the institutional DS, is merely an expectation phenomenon fostered by well-indoctrinated care staff. The observers for the second study were 210 college students who applied the Sonoma checklist to 21 matched pairs, one member of each pair being DS. Of the 210 test items, 56 differentiated significantly between the DS and non-DS patients. Considering just the socialization items, the DS series appeared to be more hostile, shy, cooperative, show-off, pleasing, unfriendly and so on. The non-DS series excelled as out-going, rude, withdrawn and unsociable. Domino conceded that their hospital ward was unusual in that it was 'open to visitors', and the residents were likely to be screened against serious behaviour difficulty and inadequate personal habits. While Domino interpreted his findings as a confirmation of the classical social stereotype for DS, i.e., as having 'a substantial empirical basis' and as well bounded (definable and identifiable to naive observers), the data permits no firm conclusions.

The foregoing investigations have depended on institutional samples. Blessing (1959) rejected the institutional behavioural stereotype of DS as probably distorted, a product of hospital care routines and propagated by staff training manuals. He chose to test the social reputation using 83 community DS school children and teacher ratings. The sample was representative of community DS in the state of Wisconsin and within the ability range required for special schooling. The intellectually less promising cases, the more difficult multiply handicapped and those below the legal age for formal schooling, are thus not included. An advantaged group might well exhibit the traditional social stereotype, if it exists. Teachers were sent a questionnaire which required the scoring of each DS child for 11 favourable behavioural traits and 19 unfavourable traits. Table 9 shows the most and least frequently occurring 'satisfactory' traits, and Table 10 the least and most frequent of the 'problem' traits. Clearly, the social picture for community DS, despite the favourable ages and conditions, is a mixed one. Working against the emergence of the appropriate social image are a number of factors not obvious in the previous studies. These include (i) a physical fatigue threshold for DS such that good social behaviours are not easily sustained, and (ii) poor communication facility serving to subvert the more complex social behaviours expected of community-placed Down's children. Some of the social antics of DS, considered by many as cute, were attributed by Blessing to attention seeking while positive social performance (when seen) was linked to temperamental predisposition. Social interaction skill or evidence of social sensitivity was not abundant. Blessing concluded that type and quality of social responsiveness in DS varies widely, perseveration, stubbornness, hyperactivity and short attention span being mentioned prominently. Yet when teachers were subsequently asked to rate the five aetio-

Table 9. *Counting behaviours in DS subjects*

Satisfactory aspects mentioned most frequently	Satisfactory aspects mentioned least frequently
Amenable, good-natured Gay, happy, cheerful Obedient, docile (With considerably less frequency) Independent	Good communication Special talents in music, art (With somewhat greater frequency) Good motor ability Orderly

After Blessing (1959).

Table 10. *Counting behaviours in DS subjects*

Problems mentioned most frequently	Problems mentioned least frequently
Short attention span Poor communication Stubborn (With less frequency) Attention seeker Tires easily	Selfish, egotistical Perseverates Hyperactive (With slightly greater frequency) Annoying, undesirable habits Shy, fearful, tense

After Blessing (1959).

logical groups most commonly found in community special schools, in terms of their ease of management, DS ranked first and cerebral palsy last. The teacher's partiality to DS, in the face of their own evidence against any special social ability matrix, might be explained in terms of personality artifacts, stereotype projection, syndromic contrast effects, or wishful thinking.

A similar study by Connor and Goldberg (1960) supports this. They contacted 200 teachers of the 'trainable' mentally retarded from 40 US states, representing public and private residential facilities and private and public day classes. Ninety-two teachers responded and 15% of all replies were for DS subjects. The 2700 behavioural items were catalogued by five educators as representing either 'satisfactions' or 'problems'. The tendency was for teachers to focus on problem areas and for these to relate more frequently to emotional and social, rather than to learning disturbances. The 'satisfactions', more often than not, reflected learning 'ability' rather than socialization potential. It was found that of 350 DS individuals, 54% manifested 'characteristics not conducive to good classroom management' (p. 662). Most frequently used positive descriptors included placid, pliable, active, affectionate and communicative. The negative social characteristics were predominant for the majority of DS cases studied.

Although the large-sample trait surveys have not settled the question of whether or not there is a distinctive social quality to DS, they have exposed the complexity of the issues in relation to criteria selection, sample age, sex, care status and the problems of scaling. Specific social behaviours will need to be considered across aetiological groups of MR and under standardized conditions. Controlled tests of the behavioural competence of DS and matched non-DS mentally retarded subjects, have begun to appear. Three studies (Moore, Thuline and Capes, 1968; Johnson and Abelson, 1969 a, b; Francis, 1970) are relevant.

Moore, Thuline and Capes (1968) criticized the previous work as being entirely dependent on *post hoc* ratings of DS behaviours. These authors put a greater emphasis on direct observation of the specific attributes to be explored. A total of 536 DS and matched controls, drawn from four institutions, were examined with the expectation that 'mongoloids would exhibit less behavioural maladaptation'. Only ambulatory cases were included, these being matched with non-DS controls for sex, age, level of retardation, regional origin and length of institutional residency. Aetiological content of the controls was wide-ranging; from the relatively benign cultural–familial retardate to the more heterogeneous causal groups, e.g., kernicteris, and the cerebral degenerations. Social quotients (SQ) were reported separately for the Arizona and the Washington sources. Results, based largely on adults, indicated little difference (about 4 points SQ) between DS and control groups, favouring the controls. Specific items of behavioural adjustment were subsequently compared for the two groups (Table 11). Similar frequencies of socially maladaptive behaviours were found for control and DS subjects. Regional differences point to a possible distortion of previous findings resulting from the sampling of single institutions.

Moore (1973) has more recently published an index of social (self-help) skills for 2748 Down's cases. The majority were in the 11–30 year age range. Their self-care status is impressive, the major limiting factor being a disparity between receptive and expressive language. Companion figures for a large sample of community DS and controls are not available.

Johnson and Abelson (1969 b) focussed on the frequency of adaptive rather than maladaptive social patterns for DS. Their hypothesis was derived from

Table 11. *Social quotients across regions for DS subjects*

	Arizona		
	Mongolism $N = 112$	Control $N = 112$	Total $N = 224$
Chronological age	16.7	16.2	16.4
Social quotient	33.8	32.8	33.3
Years of residence	8.5	7.0	7.7
	Washington		
	Mongolism $N = 424$	Control $N = 424$	Total $N = 848$
Chronological age	22.5	22.3	22.4
Social quotient	26.0	31.9	28.9
Years of residence	13.3	11.9	12.6
	Combined		
	Mongolism $N = 536$	Control $N = 536$	Total $N = 1072$
Chronological age	21.3	21.0	21.1
Social quotient	27.6	32.1	29.8
Years of residence	12.3	10.9	11.6

After Moore, Thuline and Capes (1968).

Spreen's (1965) evidence that communication disorder or speech lag is commonplace in DS and that this deficit corrupts social growth, particularly as age increases. In other respects, the study is an extension of that by Moore *et al.* (1968). The subjects were 2606 DS and 20605 MR controls taken from a regional census. The mean age of the DS subjects was 21 years and of the other aetiologies, 24.45 years. The mean IQ for the DS group was 28.6 points against 32 points for the controls. The selected indicators of social competence included self-sufficiency in dressing, satisfactory communication, self-feeding, grooming, hygiene control, toileting and helping others as a ward assistant. The two general classes of social competence comprised self-help and other-help items. Despite being both younger and more retarded, the DS subjects exhibited significantly higher percentages of achievement on seven of 11 categories of social adaptation. These were mainly the rudimentary self-help items (toileting, dressing and feeding) and involved little other-help content.

The most striking deficiency was in the social aspects of communication. Here the Down's were notably inferior, supporting the conclusions of Spreen (1965) and Moore *et al.* (1968). While a positive social stereotype for DS might be authentic for the simple motor-based self-help activities, the more complex social skills are usually absent; probably as a result of communication handicap and extent of mental retardation. A third study (Francis, 1970), showed the social contact skills of the low-grade institutional DS patients to decrease quite sharply with age. Her procedure permitted an objective test of the alteration of social behaviours, over time, and of the ingredients of social outputs for the more severely retarded. A negative correlation, of social contact with CA, was significant statistically (Kendall's coefficient). She says, 'in the other age groups, a greater proportion of the mongoloids were mobile and hence able to approach other patients and nurses and initiate social contact, and yet social contact decreased rather than increased' (p. 98). Quality and length of institutional care, and the operation (or not) of secondary organic processes for the severely retarded Down's, were not assessed.

Whatever the shortcomings of the preceding studies, they do challenge the stability of the favourable social stereotype. Moreover, the majority of DS adults are of custodial to low-trainable level intelligence such that as life-expectancy increases, for the syndrome as a whole, a greater number will be discordant with the traditional social image. Social care and training needs for DS individuals, too, will change as they are channelled into a greater range of quasi-independent community life-styles where interpersonal skills are paramount. As yet we know little about the social adjustment possibilities of DS in the adult years or how to prepare for those years. Open, to this point in the review, are the following questions:

(i) whether or not quality of social responding is unique to the syndrome;

(ii) the extent to which social behaviours, negative or positive, are a result of the intellectual and affective characteristics of the disorder;

(iii) the age specificity of the social features of DS, in relation to the maturational timetable.

These issues are examined now.

The interaction of social and intellectual performance
Intellectual and social capacities: hypotheses

The reputedly good social performance of DS individuals is centred on children of school age who display average or better intelligence for the syndrome and who are easily accessible in institutional settings. These are a minority of all cases. Speculations about the origins of the social stereotype, dating from 1866, are briefly considered because they provide the hypotheses which form a basis for much of the current psychometric and experimental research.

Social potential as inborn and special

Social responsiveness, supposedly more evident for DS than for other classes of MR, has been linked to racial retrogression. Langdon Down (1866) and Crookshank (1925) are the most notable proponents. Superior social imitation facility is thus atavistic and instinctual; unrelated to general intellectual capacity or learning ability. A compatible view is that 'social' imitation for DS is centred in nervous system impairment, e.g., echopraxia. Echopraxia is described as a characteristic neurological fault of DS equated with the origins of repetitive mimicry. Supporters of both explanations, however, consider the phenomenon to have no practical treatment value. Tredgold (1947) agrees that socialization and mimicry facility are characteristic of DS but not especially reflective of overall learning and adjustment capacity. The developmental argument for a special social status is less mysterious. The reasoning goes that DS individuals enjoy an imitative talent which is a maturationally set form of social imprinting seen in normal children between 2 and 4 years of mental age. This period of maximum susceptibility to imitation is perhaps extended in DS because mental growth is slow and frequently terminal within the 2–4 years mental age range. While the atavistic and inherent abilities notions have excited little research interest, impairment and developmental hypotheses continue to be pursued.

Social potential as a by-product

Socialization facility for DS has been coupled with good rote memory, observational ability, motor ability, over-achievement and sex status. For example, ease of acquisition of elementary social habits, such as toilet-training, has been explained as a need for the repetitive experience. A number of writers have commented on the relative absence of anxiety surrounding early social habit training in DS and on the possibility that these basically motor skills are less strongly related to emotional and cognitive development than for other categories of MR. A problem mentioned earlier, however, is that most cross-aetiological research has used comparison groups with a wide range of causes. An effort to circumvent the difficulty was made by Gratz, Henderson and Katz (1972) using clearly defined controls (e.g., phenylketonuria and cerebral anoxia). An index of independent activities of daily living was administered to 15 cases in each group. The test is not unlike the Vineland social maturity scale and includes measures of independence for bathing, dressing, feeding and toileting. The DS subjects, even though less intelligent than the other MR samples, were significantly more independent. Conclusions for the relative importance of social skill over IQ, for the results, are not possible because there was a significant F-ratio of CA and diagnostic category. Uncontrolled MA and physical maturation differences, between groups, could alone account for the main finding.

Reference has been made earlier to social over-achievement in DS as a compensatory phenomenon. The argument is that since DS is characteristically impaired intellectually (e.g., concreteness of thought, inability to relate events, poor conceptualization and cognitive transfer facility, failure to ingest and use symbols) but relatively intact emotionally, achievement drives will be disproportionately channelled along social–behavioural lines. This position, if sound, would have remedial value only within the age span of unimpaired emotionality. The literature is suggestive but by no means conclusive.

Oster (1953) invented good powers of observation for DS in order to account for their mimicry and socialization potential. No experimental evidence was provided that DS possesses superior observation talent, or that superior observation is a foundation for social mimicry. Unsociable behaviours were claimed to have subsidiary origins in the parent practice of isolating the DS offspring from outside contact so as to protect him from anticipated ridicule and neighbourhood curiosity.

The fixed social stereotype for DS is further confused by the disparate findings for males and females. The traditionally positive picture is possibly more suited to the young female. Data has been presented contending that institutional and some home care regimes might differ by type and quality according to the sex of the child and that early mortality rates are sex and IQ selective. There has been little direct study. A beginning has been made by Schlottmann and Anderson (1973) who inspected the social behaviour of DS subjects in sexually homogeneous and heterogeneous dyads. Girls engaged in more sedentary activity, socially, than boys. Boys were more influenced by peer-sex than girls, especially in respect to type of social interaction rather than to extent. A second study by Schlottmann and Anderson (1975) compared DS and non-DS retarded subjects (mean age 10 years) for peer-specific social behaviours. The DS males were more sociable and gregarious than controls. Other factors, of possible importance to understanding the differences, were cottage placement policy and the assignment of drugs across aetiological groups. The authenticity of the stereotype is thus uncertain because (i) non-DS custodial and trainable grades of mental retardation are too heterogenous to have much value as a comparison index, (ii) sex-linked behavioural characteristics for DS have been frequently ascribed to differences in intelligence, somatic factors and mortality or survival rates by sex, and (iii) most of the relevant research is from atypical institutional populations.

Social potential images as bias

Throughout the present discussion, the interpretation of research findings has depended on the comparability of institutional and non-institutional samples. Most past research has taken advantage of the easy accessibility of institutional populations. Generalizations are then made to the entire DS population, most of whom are resident in the community. The validity of the assumption of sample comparability has been questioned by Saenger in his *Factors influencing the institutionalization of mentally retarded individuals in New York City* (1960). Samples were predominantly in the trainable mental retardation range and included many instances of DS. Saenger reported that 91% of the hospital residents had had serious behaviour problems as against 59% of the otherwise comparable non-institutionalized community sample. The most obvious differences occurred in the areas of social control. Parents institutionalized their retarded child in part because of home and community socialization difficulty, or else rationalized their action in this way. Or are these parents less tolerant of the social stresses surrounding the care of the retarded? Taken at face value, the findings indicate that the social behaviours of institutionalized DS individuals are not representative of the syndrome and need not, moreover, be a product of hospitalization.

Whether or not the social features of DS are real or apparent, negative or positive, artifactual or focal, is impossible to determine from the early literature. An alternative approach would be to examine socialization developmentally and in relation to other graded capacities, e.g., intelligence. To do so successfully will require a definition of the socialization parameters of DS and some concern for how these parameters are to be assessed.

Defining and measuring social capacity

A first systematic attempt to record the social responses of DS subjects was made by Pavlov who, in 1932, presented a film sequence at the International Congress of Physiology in Milan. He compared the feeding responses of DS young adults with normal children. The DS fared poorly, being seen to equate socially with an 18-month-old normal. Despite the experimental beginnings, the approach most often used is psychometric. The premier device has been the Vineland social maturity scale (VSMS) designed by Edgar A. Doll. The method was described initially in 1935 and more fully in Doll's *Measurement of social competence* (1953). Devices in current use are geared to monitoring treatment rather than to prediction and have not had much use as a research tool. An example is the *Progress assessment chart of the social development of 'mongol' children* by Gunzburg and Sinson (1973).

Curiosity about the contradiction between an ostensibly stronger early social than intellectual growth for DS children, helped inspire the VSMS. The only clinical class of mentally retarded included in the standardization of the VSMS was DS (39 cases). Doll's normative DS subjects were, however, culturally selected; as determined by measures of parent occupational class. The choice of high socio-cultural level parents was defended by arguing that DS is derived disproportionately from the upper strata of society. That position has since been questioned, except insofar as there might be a slight tendency for better placed parents to have married late thereby increasing the risk of standard trisomy offspring. At the outset, then, there is a danger that the 'social age' norms developed for the VSMS are weighted in favour of higher social expectations than are realistic for the syndrome when taken across all social classes.

The mental and physical ages of the standardization samples are also problematic. A median CA of 21 years (and as high as 38 years) was not characteristic of the period. Nor was a median mental age of 4.9 years. Accordingly, the construction of the Vineland test, at least from the DS data, has been warped for intellectual status as well as for CA and socio-cultural background. Notwithstanding, a reliability coefficient of 0.76 was obtained between mental age and social age but dropped to 0.73 when corrected for CA interaction. Doll (1953) said of the qualitative aspects of social performance for DS, 'this means that these subjects were below the level of significant literacy, useful occupation, self-direction and socialization; that is, they received most of their item credits in the categories of self-help and the early stages of communication, occupation and socialization' (p. 447). Two conclusions are provisionally possible; that MA and SA co-vary and may be rooted in common factors, and that 'social success' for DS is achieved more obviously for the simple, discrete and motor-based behaviours than is the case for normal children of similar MA or CA. These observations are in line with modern findings and warrant elaboration.

The VSMS is segregated into eight categories. The self-help category includes various motor items (balances head), feeding items (does not drool), dressing items (goes to bed unassisted), communication items (follows simple instructions), self-direction items (makes minor purchases), locomotion content (moves about on floor, occupation skills), and general social interaction (plays with other children). These criteria are age graded from 0 to 25 years. All categories of test behaviour were standardized for each age level. Comparison of Vineland test items with the item content of standard infant schedules, as well as with the early years of the Binet scales, revealed a considerable content overlap. What is described in the VSMS as self-help growth, is catalogued in infant development schedules as psychomotor growth. A high correlation between SA and MA or developmental quotient, for behavioural competence in very young DS, is thus guaranteed. It is hardly evidence for any real connection between social and intellectual facility, especially for older DS children. Only at the upper performance range of the Vineland and Binet scales is there a separation of item demand with discernible social and intellectual modules. Evaluation of the validity of the VSMS for DS, against measures of IQ, would thus show good IQ–SQ congruence in the early years and less in later periods of growth and decline.

The forecast power of Vineland social quotients has been seldom tested on DS alone. Johnson (1970) reported on the 'prediction of independent functioning and of problem behaviour' from SQ scores for hospitalized MR subjects but did not separate the trends for DS subjects. Data included social quotients, independent rating of capacity for self-help, and frequency tabulations of various anti-social behaviours. Analysis was correlational, comparing SQ with the two other approaches. Mean scores were in the order of 28.20 points IQ and 31.11 points SQ. The relation of SQ scores to specific real life behavioural indices was better than chance, the highest forecast coefficients appearing for the self-help items. Prediction from global SQ to specific behavioural deviation was not so strong and the combination of SQ and IQ did not apparently enhance behavioural prediction.

Johnson concluded that while neither SQ nor IQ scores predicted deviant social behaviours to any remarkable degree, IQ alone was able to forecast social competence and independent functioning about as well as SQ. The tendency for SQ scores to be about 35% greater, than same-sample IQ scores, might indicate that social maturity scale items are less rigorous than age equivalent intelligence scale items; or that parents and ward aides over-estimate the precision of social performance for DS. Feeding cleanly might be less difficult for Down's than making an age equivalent verbal response. The former response would be more highly valued in an intensive care situation. Another difficulty is that the VSMS is not dependent upon direct behavioural sampling. These several considerations provide, for the moment, a simple explanation for high SQ over IQ ratings in DS, without appeal to special abilities, social or otherwise. Additional complexities will be introduced in the section to follow:

The relation of SQ and IQ

The SQ–IQ comparison research has provided a few clues to the nature of social growth in DS. Doll (1935) observed that SQ is consistently higher than IQ for Down's. Pototzky and Grigg (1942) agreed, adding that (i) social ages are in advance of those of non-DS retarded at similar mental ages, (ii) social age is an average of 3 years 4 months ahead of mental age, and (iii) social age accelerates beyond mental age, with increasing CA, particularly in the early years. Pototzky and Grigg resisted any hasty conclusion, saying 'no doubt the marked tendency to imitate found among mongoloids plays an important role. Also, such children are often given special attention by their teachers and nurses because of their likeable qualities; such added attention is, in effect, additional training which less attractive children do not receive' (p. 505). The rigorous intake selection criteria, in effect at the private institution where the study was conducted, also ensured a higher intellectual level and socio-economic origin for their sample than is usual in the public care sector.

A community sample, somewhat younger than the previous hospital group, was examined by Quaytman (1953) for comparative social and intellectual growth. Her 40 clinic cases ranged from CA 2 years 8 months to CA 16 years 7 months, with a mean CA of 7 years 7 months. The mean Binet IQ score was 44 points (from 23 to 77 points) with a mean mental age of 3 years. The mean social age (SA) was 4 years and the SQ 55 points, with a higher SQ than IQ displayed by 35 of the 40 children. Somatic and psychological profiles of the five cases showing a lower SQ than IQ would be of interest. The IQ–SQ and SA–MA differences, reported by Quaytman, are less dramatic than those offered by Pototzky and Grigg. Quaytman also charted early developmental achievement along with social quotients (Vineland). A positive relation between quality of early growth and magnitude of social quotient was obvious enough. Still, many of the motor coordination and habit training items of developmental schedules are shared by the Vineland (at early ages) such that high correlations between scales are little more than replicated measures. Taking Quaytman's results uncritically, community-based DS children of school age exhibit a 'trainable' intellectual status and an 'educable' social status.

Hospital and community samples were compared by McNeill (1955) for IQ and SQ across various CA strata. For hospital samples of 3 years CA, MA was found to be 10.84 months and SA 10.37 months. By 6 years CA, MA was 21.11 months and SA 22.56 months, while by CA 9 years, MA was 23.25 months and SA 30.17 months. At 12 years of CA, the MA and SA scores were 28.65 months and 33.23 months respectively. Finally, by 15 years CA, mental age was 36.77 months and social age 47.11 months.

Differences among IQ–SQ ratios, across age levels and between types of care, might be a result of selective hospitalization practices; the more retarded, difficult or physically complicated children being institutionalized early. In addition, the home-reared sample would have enjoyed those community opportunities for socialization which closely parallel the test items of the Vineland scale. Home resident DS children were in fact superior, both for social age and mental age, to the institutional cases at similar chronological ages. The home sample yielded a mean mental age of 40.10 months and a social age of 50.60 months, at 9 years CA. By 12 and 15 years of CA, a mean mental age of 46.11 and 51.40 months and a social age of 57.78 and 68 months were recorded. Interpretation appears to favour (i) the superiority of home environments and (ii) a high degree of plasticity for the socialization potential of DS. Institutional selection bias and the use of instrumentation derived from community social norms (versus institutional) could account for the findings equally well.

Centerwall and Centerwall (1960) attempted to manipulate both selection and disposal bias. These writers compared IQ and SQ for DS subjects placed in foster homes from birth and for those kept at home until 2½ years of age, or longer. The average IQ was 16 points for the fostered group and 23 points for the home-reared group. Average social quotients were 24 and 32 points respectively. Both home and fostered children were later hospitalized, at which time SQ ratings were repeated. Assessment of IQ was done before admission to hospital (average CA 2.75 years) and again after hospitalization (average CA 7 years). One group had been placed outside the home 'soon after birth', while the other remained at home until at least 2½ years CA. The foster placements ranged from private homes to institutions. Fostering is thus not a homogeneous 'treatment' variable. Reasons for placement of certain children away from the family unit early is unexplained. Difference in height and weight, in favour of the home group, could indicate an initial physiological advantage for the home-bound sample. Centerwall and Centerwall observed generally better nutritional status for the home-reared DS children, the benefits persisting even after separation. Accordingly, the SQ advantage reported for early home-reared, over the early fostered sample, does not support a psychological hypothesis for the origins of social performance in DS nor for the superiority of any given care regime. Of primary interest is the constancy of SQ–IQ differences across care conditions. The ratio of SQ to IQ for the two nurtural conditions is 0.66 for the fostered cases, and 0.71 for the home-reared sample. The mean IQ appears to be two-thirds of the SQ mean, on the average, regardless of type of care situation or magnitude of initial SQ or IQ. It has been indicated that these ratios can shift across age levels, although Domino and Newman (1965) reported about the same magnitude of SQ to IQ for 15-year-old samples. More interesting is their finding of IQ/SQ ratios of 22/34 for males and 27/39 for females; or 0.65 and 0.69 respectively. The suggestion of a sex factor related to magnitude of mental and social growth indices could be important for future study as could the indication that higher IQ scores, for the female DS patients, are accompanied by greater congruence of IQ–SQ levels. This phenomenon was first detected by Stickland (1954) and has been discussed elsewhere.

The likelihood that intellectually 'advantaged' DS individuals will show proportionately higher SQ than IQ, was examined by Dunsdon, Carter and Huntley (1960). Dunsdon *et al.* selected the intellectually brightest of all DS subjects enrolled in a community hospital clinic between 1945 and 1950. Intelligence quotients ranged up to 65 points, most falling between 35 and 54 points. Social maturity was assessed using the Vineland scale. These exceptional community-based DS children (mean CA 10 years) achieved similar IQ and SQ scores. Only with the intellectually most advanced was there any significant tendency towards lower SQ than IQ scores. The findings for the lower IQ children were more consistent with conventional expectation, e.g., a mean IQ of 38 points and a mean SQ of 51 points. One conclusion would be that relatively good social habits, for DS children around the IQ median, are more or less independent of intellectual facility; surviving chiefly on the basis of perseveration quality, temperament, mimicry, motor ability, or other discrete non-cognitive characteristics of the syndrome. Alternatively, the brighter DS children would have matured beyond psychometric demands of a primitive self-help nature and would now exhibit a closer correspondence between SQ and IQ levels. There is demonstrably increasing cognitive demand involved in adequate social expression as age

advances. Overall, then, a reasonable prospect would be for a closer correspondence of IQ and SQ at the low and high deficiency range, and for the
quite young and the adult members of the syndrome. The greatest IQ–SQ
disparities would be most evident among school-age DS children having
median IQs for the condition. Cutting across both explanations is still the
issue of nurtural effects on both IQ and SQ.

Shotwell and Shipe (1964) pursued the origins and durability of SQ score
for DS according to nurtural conditions. Their family and non-family samples
displayed an IQ of 48.9 and 34.5 points (pre-institutional), in favour of the
home-reared cases. At time of subsequent admission to institution the home-
reared children had an SQ of 45.1 points and the out-of-home, 29.6 points.
Some time after admission, the comparative SQ scores were 40 and 26.1
points. Methodological problems, discussed previously for the Centerwall
and Centerwall investigation, also influence the Shotwell and Shipe results.
The questions are whether there was initial neurological and somatic equivalence of the two 'treatment' groups and the comparability of the pre-
institutional nurtural conditions for each group. Pre-admission IQs were
assessed between 3 months and 3 years of CA, approximately, yielding IQ
means of 52.9 and 41.4 points (corrected for age differences) in favour of the
home-reared sample. Large disparities of intellectual promise, evident
so early in life, suggest an initial maturational difference between groups.
To accept an exclusively nurtural hypothesis, for the origins of socialization
facility, one would have to contend that the average family regime is
markedly superior to the usual foster home. The Shotwell and Shipe findings
indicate only that poor institutional care has an especially negative effect on
DS children or that an institutional placement or fostering decision, taken
soon after birth, might reflect the presence of special care and health
problems. These could include more profound amentia, serious secondary
physical handicap, and behavioural disorder. Otherwise, it appears that social
growth for DS is dependent upon initial IQ, CA at time of measurement, and
type or quality of nurtural background. Assigning relative weights to these
three major sources of variability, for SQ, is not possible on the basis of
the Shotwell and Shipe data or those of most other studies which have not
been designed to account for selection and maturational events.

The relation of maturational variables to social quotient

The shape of social growth, with changing CA, has been a special concern
of Kostrzewski (1965). Mental age and social age appear little different by
1 year of CA but became progressively disparate with time. By CA 22 years,

and at an average MA of 40 months, the average SA was between 80 and 90 months. There was little evidence of a radical deceleration of social growth curves, as is the case with mental maturation over time. Absolute increments of social age did slow somewhat with advancing CA. The movement of SQ was negligible between CA 2 and 5 years; from 51 to 57 points between CA 6 and 10 years; and from 41 to 47 points between CA 11 and 14 years. Initially, SQ appeared to rise; 45.6 points at CA 1 year, 53.2 points at CA 2 years, 55.56 points at CA 3 years and 61.25 points at CA 5 years. A serious eroding of social growth rates was first evident at about CA 5 years, coincidental with the changing task demands of intelligence tests at higher ages. These demands evolve across the early years from simple, concrete and motor-based to more conceptual responses requiring the forming of comparisons, abstractions and generalizations. The early and increasing advantage of social age over mental age can be understood, once more, in terms of test content; routine and early self-help skills being little dependent upon complex intellectual operations.

Whereas Kostrzewski had found a reliable advantage of SA over MA in the early years, Cornwell and Birch (1969) were not so sure. They examined the differences between social and intellectual maturity patterns in DS as age increased. Institutional samples were rejected for their purpose because they represent the lower ability range of DS and are constricted for social expression. The Cornwell and Birch investigation is one of the few to compare intellectual and social growth for DS using quasi-longitudinal methods. The sample was comprised of 44 cases aged 4–17 years. These individuals were VSMS tested on first contact with a community clinic, and again 2 years later (see Fig. 5). The data demonstrated 'a greater correspondence between CA and social age (SA)...in the younger age groups (4–8 years old), than in the older group (9–17)' (p. 344). Thus, social growth slowed as socialization indices demanded higher levels of communication and cognitive involvement; apparently despite the quality of previous or current family and community care. Fig. 6 from their study traces the close parallel of IQ with SQ at various chronological ages. The spread is comparatively minor by CA 4 and 5 years, growing notably between 5 to 10 years of age, and narrowing again past CA 12 years. A spread between IQ and SQ is again evident during the 13–16 year CA range, closing finally as adulthood is reached. The age stages exhibiting the greatest IQ–SQ disparity could represent merely a measurement bias attributable to the DS child's early success with the simple motor self-help content of the VSMS scale and the regression of IQ scores with age as conceptual content of standard tests is strengthened.

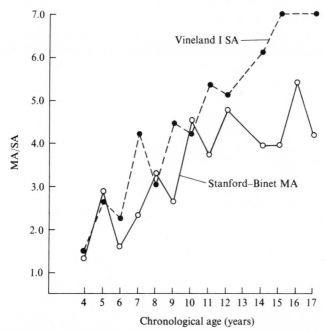

Fig. 5. Mental age (MA) and social age (SA) of children with Down's syndrome by chronological age. (From A. C. Cornwell and H. G. Birch (1969). *American Journal of Mental Deficiency*, **74**, 345.)

Certain qualitative aspects of social competence for DS were said by Cornwell and Birch (1969) to be increasingly uneven as CA increased. Some social skills improved with age while others related to communication, group socialization, and social direction or decision functions, did not. What acquisition of social skills occurred, from first to second testing, is credited to ongoing parent counselling at the clinic. No controlled comparisons are available and so the 'treatment' effect cannot be evaluated. Performance analysis of discrete categories of social competence, with CA, was done for general self-help items, self-help in eating, self-help in dressing and self-direction, and for particular occupation, communication, and locomotion items of the VSMS. The three self-help categories showed most improvement with age, a few of the group achieving the highest score possible. General self-help scores were most elevated, followed by eating and dressing. Fewer successes for eating and dressing items are, in part, explainable by the finer visuo-motor coordination required for tying shoe laces, cutting meat at the table and so on. Otherwise, the self-help items comprised mainly the more simple or mechanical processes requiring little conceptual ability or foresight. The occupation and communication categories ranged more widely with CA and varied between 50 and 75% of normal expectation, generally dropping more markedly with increasing CA. The decline is attributed to the inability of most Down's to read, write, or self-direct.

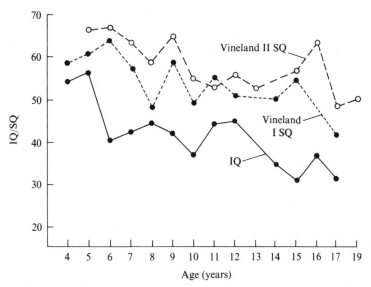

Fig. 6. IQ and social quotient (SQ) of children with Down's syndrome by chronological age. (From A. C. Cornwell and H. G. Birch (1969). *American Journal of Mental Deficiency*, **74**, 344.)

Cornwell and Birch concluded that while SQ scores differ greatly, from case to case, they do not decline at the same rate as does IQ. It also appears that while older DS children fall mainly in the TMR category, whether resident in institutions or at home, social quotients for at-home DS children are higher than for institutionalized cases. Differences between SQ narrows as both care groups face the increasing interdependence of cognitive and social capacity with age. Finally, these authors conceded that 'the interactive effects of selective retention or institutionalization on subsequent development are not clear from these data' (p. 348). The extent of reciprocity between social and intellectual maturation, at various age stages of DS, will need to be viewed in the context of the origins of both.

The origins of social adaptation

It is clear that the socialization profile for DS is multidimensional, dependent on level of intellect, temperament, age, sex and environmental conditions. It is not so obvious how the social stereotype is expressed across individual cases. An appreciation of the probable antecedents of social behaviour might help. The materials to follow concern social behaviour for DS related to intellectual status; in the context of various environmental influences; as a function of varieties of temperament; and as a product of physiological status, both initially and ongoing. Physiological factors include cytological subclassification, general health and extent or severity of secondary handicap. The interaction of temperament and social capacity for DS is touched on also in the chapters on personality and intelligence.

Social behaviour and intellectual status

Debate about the nature of social capacity for DS is a result of investigations into its affective and cognitive aspects. These studies have identified particular social performance qualities as correlates of (i) degree of intellectual deficit, (ii) the nature of intellect and temperament at various mental and physical ages, and (iii) the instrumentation employed to measure social, intellectual and personality outputs.

Psychometric evidence has supported a reliable if decelerating mental growth to approximately 2 or 3 years of MA, followed by a levelling. Past 4 years of MA, intelligence tests demand conceptual abilities which do not emerge strongly across the syndrome. The DS child cannot now so easily collect test credits for the more sophisticated social performance items, most of which are dependent upon an ability to manipulate language symbols and an appreciation of social consequences (anticipation and prediction). If socialization ability is defined, in part, as a product of intellectual capacity, it is not difficult to understand why (i) social behaviour is not especially ahead of intellectual status for the more severely retarded DS individual, (ii) social and intellectual scores are not so different for very young DS cases and (iii) social performance is significantly advanced over intellectual performance during the early more rapid maturational period. Otherwise, much of the aura of good social habits for DS is derived from its comparison with the more capriciously damaged categories of MR, or is a side-effect of personality status. In the latter case, a separation must be made between social competence and social attractiveness.

Whether or not any particular intellectual features of DS can predict social competence, is not established. Supposed memory and observational facility have been implicated as contributors to social performance capacity, as have the suggested imitative propensity and some features of psychomotor development. The apparent superiority of visual over auditory intake and the low arousal–anxiety characteristics of the condition have also been mentioned as facilitating specific positive self-help behaviours. The scientific value of these positions has been elaborated in other chapters.

Social behaviour and personality

The inflated social promise of DS is a result, partly, of a failure to separate temperament, intelligence and activation styles from social performance. Research already examined supports a distinction between gross approach behaviour (frequency, vigour and direction) and particularized social skill in DS. The largely favourable emotional reactivity of the moderately retarded DS child, when compared with other TMR groups, had tended to enhance the traditional social stereotype. Moreover, some of the positive social image of DS can be re-interpreted in terms of the social–behavioural consequences of 'extroversion' and imitation. If temperament is somehow more intact for DS children, than for other MR children, social conditioning would be more reliably established. These themes were expanded in the chapter on personality.

Social behaviours as a function of environment

The DS individual appears socially more pliant than MR subjects of other origins, on the whole. The effect could be largely contextual. The traditional institutional system was regimented for administrative convenience and became, consequently, depersonalizing. It provided few opportunities for misadventure or for novel or intimate personal transactions which could expose a paucity of social capacity. Further, sparse environments elicit, quite often, a vigorous competition for attention (or affection) among those able to compete. The young DS child, because of his relatively uncomplicated neurophysiological and emotional status, was able to command positive attention and did so. Ward staff acquired a favourable impression of social drive and capacity for this group, especially when they were housed with other MR children of similar IQ. Reports by mothers, raising their DS children in normal family and community situations, are less enthusiastic about the social gains of their DS offspring.

The brighter DS child (in the lower educable MR range) is most often singled out for favourable comparison. Appearance can be deceiving: Educable retarded children of unspecified aetiology originate disproportionately from lower socio-economic strata (Gibson and Butler, 1954). It has been argued, moreover, that the social origins of DS are superior to those of the general population of retarded insofar as the syndrome (i) is often a manifestation of the late child-bearing period, (ii) tends to have older siblings as agents of socialization, (iii) has, conceivably, more mature and experienced parents, or (iv) has parents who left school later and married later. The DS child, coming to institutional care, on the average at about 9 years of age, seems better socialized than intellectually similar non-DS children and might maintain some significant part of his early good social habits. The initial socialization advantage, of whatever source, is subsequently reinforced by care staff. Socialization data, derived from the study of continuing home care for DS, is less encouraging. As the afflicted grow older, parents more easily identify the inflexible, impulsive and negative qualities of social output. To compound the matter, there are apt to be normal siblings for comparison purposes, as well as opportunities (in a usually more permissive and more personalized home care regime) for the expression of a broader range of social behaviours, including the negative. The greater tolerance of deviancy, inherent in family environments, has other explanations including the operation of parental guilt and a tendency to compensate at home for the effects of rejection by some neighbours and relatives.

The negative socialization effects of family care must be recognized as well. The home-reared are, in many instances, still an object of shame. A common means of protecting the DS individual, his siblings and his family, it to withdraw from full community participation. Some parents create an environment so arid that the retarded child becomes internalized, shy, fearful, neurotic and unattractive in a social sense. The problem is complicated by poor agreement on the proper goals of socialization; whether for terminal institutional care, community fostering, industrial or agricultural 'village' group living, or continuing family care into adulthood. An imminent need is to identify the extent, origins and pliability of social capacity in DS so as to match training styles with projected life-styles.

Social performance and physiological status

A variety of somatic factors contribute to the undesirable or declining social habits of DS. These include communication handicaps, progressive intellectual decline, sensory disorders or limitation, circulatory defect, easy fatigue, finer motor control handicaps and the many structural problems associated with feeding, dressing and play activity. Some of the structural limitations are correctable or abate with time. The neurophysiological constraints to adequate socialization are more troublesome.

Down's syndrome individuals, at their worst, are described as restless, stubborn, aggressive and destructive. These psychological signs are found especially among the seriously retarded cases and at more advanced ages. Since the more severely retarded members of the syndrome are at higher risk, the statistics determining the behaviour stereotype are partly a product of the numerically inferior but stronger survivors. Therefore, as the severely handicapped benefit increasingly from modern medical and other new support technologies, to survive infancy and childhood, the more pleasing behavioural stereotypes will be strained. It is also reasoned that many suffer secondary central and peripheral nervous system damage, not assignable directly to the karyotype; a matter of the chaining of risks. Whether or not the damage is primary or secondary, progressive deteriorative effects are cumulative and have serious consequences for the quality of social behaviour with advancing years. Hyperactivity, poor attention level, aggressiveness, perseveration, conceptualization deficiency and language deficit are a few of the less pleasant sequelae. Ongoing somatic decline corrupts, as well, a reasonably intact emotionality, slows the learning process and disrupts rudimentary but workable social and self-care patterns. Several workers have extended a 'hyperkinesis' hypothesis to cover even the apparently positive social outputs of DS individuals, e.g., hyperactivity masquerading as vigorous approach behaviour, defective arousal seen as placidity and emotional lability interpreted as enthusiasm. Yet, most trainable level DS pre-adolescents appear better socialized than non-DS retarded and many DS adults hold their socialization gains despite obvious physical reversals. The failure to prove more precise relationships between neuropathological and behavioural events in the young DS adult is a paradox which deserves further study.

Evaluation

The social image of DS is in transition. Improving investigative techniques have fractionated the classic social stereotype, across ages and stages of development, and against various environmental and somatic variables. The traditional stereotype has credence for younger DS children, within limits, and especially for those having few secondary physical complications, median or better intelligence, and under suitable care conditions. While these are a minority of the members of the syndrome, across all grades and ages, they are the most visible and contribute disproportionately to the propagation of a positive social image. The components of the image extend very little beyond easy personal habits acquisition, reliable motility, relatively unimpaired motor imitation and reasonable emotionality by middle childhood. These latter properties are evident chiefly in comparison with other mentally retarded who have a similar degree of gross intellectual handicap. There has been no serious test of the permanence or long-range adjustment value of particular social skills, for DS, nor any extensive comparisons of these skills against socialization indices based on normal children along a mental or motor age continuum. Possibly, the stereotype survives more strongly than the research data would justify because we who work with the condition value it.

Social ages and quotients for DS are described as eroding with time as psychometric criteria become more rigid for language and conceptual skills, and as neuropathological effects mount with advancing years. Social quotients rise above IQ and motor quotients as infancy extends into childhood, declining subsequently to approximate IQ as childhood advances into the adolescent and adult range. The less attractive social status of some DS individuals throughout life is a product, we think, of low intellectual status, meagre energy outputs (whether motivationally or physiologically viewed) and rate of CNS deterioration. 'Intelligence' and drive control decline with time and appear to parallel metabolic and neurophysiological changes. Notwithstanding, many DS adults manage to maintain comparatively good social quotients. It might follow that intensive sensory and motor training, during the susceptible early months and years, can provide a basis for socialization patterns capable of resisting physiological and psychological reversals later in life.

While much of what has been discussed is supported by the research, in a consensual way, there are too many exceptions to permit comfortable conclusions. Important sources of individual variation for socialization status have been identified with developmental timing, quality of physical and psychological care, variation of abnormal karyotype, sensorimotor and cognitive abilities, and rates of deterioration of the neurological and metabolic systems with advancing years. Quality of temperament was isolated, second only to extent of intellectual capacity, as central to the favourable social stereotype. The equation is supportable for institutional samples but less clear, as yet, for those remaining in the community. Overall, the evidence does not support the belief that DS has numerous, special and uniform social propensities, except when compared with aetiologically heterogenous MR populations. Even so, the positive image holds only for the middle childhood years and is substantially dependent upon quality of intellect and temperament.

7

Ability profiles

Witmer (1896) is credited by many as being the first to urge social scientists to undertake applied research with the atypical child. His message was that human data should be processed empirically and related to living environments. The result was a measurement orientation to mental retardation, having its origins in Goddard's translation and elaboration of the Binet scales and in Wallin's (1909) talent for overview. Thus emerged a problem-solving role for psychologists which could be clearly demarcated from the established positions and practices of medicine and education. Mental tests permitted the grading of mental retardates for appropriate group management and the identification of qualitative differences related to individual remediation. Retardates of approximately similar gross MA and IQ levels were discovered to vary in many behavioural directions (on sub-test, profile and scatter analyses). These distinctions appeared, often, to reflect biological and aetiological variables and tempted the tester to make causal inferences, e.g., that an MR child was of endogenous or exogenous origin. So it was that two major theoretical biases developed; (i) an attempt to extract bio-behavioural links for MR and (ii) the functional position, i.e., that since psychological effects are measureable and capable of some modification through learning, mediational constructs are largely irrelevant. Both approaches have survived into the present abilities literature concerning Down's syndrome.

Earlier chapters have examined the quantitative aspects of intelligence for the syndrome – with age, care condition, somatic status and sex. This chapter explores the qualitative aspects of intelligence and the validity of the special abilities attributed to the syndrome. These include a number of distinct cognitive features and a supposed special status for musicality, memory, mimicry and temperament. An effort is made to identify the contradictions within the literature on psychometric profiles and to provide a framework for understanding the contemporary experimental material on learning and arousal, which is considered in a subsequent chapter.

180

Mental ability: psychometric research

Preamble

Belmont (1971) proposed the view that our curiosities about the apparent disparities surrounding the mental abilities of DS have sometimes been satisfied by drawing upon infrahuman analogy. He says,

Clinicians are divided as to which species is best suited for comparison with mongoloid children. Crookshank (1924) favoured simian allusions, while Benda (1946) preferred the image of a puppy. West and Ansberry (1968) explicitly considered mongoloids to be subhuman, finding chimpanzees, dogs and parrots to have illustrative value, while Engler (1949) was sometimes content merely to call them 'creatures'. (p. 33)

Crookshank's (1925) preoccupation with 'simian allusions' is a product of an intent to trace varieties of evolutionary descent. His atavistic causal concept for DS encompassed numbers of intellectually normal individuals who were regressed racially, i.e., were 'mongoloid' in appearance. The criteria were quite generous. Their other distinguishing characteristic was an intellectual cunning untempered by moral or abstract concerns; features which modern European peoples are said to have acquired in the general biological advance. While Crookshank's view was not based on satisfactory data, his description of mentality for DS ranks among the first, other behavioural accounts having dwelt heavily on temperament and the special traits. Otherwise, the absence of a body of naturalistic evidence concerning learning and thinking in DS can be attributed to (i) an unsympathetic cultural climate within western society (that the afflicted were 'creatures') and (ii) a lack of suitable instrumentation. Not until 1967, and the publication of *The world of Nigel Hunt: the diary of a mongoloid youth*, was there any first-person account of cognitive patterning in DS; along with a compelling conclusion that simple reflexive or atavistic explanations are insufficient. The new psychometry served first to give numbers to the clinically obvious gradients of retardation. Later work used test pattern inspection and item-by-age scatter analysis to expose the extent of IQ variability within the syndrome in relation to CA, type of care regime, and various demographic factors.

Within-syndrome findings

Brousseau and Brainerd (1928) pioneered the argument that Binet test patterning across mental age levels (pass–fail distribution and extent of item scatter) does not differ between DS and other mentally retarded children. Examination of their sample of mental test profiles, however, indicates that a representative segment (12 cases of MA 3 years) performed appropriately to mental age for the identification and naming of various items but poorly with materials requiring the sequencing and relating of events. At higher MA levels, failures were a function of the extent of item language content. Pototzky and Grigg (1942) proposed that arithmetic test items, specifically, were about as equally difficult for DS subjects as for other mentally retarded children. Of the cases examined by them,

50 per cent could perform simple additions; 30% could perform long additions of three-place numbers; 35% knew their multiplication tables, but only 5% could perform long multiplication; 30% can perform simple subtraction of digits, but none of them can perform subtraction of three-place numbers. (p. 509)

These frequencies are difficult to credit in the light of Kostrewski's (1965) careful observation concerning the temporal phasing of number sense in DS and his belief that number sense is one of the most limited areas of mental growth for the disorder. Kostrewski recognized a 'first' phase which he says includes understanding the notion of general size and sequence, e.g., more or less, mechanical rote counting. The concept of 'one' versus more than one is not observed for DS in the first phase of arithmetic development (between 25 and 36 months of mental age). For the average DS child the foregoing MA span would represent 5–7 years of CA. A second phase of arithmetic understanding is described as including true, although rudimentary, number appreciation (at mental ages between 37 and 48 months). During this period memory to four digits, counting to ten digits, and a genuine appreciation of the distinction between the concept 'one' (as opposed to more than one) make their appearance. Phase three of developing number sense incorporates MAs ranging from 49 to 72 months with the unfolding of rote counting to about 21 and an appreciation of between three and seven distinct objects. For example, the DS child could give the examiner up to seven objects in the manner of a Binet test requirement. Phase four required a command of simple addition and subtraction skills (numbers up to ten) and an MA range from 73 to 84 months. Very few achieved these higher mental ages. Kostrewski mentioned the brighter DS child's appreciation of the decimal concept but recorded no instance of successful multiplication or division. Many writers have observed a deficiency of symbolization facility in DS. Kostrewski speculated that symbolization deficiency could be derived from limitations of auditory–perceptual patterning, attention deficit, and/or some more inherent cerebral inability respecting the abstract attitude. Number manipulation is possibly more revealing of abstraction deficit than letter or word manipulation. In short, DS is deficient in symbol management and generally more so than other forms of mental retardation at similar maturational points.

Wallin (1944) also doubted that arithmetic proficiency for DS could match the arithmetic proficiency seen in other MA comparable mentally retarded individuals. His DS clinic subjects nevertheless achieved reading levels higher than expectation based on Binet MA scores. The psychometric advantage is attributed to Wallin to the simple 'mechanics of word calling' as distinct from comprehension facility. He offered that DS children are especially intact for visual-receptive ability and rote memory.   Rollin (1946), acknowledging some psychometric individuality for the syndrome, preferred an activation-temperament explanation of the proposed differences. Simple repetitive tasks are presumably more ably handled by DS subjects because of their comparative (to other 'imbeciles') self-assurance and, he says, their good reaction time. The majority of his DS cases were catalogued as extroverted, given to brisk responses but displaying little reflection or concern regarding the quality of the response. The response of the introverted DS child (a minority, according to Rollin) to mental test situations depended on the extent of examiner assurance. The introverted were less obviously alert in test situations but, when given suitable encouragement, performed at levels superior to the extroverted DS subjects. The typically extroverted displayed psychometric strength only when speed of response was a major scoring criterion. Rollin attributed their facility for the rapid management of routine non-conceptual test material to impulse disorder, associated with classical extroversion; an innate behavioural feature of the syndrome, he claimed.

Other impressions of psychometric uniqueness for DS have been recorded by Stickland (1954). He was drawn to the similarity of Binet test scatter and patterning for two quite intelligent DS adults reared in culturally and educationally superior homes. Similarities of test failure pattern were accounted for in terms of a deficiency of abstract or conceptual vocabulary skill; a much-mentioned deficit in the pre-experimental literature. He contended that the high IQ and test-pattern congruence of his pair was a function of intensive home and school training which had been directed to exploiting memory facility as a compensatory device and to forcing academic and social skills. There is no assurance that other mental retardates would not display similar results in equally advantaged environments.

The manifestation, or not, of special mental abilities for DS has been pursued by McNeill (1955) in the realm of psychomotor behaviours. He concluded that eye–hand coordination and self-help skills are generally superior to global mental age. He cautioned that the kind and distribution of special mental abilities can be a function of type of care regime, somatic differences within syndrome, and chronological age. Secondary explanations aside, both Stedman and Eichorn (1964) and McNeill agree on the better performance of DS subjects on psychomotor than symbolic test items. The Cornwell and Birch (1969) and Cornwell (1974) studies offer corroborative evidence. Cornwell and Birch confirmed (i) that increasing language item failure coincides with increasing physical age, and (ii) that social growth (Vineland scales) slows as the language demands of mental test content increases with age. Of particular interest was the finding that self-help growth decelerates with advancing age especially as progressively finer visual and motor-manipulative skills (tying shoelaces, buttoning) are required to meet age-graded test norms. The middle childhood psychomotor advantage is apparently short-lived. Cornwell (1974) concluded that DS reveals 'a slow accretion of certain rote skills and progressive improvement of other abilities but severe limitation in concept formation, abstraction and higher level integrative abilities regardless of age'.

The intra-sample psychometric studies have identified a number of specific mental abilities as possibly characteristic of DS. The most favoured psychometric abilities picture depicts DS as relatively high-scoring on tests loaded for rote memory, psychomotor, visual-motor, and non-conceptual components. Difficulty is experienced for MA-equated test materials having significant abstract, symbolic, verbal and recognition vocabulary content. The profile might be reliable for DS but is not necessarily distinctive among the mental retardations.

Across-groups mental abilities patterning

From 1955 onwards most psychometric profile investigations compared mental ability in DS with other retardates of similar IQ level, or with normal children of similar mental ages. The study of performance quality was undertaken with a variety of psychometric devices and categories. Work by Murphy (1956) and by Lyle (1959) provide two of the best illustrations of the promise and the problems of the comparative approach.

Degree of eye–hand coordination, neuromotor efficiency, and verbal performance for DS and non-DS imbeciles concerned Murphy (1956). Using the Cattell, 'draw-a-man', and Binet scales she concluded that test pattern differences for DS, familial retardates and exogenous retardates were not striking. The DS sample displayed similarities with the CA-matched familial sample by exhibiting less performance variability for both verbal and non-verbal test items. Down's subjects were said to be more like the brain-damaged group in a qualitative sense, a possible reference to the conventional notion that the exogenous mentally retarded are more concrete, perseverative and impulsive than are the endogenous types. A controlled comparison of verbal and performance components of mental test-patterning, undertaken by Lyle (1959), produced similar results. His sample included 34 hospitalized and 76 day-care retardates tested with the Minnesota pre-school scale of intelligence. Down's children were less proficient on the verbal components of the test than were other imbeciles. The hospitalized were, in turn, less proficient than the day-school DS. Lyle argued that these mental ability deviations were a product of the separate effects of hospital and community care systems. The point is a difficult one since there was a mean difference (between hospitalized DS and non-DS subjects) of 9 months of verbal mental age, whereas no significant verbal score difference obtained for the DS and non-DS MR day-care samples. The influence of selective institutionalization provides an alternative explanation for verbal performance disparity between DS and other comparable MRs and thus cognitive distinctions attributable to syndromic factors cannot be eliminated.

Both the Murphy and the Lyle conclusions suffer from having compared causally mixed control groups against a specific clinical aetiology and from the failure to control for type of care regime between groups. As well, mental abilities for DS are likely to shift quantitatively and qualitatively, over time. The across-groups evidence to follow will be graded for age of sample, beginning with the pre-school DS child.

The infant scales

Kralovich (1959) screened 28 DS children through 113 subtests of the Cattell infant scale. Only five items separated DS and non-DS 'organic' controls. Samples were matched for CA, sex and socio-economic condition. The few significant test items favoured DS in the area of motor manipulation and were all representative of the first 22 months of the test schedule. While the frequency of significant items exceeded (barely) chance expectation, interpretation is seriously restricted by the unusually low IQ of the DS sample (17.2 IQ points), the predominantly motor content of first stages of infant schedules, and the extent of motor anomaly likely to be exhibited by severely damaged non-DS retarded children (IQ 15 points for the Kralovich sample). The higher IQ samples, examined by Fishler, Share and Koch (1964), implicated only language item performance as consistently wanting (Gessel scales) for DS. Self-help items (e.g., toileting) were observed to be least lacking against age-graded test norms. To the extent that simple self-help training success is based on motor facility, Kralovich's finding of comparatively good early motor performance for DS is supported. Dicks-Mireaux

(1966) reported, however, that motor growth lag accelerates for DS as age advances and that motor status is initially unpromising (1972).

Dicks-Mireaux ordered the Gessel scale items for DS in terms of motor, adaptive, social and language content for subjects 12 to 82 weeks of CA. Carr (1970) documented the early strength but subsequent quick decline of motor indices for DS. Shotwell (1964) explored the proposition that mental ability configurations for DS (derived from infant scales) are little more than a test of landmark heterogeneity against aetiologically mixed control groups. Using the Kuhlmann–Binet scales, she contrasted psychometric patterning for DS, post-traumatic, familial and undifferentiated mentally retarded. No exclusive pass–fail pattern was supported for DS beyond an indication that the age-related difficulty of particular items varied by aetiology. The prospects are that developmental timing, for the appearance of various mental abilities, is aetiologically specific and that infant schedules are not sensitive to the more subtle growth differences across groups.

The adult scales

Numerous ability patterning studies have indicated that where mental test content is substantially visual-motor, repetitive, mnemonic, low in language content (expressive) and low in abstraction demand, the more mature DS subject fared comparatively well. But such evidence does not prove intellectual distinction for the syndrome. The mental tests of the period did not distinguish between cognitive and delivery capacity, e.g., motor speed, arousal level and sensory acuity deficits. Share (1975) noted that the capable DS child is most easily distinguished by his co-operation, level of organization and use of good quality gestures to circumvent speech difficulty. Special test instruction was necessary, however, in tasks which incorporated spatial relationships.

Experimental investigation of the ability to copy and reproduce designs, as an expression of tactile-shape recognition facility (O'Connor and Hermelin, 1963), has shown DS subjects to be inferior to other IQ-matched MR. Down's children also proved to be slower for motor speed and lower for stereognostic recognition than were MA-matched normals. Visual perception proficiency did not obviously differ between DS and other retardates. Coleman (1960) has supported the latter proposition for brain-injured and DS children but found the DS subjects to be superior on a classification or object grouping task. Gordon (1944) had previously observed normals to have significantly superior tactile recognition ability when compared with DS individuals. Disparities between general psychometric patterning and specific abilities studies for DS are probably dependent on how precisely the various abilities are defined and on the sensorimotor circuits employed.

Whatever the discrepancies, the traditional test pattern literature has provided some interesting leads. Nakamura's (1965) Binet profile study of older DS subjects is a suitable starting point. His goal was to determine any association among cytological, somatic and behavioural variables. Item pass–fail percentages were calculated for Binet years II through VIII for 64 institutional DS subjects (16 years and older) against age, sex and IQ-matched controls. The low mean IQ (23 points) for both samples, the use of an aetiologically mixed 'organic' control series, and the lengthy institutional history of the samples were acknowledged as problems. Items were re-grouped for memory content and for non-verbal or low-verbal characteristics. Significance between correlated proportions was obtained for four of the 60 Binet items across all age levels. These items were formboard, block-bridging and circle-drawing proficiency, and performance on repeated digits. All but the latter favoured the DS sample. Memory content and low-verbal content (as a class) did not separate causal groups. Although a finding of four significant subtests (from a total of 60 comparisons) is hardly impressive, the skills identified with DS are similar to previous reports. The argument would favour visual-motor (psychomotor) strength for DS superior to that observed among brain-damaged MR controls. The isolated success of the controls, with digit repetition tasks, is interpreted by Nakamura as an indication of selective attention or retention disorder in DS. Particular difficulty with number symbols, whatever the receptive or expressive mode, has been frequently mentioned.

Data from standard psychometric devices do not permit critical hypothesis testing and are not always representative of ability extremes. Further, ability levels for DS are frequently below the range of the older mental tests. There have been a few instances of DS individuals who are sufficiently intact intellectually to produce test profiles which will support complex analysis. Some, though, have been provocative single case observations where DS is not clearly established or is clinically atypical. An occurrence of confirmed translocation DS with a Wechsler intelligence scale for children score of 82 points, averaged over a period of time, was reported by Rosecrans (1971). Performance IQ was 68 and verbal IQ 86 points. Arithmetic subtest was particularly low. Other tests such as the Bender–Gestalt indicated performance distortion, perseveration, directional difficulty and poor visual–perceptual organization. A high level of distractability was observed. The foregoing signs are usually taken as indicators of cerebral insult, and are 'more frequently associated with right hemisphere disturbance than left hemisphere, although a generalized cortical deficit is evidenced' (p. 293). Chronic brain syndrome has been widely documented for DS as early appearing and as a correlate of progressive personality and intellectual deterioration. Fishler (1975) examined mosaics against age-matched and sex-matched standard trisomy cases. In addition to being generally more intelligent, the mosaics displayed a better number sense, less visual– perceptual handicap and more normal voice intonation compared to the hoarse, flat, poorly articulated speech of the trisomy cases. Differences were not detected for social or personality status.

The new psychometry and ability profiles

The pursuit of special mental abilities profiles for DS had by about 1965 outgrown dependence on test scatter analyses. The newer tests are designed to sense a wider range of intellectual qualities, to represent factorially pure item content and to trace input–output or receptive–expressive patterns involving different modes. Several are examined now.

The search for a 'characteristic cognitive style' for DS was extended by Bilovsky and Share (1965) using the Illinois test of psycholinguistic ability (ITPA). Nine discrete ability subtests were inspected for 24 community cases (up to 23 years CA, and IQ range 31–86 points), having a mean IQ of 46.6 points. The subtests of the ITPA permit grouping for decoding content (receptive language ability), encoding content (expressive ability), and 'understanding' level. Interpretation favoured comparatively strong performance for visual decoding (understanding pictures–low verbal content) and motor encoding (expressing thoughts by gesture). Auditory–vocal items, both sequencing and automatic, were most depressed from individual subject means. Auditory channelling (encoding or decoding) was most afflicted, whereas visual decoding and motor encoding emerged most strongly. It could be claimed, in the absence of a control series, that non-DS retarded groups might produce similar patterns. Against this position is the overall similarity between these findings and related Binet studies which did employ controls. The relatively small intra-sample variability also favours a syndromic hypothesis for the ability patterns observed. Bilovsky and Share concluded that DS appears deficient for the management of non-concrete symbols and displays poor vocal or auditory processing skills. The DS subjects exceeded their overall performance mean for the use of representational material, visual receptive tasks and motor expression. Two unpublished doctoral studies support this (Strunk, 1964; McCarthy, 1965).

Clausen's ability structure project (Clausen, 1966, 1968) provides a second example of the power of the newer psychometry for study of general mental abilities in DS. The 'ASP Mongolism Report' involved a battery of 34 tests yielding a total of 50 variables and covering the domains of sensory, motor, perceptual and cognitive functioning. Twelve DS subjects were compared with 196 other mentally retarded and subsequently with a refined control of 24 non-DS mentally retarded (matched for IQ, CA, MA and sex ratio, where appropriate). Two apparent strengths for DS, grip measure and time interval estimation, were attributed to age differences across samples. McNeill (1955) had previously identified grip strength as high in the ability structure of DS children. Table 12 of the Clausen report is ordered such that high scores correspond to high performance levels. Only the columns for DS and matched controls are of concern here since the unselected controls had a higher IQ level than the DS subjects. Significant differences were obtained for six variables, as shown. Clausen (1968) observed that no differences existed 'with respect to motor functions, to intelligence measures, or to the majority of perceptual variables', but that 'the sensory modalities of vision and audition tend to be more impaired' (p. 123) for Down's cases. These conclusions are not necessarily in conflict with previous findings insofar as speed of perceptual and sensory functioning was identified as the deficient component. Other differences could be explained as a function of incomplete matching.

Further attempts to prove that DS is a psychological entity have been made by Neeman (1971) who dismembered the Purdue perceptual-motor survey and by Reinecke (1973) using the Lutey schema for the differentiation of cognitive functioning (Stanford–Binet Scales). Neeman compared the Purdue items (walking forward, sideways and backward, jumping, writing, ocular pursuit, form perception, etc.) for DS and non-DS retardates. The DS cases scored less than the controls on all items except 'imitation of movement' where they exceeded controls. Perhaps findings can be explained in terms of an 11 point IQ difference favouring the control sample. Reinecke found no difference between DS and undifferentiated controls for any of 13 areas of cognitive functioning or at any of three age levels. Older DS subjects were, however, less variable than controls. Clausen might view the negative findings as a failure to control for arousal potentials across aetiological groups. His point is that activation–performance ratios, rather than areas of cognitive potential, are more likely to be syndromic. Carter and Clark (1973), applying operant conditioning to a discrimination task, with DS subjects, found faster discrimination to be associated with mental age. Drive property might have special importance for predicting cognitive ability for the syndrome. The inability of the psychometric literature clearly to define DS as

Table 12. *Comparison of the DS group with the total and the matched non-DS groups for fifty variables*

	Non-DS total M	t	DS M	t	Non-DS matched M
Hand dominance	49.9	0.20	49.5	0.88	47.2
Eye dominance	50.2	0.13	49.8	1.18	45.8
Visual acuity	42.0	4.91***	22.9	2.54**	35.9
Colour vision	46.4	2.28*	36.0	1.52	43.6
Audiometric left	18.9	1.70	−7.2	0.90	9.0
Audiometric right	27.8	1.44	6.8	0.59	14.2
Threshold for speech	49.6	4.51***	26.8	3.86***	48.1
Kinaesthetic left	23.4	1.33	46.3	2.31*	39.5
Kinaesthetic right	41.9	0.76	43.9	1.25	39.7
Two-point left	41.4	1.20	44.2	1.13	39.7
Two-point right	40.9	0.25	45.1	0.29	40.0
Two-point R–L	50.8	0.90	52.2	0.07	52.1
Ataxiometric medial	55.5	0.35	57.3	0.63	53.4
Ataxiometric lateral	49.3	2.21*	42.2	1.30	46.7
Grip left	79.2	1.18	74.4	0.45	78.0
Grip right	82.9	1.35	71.1	0.95	78.6
Lower arm movement	26.6	3.43***	−18.9	1.50	5.3
Tapping	44.9	2.87***	30.4	0.01	30.3
Visual reaction time	38.4	2.39**	14.4	0.08	13.4
Auditory reaction time	41.1	2.91***	−1.3	1.15	17.0
Auditory choice reaction time	44.4	2.20*	20.9	0.89	30.6
Scramble foreplay reaction time	44.8	2.21*	16.2	1.15	31.1
Hand precision hits	42.0	0.13	41.5	1.93	31.5
Hand precision errors	57.2	3.38***	45.3	1.82	52.9
Pegboard right	48.5	5.01***	31.0	0.58	33.5
Pegboard left	51.0	5.47***	31.0	1.14	35.8
Pegboard both	49.0	5.78***	29.2	1.36	34.9
Mirror drawing errors	46.9	1.58	41.2	1.33	32.3
Mirror drawing error range	51.1	1.85	56.9	1.89	49.3
Mirror drawing total time	52.8	0.10	52.1	1.55	44.4
Railwalking	37.1	4.32***	21.5	1.12	26.3
Word association	43.0	2.97***	32.0	1.19	37.7
Reaction time to pictures	41.4	4.48***	16.6	2.50**	33.8
Span of apprehension	41.6	2.76***	30.5	1.53	37.4

Table 12. (*cont.*)

	Non-DS total M	t	DS M	t	Non-DS matched M
ID threshold	35.4	2.05*	14.0	2.49**	39.2
Recognition non-meaningful	40.7	3.19***	30.8	1.11	34.7
Azimuth arithmetic	38.6	1.33	34.7	0.40	33.3
Azimuth reversal	35.8	0.37	32.8	1.20	22.2
Brightness discrimination	53.5	2.93***	44.8	2.42*	54.0
CFF	37.0	4.51***	25.3	1.58	32.8
Stereognosis	43.4	2.43**	28.0	0.14	28.9
Time interval estimation	43.6	0.50	38.2	0.58	31.2
Weight lifting	53.6	2.70***	63.6	0.32	65.3
Muller–Lyer extent	52.1	0.73	48.2	0.67	52.1
Muller–Lyer anticipation	49.4	0.51	47.4	0.18	46.3
Porteus Maze MA	41.9	1.86	34.6	0.39	33.0
Porteus Maze IQ	30.8	1.86	25.6	0.32	24.6
Ravens	39.4	3.68***	34.5	0.04	34.6
Primary mental ability – IQ	10.5	6.18***	0.7	0.61	1.7
Primary mental ability – MA	30.4	5.97***	16.4	0.52	17.6

After Clausen (1968).
* Significant at 0.05 level.   ** Significant at 0.02 level.   *** Significant at 0.01 level.

a psychological entity probably also represents a failure to separate the power, speed and modality components of cognitive tasks. The experimental literature, examined in the chapter to follow, does attempt to isolate the particulars of intellectual process for the syndrome and to relate cognitive and affective processes.

The psychometric evidence: consensus and conflict

The mounting contradictions within the clinical and psychometric studies of mental process for DS have a number of sources, which will now be reviewed:

(1) Surveyed against causally mixed MR control groups, range and scatter of intellectual characteristics for DS has seemed comparatively narrow (Murphy, Bilovsky and Share). A greater degree of cognitive homogeneity for DS, over other discrete clinical entities of MR, is however not established in the measurement literature.

(2) Language lag, more evident with increasing CA for DS than for non-DS control samples, has been a popular conclusion of the psychometric studies (Lyle; Fisher, Share and Koch; Brousseau and Brainerd; Bilovsky and Share), but not universally so (Nakamura; Wallin; Butterfield). There are CA and IQ differences across samples, variable aetiological make-up for the control groups, and poor comparability among the vocabulary test items used, e.g., simple repetitive word-calling versus a relational or interpretive requirement. Stickland had drawn a distinction between abstract–conceptual and rote vocabulary activity for DS. Benda has speculated whether or not vocabulary and vocal retardation in DS is centrally, modality, or mechanically founded. These issues will be explored in a later chapter on language. They are important here because decisions about cognitive quality and capacity for DS are tied to the nature of output or release mechanisms, sensory threshold levels, circuiting facility, and to the speech apparatus itself.

(3) Number sense is usually described as poor in DS, especially when compared with other academic skills and against matched non-DS mentally retarded subjects (Kostrewski; Wallin; Butterfield; Nakamura). Pototzky and Grigg, alone, concluded otherwise. Number management is a multidimentional behaviour so that interpretation of the nature and source of the deficiency is difficult. The most simple present explanation probably implicates the difficulty DS children have with the abstract or relational requirements of primary arithmetic operations such as addition and subtraction. These operations are less important for the grouping and identification of letter and word symbols in the early learning stage. Particular frustration, however, is experienced by older DS children with abstract word concepts, especially those having no practical reference point. Attention and retention disorders have been mentioned as determining factors for deficient number sense in DS (Nakamura), but this limitation too is perhaps a sign of a deficient conceptual ability. Relational, conceptual, and other internal cognitive operations, involving the manipulation of symbols (where rote memory and motor facility are not major factors), are particularly lacking in DS (Crookshank; Butterfield; Brousseau and Brainerd; Kostrewski; Wallin; Stickland; Bilovsky and Share). Many of the same observations have been made for other clinical syndromes and types of mental retardation so that no special claim

can be made for distinctive conceptual deficiency on the basis of the evidence considered thus far.

(4) An intact or only slightly impaired rote memory facility has often been attributed to DS, although not uniformly so (see Nakamura). Explanations have varied from proposed 'savant' abilities and selective impairment hypotheses, to skill substitutions and compensations through specific training and environmental enrichment. Similar propositions have been advanced to account for the uneven psychometric profiles of the exogenous learning handicapped, aphasics and other 'injury' classes of developmental disorder. Storage facility is, in any case, highly dependent on extent of secondary CNS deterioration in DS as age advances.

(5) Most enduring of the special performance abilities alleged for DS in the psychometric literature is the combined area of psychomotor, visual-motor, eye–hand coordination, grip strength, and motor encoding facilities. These components of mental processing have been viewed as keys to improving intellectual outputs for the syndrome. This optimism is premature. No study has thus far successfully identified or manipulated the numerous variables implicated for general motor development in DS. While the psychometric evidence supports comparatively good visual-motor performance, slower motor speed, good motor strength, superior early self-help skills and efficient motor encoding as compared with other ability areas and with the general motor functioning of non-DS trainable and custodial MR, these data hold most convincingly only for the young DS subject. Results using older subjects (late adolescence and adulthood) are more equivocal.

(6) Findings with DS infants usually support good initial motor potential but rapid erosion of the promise during the first year and beyond. Responsibility for the rapid decline has been attributed to an ongoing hypotonia, delayed myelinization, faulty circulation and the immature cerebellum. Crome, Cowie and Slater (1966) speculated (i) that the reduced size of the brain-stem and cerebellum for DS may relate to low muscle tone and (ii) that an increasing degree of hypotonia could be a major factor in progressively depressing psychomotor performance. Jebsen et al. (1961) classed infantile muscular hypotonia as originating in the central nervous system. Cowie (1970) demonstrated that low motor development scores overlap the main neurological effects and that, together with hypotonia, comprise a common statistical factor particular to DS. The rapid decline for motor development quotients over time and the general 'clumsiness', often attributed to the syndrome, seems inconsistent with psychometric evidence for higher psychomotor than other behavioural indices and with evidence for good proficiency of eye–hand coordination and of general visual-motor functioning

seen on tracing tests, manipulative games and self-help tasks. K. M. Gibson (1972), employing motor training for the treatment of speech disorders in DS, indicated that quality of motor functioning is conditional. General clumsiness and poorly differentiated gross coordination in DS individuals involves mainly the large muscles where the circulatory–nutritional and innervation demands are high in comparison with the small muscle groups engaged for finer visual-motor functioning. Performance for DS holds better on the latter than the former. Brief displays of good muscle strength, on the other hand, might relate to the compacting of skeletal structure – especially in the extremities. In any case, easy fatigue of the large muscles is often mentioned. While gross motor expenditures appear efficient, they are briefly sustained.

Evidence supporting a specific mentation for DS, e.g., differences of behavioural efficiency as among visual-motor, tactile-motor and auditory-motor loops, is incomplete but promising. Other questions raised by the psychometric literature remain unresolved; especially those associated with Brousseau's notion that behavioural handicap in DS is more centrally than peripherally controlled. Issues of mediation and locus of control are the province of the experimental literature.

Special abilities

A potent special abilities stereotype for DS has survived from nineteenth-century clinical mythology. The image includes a general acceptance that musical and rhythmic potential, mimicry, mischief, imitation and memory facility, stubbornness and affectionality, are all characteristic of DS and exclusively so among the mental retardations.

Music and rhythmic activity

A high point on any tour of a large mental retardation institution was the visit to a ward suitably outfitted with a percussion display – drums, tambourines, triangles – manned entirely by DS patients. Some care facilities treated the visitor to DS girls twisting or dancing to recorded music. The view that DS children are particularly adept musically was not shared by Down (1866) who, in apportioning behavioural characteristics to various 'ethnic' classes of idiocy, associated musical responsiveness with the traumatic disorders. Possibly he was impressed by the systematic rocking and other drive qualities of the brain-damaged retardate. Responsibility for the musicality stereotype for DS belongs therefore to Fraser and Mitchell (1876). Other early clinical opinions support this (Shuttleworth, 1895; Sherlock, 1911; Tredgold, 1914).

Elaboration of the notion of special musical abilities for the syndrome belongs with Apert (1914). He invited the use of music for the management of attention disorders, noting the ease with which DS children responded to rhythm. With musical accompaniment they are able, he claimed, to sustain effort over long periods and with appropriate and vigorous motor expression. Shuttleworth and Potts (1916) offered that DS children excel especially in timing, sense of melody and motor expression, when required, for drill and dance. The most enthusiastic supporter of this view was Brushfield (1924) who declared his DS subjects ($N = 177$) 'supersensitive' to musical sounds at all mental ages. They readily imitated tunes by humming them; accurate both for note and timing. The more intelligent acquired songs easily and seemed adept at drilling and other coordinated motor activity. Brousseau and Brainerd (1928) agreed that, despite a number of possible sensory deficiencies in DS, those stimuli having a musical or rhythmic quality were most alerting and attention sustaining. The multiplication of clinical opinion led inevitably to contradictions. Penrose (1933) found in favour of a love of music for DS, but counted many exceptions to the rule. Wallin (1949) acknowledged a fondness for music and 'fairly good' rhythmic sense, claiming that they nevertheless sang poorly and danced awkwardly. Engler (1949) found the more retarded DS patients to be uninterested in music but saw, among his fewer bright cases, an excellent musical facility and for some a liking for dancing; especially the females. Benda (1949) contended that only rhythm was attractive to DS and that a limited hearing discrimination ability would reduce their appreciation of melody. Engler (1949) observed that a few could play a note or two on the piano but that poor finger dexterity precluded any significant skill. Launay and Bayer (1964) recorded the case of a DS youth who had developed a taste for classical music, especially Chopin, Beethoven and Mozart but who showed disdain for popular or experimental music. Rollin (1946) required a group of DS patients to audit dance music, and found none would dance spontaneously. Only a minority could be induced to dance and standards were poor for maintenance of motion to tempo and for quality of coordination. These widely ranging opinions are based mainly on single case reports or those offering no comparisons with other diagnostic classes of mental retardation. Criteria for musicality are unestablished.

Sample-based research on the musical and rhythmic ability of DS dates from Blacketer-Simmonds (1953). Comparing 140 DS and 100 suitable non-DS subjects, a fondness for music could be confirmed for 8 and 7% of DS patients and controls respectively. A more detailed examination employed 42 DS and 42 non-DS controls. They were required to sit through a quick, strong rhythm and a soft, flowing rhythm. Facial expressions, gestures and movements were monitored by an 'expert'. Only 14% of each group exhibited obvious enjoyment, as gauged by facial expression and sustained attention. No preference, for one or other type of music, was shown. Most were apathetic or restless, regardless of the aetiological label they carried. Rhythm was tested by allowing subjects three trials to imitate each of three drum-beat patterns performed by an instructor. An adequate performance was achieved by 43% of the DS patients, whereas 33% of the non-DS controls performed equally as well. The balance, in each group, was described as having no sense of rhythm. A chi-square test of group differences fell below significance levels. Timing sense was tested by requiring subjects to march in line, body bend and so on, to musical accompaniment. Of the DS group, 43% were judged to be good timekeepers, whereas 33% of the controls, achieved the same level. The same subjects scored high on both time and rhythm tests. Only four of the six Down's cases, who had previously registered a pleasurable reaction to music, were also in the positive range for rhythm and timing. Lastly, both groups were encouraged to sing or hum nursery rhymes and popular songs, but no approximation of a melody emerged from the ensuing noise. Blacketer-Simmonds knew of no DS patient able to imitate a tune on a piano, although enthusiastic key-banging was not uncommon. The use of institutional populations for these studies could account for the overall findings as could the rather crude measures employed.

Cantor and Girardeau (1959) required normal and DS subjects to distinguish two different rates of metronome beat, on the assumption that subjects having a superior rhythmic sense would discriminate more easily. The appropriateness of kinesthetic cues was studied by having half of each sample tap with a metronome beat, prior to indicating a discrimination response. Out of 59 DS subjects, 44 usable scores were obtained. Comparison subjects ($N = 24$) were considerably younger and superior for MA (approximately 66 months versus 52 months). Mean IQ levels were 117 and 37 points. Subjects were asked to identify the beat of the hidden metronome as either fast or slow. Number of correct responses, taken over 60 trials, constituted the criterion measure. The DS subjects performed significantly more poorly than normal children. The additional tapping cue did not improve performance for either sample. The authors urged that additional study be undertaken using more precisely MA-matched normals and non-DS retardates.

A similar study of rhythm sense was undertaken by Fitzpatrick (1959) using 20 young adult retardates, half of whom were DS. The tasks included making bilateral folding movements to a metronome beat in order to determine (i) if DS would evidence a superior sense of rhythm, and (ii) whether severely retarded young adults could perform rote work assignments faster with rhythmic background encouragement. Neither sample displayed enhanced output which could be attributed to the intervention of a metronome beat and, indeed, there was a tendency for performance under these conditions to become progressively more erratic regardless of diagnostic grouping. The DS subject in the long run worked less effectively, with metronome pacing, than did the other retardates. Fitzpatrick proposed that the reputation for imitation in DS is originated in the area of socialization to create an unearned impression of companion skills. Otherwise, the inability of DS subjects to perform in time to a metronome is related by Fitzpatrick to difficulties in auditory perception and time interval estimation, which are said to be pronounced for the syndrome.

Differences between the recent experimental and older clinical findings, on the musical ability of DS, are considerable. If DS children suffer less upset of neural integration than do other young severely to moderately retarded, or exhibit a syndrome-specific muscular hyperflexibility attributable to hypotonia, or have some prolongation of the normal imitative facility present in pre-school children then an impression of unique musical and rhythmic skill might easily be sustained. There would be no need to hypothesize about an innate rhythmic or melody sensing talent. The opinion for superior miming and musicality is most insistent for younger DS children. It is possible, too, that the disclaiming studies have not successfully isolated the relevant components of musicality, or that rhythmic sense is not elicited in experimental situations which fail to breach the high auditory thresholds of the syndrome. Finally, a favourable temperament status (affect and impulse qualities), which dispose to a generally cooperative attitude among DS children, is often in contrast with the behavioural and motor inflexibility exhibited by many young brain-damaged imbeciles. Reactions to rhythm and melody are essentially social, the unsophisticated quality of the output of the DS child being cloaked by his enthusiasm. Even the failure of DS children to make articulate sounds to music is often overlooked, a handicap which will be explored later when dealing with language ability.

Ongoing research into musical and rhythmic ability for DS individuals should explore the contribution of mimicry, hypotonia, temperament, social propensity, IQ level and language skill. At this time, the appearance of musicality for some DS children and in some circumstances is probably an artifact of other ability or deficit parameters and tied to developmental staging.

Miming, modelling and memory

Belmont (1971), summarizing a century of opinion concerning the miming quality of DS, found almost universal praise for 'trisomy-21s *joie de vivre*'. The DS child is an adept imitator and his good spirits are infectious – so the argument goes. This most readily accepted behavioural feature of the syndrome has yet to be verified. The literature abounds with amusing accounts of the light-hearted mimicry of DS, ranging from Down's own report of the clever miming of visiting clergymen, to Brousseau's account of playing at physician and telephone operator. They systematically mock the behaviour of anyone with whom they come in contact, said Brousseau. Parents in the process of rearing young children will be reminded of the similarities between these descriptions and the heightened imitative behaviours of normal children especially in group situations where shared fantasy has bred a high degree of camaraderie. Almost all clinical accounts of miming are from institutional sources where DS children are cared for in groups. Institutional regimes have been known to shape display behaviours of inmates to meet public relations needs, the DS patient being a favourite because of his more striking physical stereotype.

The universality of the miming trait was first proposed by Down (1866). He considered the trait to be particular to the syndrome with likely significance for educational management. Brousseau and Brainerd (1928) complained that, unlike the same quality in normal children, miming in DS is superficial, rote, and of little importance for adapting to new behavioural demands. Wood (1909), and later Wallin (1949), denied that any learning advantage could be extracted from the supposed imitative habits of DS children. Tredgold (1949) and Tennies (1943) found no important transfer to social learning situations. Belmont (1971) polarized the debate: the imitation propensity for DS having either a genuine potential for creativity or being merely the manifestation of a rudimentary philominesia. The uniqueness of mimicry to DS was denied by both Tredgold (1914) and Kanner (1957), the former claiming the talent for microcephalics as well. Shuttleworth (1909) compared DS with its 'nearest' aetiological neighbour and reported that cretins do not possess the imitative facility. Shuttleworth had hoped there might be a carry over to basic learning such as writing, drawing and other copying activities.

Statistical tests of a special imitative ability for DS are sparse, except in association with other abilities. Various writers have documented social suggestibility (as a form of imitation) for between 60 and 80% of their samples. Suggestibility, in DS, was viewed by Oster (1953) as superficial and of little importance for training. Blacketer-Simonds (1953) tested mimicry, among other social traits, for DS and comparable non-DS controls. His nurses found a 10% frequency of mimicry for DS and 7% for the MR controls, hardly an impressive spread. Neeman (1971), using the Purdue perceptual-motor survey, has since found 'imitation of movement' to be the only item successfully differentiating DS subjects from other mentally retarded. A thoroughgoing study of imitative behaviour for DS would necessarily include a definition of its operational components and the relation of these components to age, care system, IQ level, rote memory facility, motor expressivity potential and temperament.

Those who have assumed a special talent for mimicry sometimes speculate about origins. Fennell (1904) considered the talent innate or instinctive. Both Crookshank and Down cast mimicry as an atavistic social propensity, claimed also for primitive man. Barr (1904) noted a congruence of imitative skill and memory facility, the miming being possibly heightened by good short-term recall. Oster (1953) related good observation and perceptual ability in DS to the imitative talent. Bilovsky and Share (1965) found self-expression to be more effective for motor than for verbal outputs; motor imitative behaviours being thus sharpened as a compensation for verbal lag. Blessing (1959) attributed the social antics (mimicry) of DS children to attention seeking and to a generally favourable temperament. Perseveration, too, has been identified as a factor and is thought to have some bearing on their taste for repetitive behavioural repertoires. Blacketer-Simmonds (1953) portrayed mimicry in DS as mindless, unoriginal and possibly echopraxic, founded no doubt in some quirk of neuropathology. Sternlicht (1966) saw the copying activity of DS as rudimentary, discrete, motorific in nature (hand waving, clapping, head gestures, facial distortions) and repetitive; much like that found in hyperkinetic or impulse-disordered children. Cornwell and Birch (1969) claimed motor behaviours in DS to be well focussed for the routine self-help items of a socialization scale, suggesting a need for achievement or satisfaction through repetition. Share et al. (1964) proposed a similar link between modelling ability and the success DS children have with specific self-help demands. Or perhaps ritual imitative activity is a security manoeuvre based in inflated needs for affection.

The most frequently mentioned source of imitative behaviour for DS children is maturational. Children between 2 and 4 years of age engage in considerable imitative activity as a device for learning and reducing anxiety, as a form of social interaction preceding suitable competence in speech and conceptual fields, and as a primitive vehicle for emotional experiencing and exploration. Since DS is especially tardy in the development of manipulative speech, the effect might be to prolong a normal MA-related phase of growth, such that gesture imitation serves a substitute communication purpose. It was Benda's (1946) belief that miming among DS individuals is an extension of a normal developmental trait, a function of the prolonged preconceptual cognitive period typical of the syndrome. Gibson's (1966) evidence for an intellectual growth plateau or pause, occurring at between 2 and 3 years of MA, supports this. Many achieve a terminal MA of between 2 and 4 years and might, therefore, exhibit MA-related imitative activity well into physical adulthood.

Most of the foregoing speculation has been derived from institutional sources which enforce uniform behavioural codes for management convenience. Further studies will need to be conducted in family and community settings. At this time, it can be claimed only that DS children exceed other retarded children in general for motor imitation facility. The source of the distinction and whether or not the facility has remedial value is unknown.

Our understanding of memory function for DS is similarly limited. Brousseau and Brainerd (1928) claimed DS subjects to be especially deficient for memory process, 38 of 53 subjects failing the memory test at year III Binet. They linked the deficiency to faulty perception attributable, in turn, to poor attention. Oster (1953) thought that DS individuals enjoy a striking memory for persons and situations but found it strange that only a few could remember a message or a brief number of items for a shopping trip. The contradiction might be understood in modality terms (the demand for visual versus auditory intake and retention) or in terms of the complexity of the abstract cognitive operations involved. Other psychometric studies, for example Stickland, showed memory items (among bright and well-nurtured cases) to survive well into the upper years of mental tests. Nakamura (1965) failed to identify Binet memory items as different for DS and matched mentally retarded controls. Wallin (1944) had claimed a good rote word-calling facility for DS children. Speculation, however, is bound to be fruitless in view of the variety of ages, IQ levels and care variables represented by these few reports. The paucity of experimental work concerning memory process is surprising but what there is serves to point out the complexity of the problem. Sinson and Wetherick (1972) compared DS and other retardates to show a retention deficit for DS subjects in terms of colour but not for shape. Further study (1973) indicated that specific deficit of short-term retention varied with different aspects of sensory information. Another possibility, mentioned by Wilcock and Venables (1968), is that DS subjects are able to employ fewer verbal mediators than other mentally retarded and thus display apparent deficit of short-term recall. Of all the interpretative difficulties, age of subjects is possibly the most important. Dalton, Crapper and Schlotterer (1974) tested short-term visual retention on a delayed matching-to-sample task for DS and matched MR controls across age groups. The older DS group made more errors than the younger DS subjects and the matched non-DS mentally retarded controls. The test was seen as an early indicator of Alzheimer's disease. Given that DS subjects are prone to develop Alzheimer's disease, and some quite early in life, it would be difficult to attribute evidence of storage deficit to the primary amentia. Intensified memory research could prove important for understanding the complexities of mental process for the syndrome; especially since appeals to superior or deficient memory are made to explain so many other real or imagined special abilities.

Stubbornness and affective behaviours

Down (1966) referred to the great obstinancy of 'mongoloids against which they cannot be coerced'. They have been known, he said, to exploit their obstinancy to achieve control of future situations. He assumed the trait to be innate and not subject to easy modification through training. He thought their positive affections to be not so strong. Brousseau and Brainerd (1928) accounted for the smiling response of infant and very young DS children as reflexive; a grimace having little to do with affect. Statistical studies of these two traits are few. Domino *et al.* (1964) and Silverstein (1964) could not vouch for stubbornness as any greater for DS than appropriate controls. Silverstein, and later Domino (1965), found DS to be more cooperative than non-DS retardates.

The age at which evidence is sought could account for their disagreement. Oster (1959) remarked on an increasing obstinancy for DS with age and relegated this to a decline, over time, of 'understanding'. Other age-related data, provided by Wunsch (1957), assigned most aggressive-hostile responses for DS to under 5 years CA and again after age 14 years. Of his sample, 14% only were aggressive-hostile, 51% docile-affective, and the balance neither, clearly. Blessing (1959) declared stubbornness and communication difficulty to comprise two of the major psychological traits of DS (based on teacher ratings), which might set them apart from other causal varieties of retardation. Domino *et al.* (1964) found hostility responses distinguishable between institutional DS patients and controls, but not stubbornness. Silverstein (1964) isolated gregariousness as significantly more common for DS than for controls. Moore *et al.* (1968) categorized close to half of their DS sample as 'aggressive'. These cases were in the adult range and had been institutionalized for some time. Like the clinical literature, the statistical studies do not persuasively identify stubbornness or its opposite as peculiar to the syndrome or as especially common.

Regardless of a general failure to isolate given affective states as representative of DS individuals, there have been numerous exercises to explain the origins of their stubbornness and affectional qualities. A mechanistic hypothesis was offered by Benda (1960) who assigned stubbornness in DS to 'inflexibility of intentions'. Volitional inflexibility was thought to be related to an inability to make easy perceptual shifts, a form of intellectual rigidity most obvious in new situations. He proposed that the central subcortical organs (governing basic emotional responsiveness) are relatively intact, whereas the so-called 'long circuiting system of the cortex, serving the evaluation of sensory stimuli and responses, and therefore, intelligent interaction with the environment, remains immature and underdeveloped' (p. 68). Sternlicht (1966) also viewed stubbornness, in DS, as a defence reaction against inherent cognitive inflexibility, or as a failure of the CNS to form adequate response sets; presumably resulting in obstinacy. Impulsivity has been singled out by some writers as basic to understanding the interactive nature of the imitative-stubbornness-affect triad. Rollin (1946) believed that a number of behavioural traits for DS have a common origin in less refined but essentially intact 'primitive modes of reaction'. The rudimentary or uninhibited quality is explained by a less mature (but essen-- tially undamaged) neurology and by the failure of custodial settings to offer active training. Hallenbeck (1960) extended the point beyond groups of behavioural traits to argue for the more uncomplicated expression of innate temperamental topologies in DS, allegedly related to somatotype sorting as a function of aberrant karyotype. In this regard, negativism was observed by Gibson and Pozsonyi (1965) to occur more frequently among trisomy than translocation Down's. Later data presented by Johnson and Abelson (1969) is not in agreement.

Neuropathological and psychiatric concepts of personality have been engaged to explain the assumed stubbornness and affectionality of DS. Many of Menolascino's recalcitrant or impulse disordered cases were identified as chronic brain syndrome; the result of a progressive secondary neuropathology said to be common among adolescent and young adult DS patients. Longitudinal investigations of stubbornness, hostility, perseveration and inflexibility, as correlates of neurological status, would be of value. A few studies, e.g., Cassel (1953), have shown progressive neurological defect to be clinically obvious as early as 7 years CA. Other studies, evaluated in the preceding chapters, found frequency for dysrhythmia (including organic irritability and negative behavioural response) as among the concomitants of declining neurophysiological status for DS. Rollin (1946) appealed to innate personality factors as an explanation for the occurrence of catatonia, regarding catatonia to be promoted by the characteristic retreat responses (stubbornness) of many DS individuals.

Developmental hypotheses have been advanced by Ellis and Beechley (1950), Benda (1960) and Menolascino (1967) to explain both stubbornness and affectionality in DS. Menolascino likened the behaviour of his hyperactive and aggressive chronic brain syndrome DS patients to the 'terrible twos' of the normal child, implicating the maturational prolongation of certain of the early growth states of the syndrome. Ellis and Beechley, like Benda, have reasoned that the lower brain centres, governing emotional responsiveness, appear less impaired for DS than for other causal varieties of middle-level MR. Rudimentary but otherwise intact approach and avoidance responses would be more visible for DS. These comparatively unmodified forms of affect, retreat and drive behaviours might survive as primitive expressions for a longer period in the developmental sequence and might also be less susceptible to modification through training because of a reduced cognitive and sensory potential. The difficulty experienced by many DS individuals in evaluating sensory inputs, because of either cortical or peripheral shortcomings, has been mentioned by Benda (1956) as a source of retreat and stubbornness.

Less pretentious explanations are available. Down's individuals, along with other mentally retarded, employ various protective devices when faced with cognitive demands they cannot meet. Stubbornness and attention-seeking are two such strategies. Children with DS might be especially susceptible to the use of these mechanisms because we tend to over-evaluate their capacity; misled by an often attractive temperament, by exhibitions of motor mimicry, and by good early habit development. The result can be an unrealistic and threatening intellectual expectation and a correspondingly disappointing delivery. Communication difficulty, identified as a more serious problem for DS than for most other MA-equivalent causal groups of MR, provides still another interpretation of the retreat and affection-seeking attributes of the syndrome. Johnson and Abelson (1969), asserted that the inability to make themselves understood was the most noteworthy handicap of the almost 3000 DS patients in their series, when compared with over 20000 non-DS mentally retarded. Stubbornness, as a defence reaction, might be a major consequence of communication frustration. Blessing (1959) found stubbornness and difficulty in communication to rate highest from among a variety of traits considered by teachers to be most characteristic of the condition. Even the easy fatigue, linked in part to respiratory and circulatory difficulty, has been mentioned as a source of precipitous recoil into stubbornness. The physical limits of DS are easily exceeded, even under routine performance demands.

In summary, explanations for stubbornness and affectionality in DS have included perceptual and motivational inflexibility resulting from a discrepancy between intact lower centres (governing affect) and immature cortical functions which serve ordinarily to modify affective behaviours. Poorly established or limited sensory equipment has been implicated as an arm of the same argument. Impulsivity and the operation of primitive modes of emotional expression (as a result of damage) have been offered by others as antecedents of affectional reactivity and stubbornness in the syndrome. Unique qualities of temperament, governed by the nature of the chromosome aberration, have been mentioned in respect to both the innate and the damage view of mediation. Growing stubbornness, with advancing age, is thought to be coincidental with progressive neurological deterioration, accompanied frequently by irritability, growing impulsivity, and attention deficit. Psychological explanations have included an unfortunate temptation to over-evaluate the cognitive capacity of DS children based on their comparatively appealing emotional and motor modelling responses. The DS child compensates, in turn, with either retreat into stubbornness or with over-developed dependency. The cycle of defence and compensation can be intensified by the growing communication, sensory, and cognitive limitations of the syndrome as age and demand increases. The interplay of these various background factors should be enough to account for the manifestations of stubbornness and friendliness in many cases of DS. The psychological result might be considered syndrome-specific but probably only in a secondary sense. However complex and uncertain the origins, the phenomena are probably exploitable for management purposes.

8

Learning and arousal

The laboratory study of behaviour for Down's syndrome began in 1904 with Kuhlmann but gained little ground during the ensuing half-century of clinical and psychometric emphases. The period was essentially one of hypothesis generation. By the mid-1950s, academic psychology had developed major theoretical positions and appropriate instrumentation for the experimental study of learning, perception and motivation in normal subjects. The elaboration of these models for subnormal subjects and children soon followed. The assumption was that mental retardates are a homogeneous group predicted to occupy the lower end of the continuum for attention, discrimination, reactivity and storage facility. The findings were often contradictory because the major causal categories of mental retardation are not behaviourally similar at given mental ages. Nor was there much attempt to understand the physiological sub-strata of the manipulated behaviours or to validate laboratory findings in the arena of remedial services. The most recent experimental work using DS individuals is corrective to the degree that specific causal groups of MR subjects are compared with one another, or with normal controls, and peripheral physiological and CNS states are controlled and manipulated against behavioural outcomes. There is even now extrapolation from research to issues of practice. The studies to be considered in the present section have most of these qualities.

Fehr (1976) offers three reasons for the anchoring of behavioural studies of MR to psychophysiological events. These are that (i) physiological responses are reasonable indicators of environmental effects, especially where there is serious verbal or motor impairment, (ii) peripheral physiological activity may serve as interoceptive stimuli influencing environmental transactions, to the extent that these stimuli feed back to the CNS, and (iii) autonomic system activity might be subject to principles which differ from those governing the traditional exteroceptive stimulus approach to understanding and aiding the adjustment of the retarded. The general thinking is that spontaneous fluctuations of autonomic system responses are related to cortical activity and skeletal-motor functions. Thus, autonomically labile subjects have faster reaction time and greater impulsivity. At the extremes, they are more hyperactive. An optimal lability of autonomic states contribute to alertness and attention appropriate to environmental demand insofar as spontaneous fluctuations of peripheral physiological response systems act as energizers of CNS activity. It is Fehr's suggestion that if these spontaneous fluctuations of the autonomic nervous system (ANS) can be manipulated then discrimination response capacity is likely to be improved.

Discrimination potential in DS is obviously complex, requiring some understanding of reaction time, attention, distraction and drive states. The identification of cognitive and drive facility for the syndrome might enlarge our understanding of the sequence of events beginning with the aberrant chromosome and ending with the problems of remediation and habilitation.

Reaction time

Previous clinical opinion (Rollin, 1946) held that DS subjects, often impulsive responders, would show comparatively fast reaction times (RTs). Others, considering the hypotonia and immature sensory apparatus of the syndrome, have supposed that RTs would be comparatively delayed. Reaction time differences related to aetiology, across the mental retardations, were first described by Berkson (1960). His study serves to illustrate the difficulties to be faced by all later studies. Two groups of Berkson's five are of interest, the DS ($N = 12$, mean IQ 31 points) and the undifferentiated subnormal ($N = 12$, mean IQ 38 points). The IQ scores were taken from case history records but there is no indication of the age when testing took place; a particularly difficult sampling problem when dealing with eroding IQ levels. The DS sample was significantly older than the 'severely subnormal group' (21.7 versus 18.7 years), less retarded (including retrospectively), and had been in hospital longer. Four simple and complex visual RT tasks were used, e.g. when facing five lights to lift a hand and press a button for whichever light appeared. The DS cases performed more slowly on all tasks, compared with the other groups and when incorporated as half of seven matched pairs (for CA, length of hospitalization and IQ). The significant groups-by-tasks interactions suggested that DS is particularly deficient for complex motor outputs. Belmont (1971) interpreted these results as indicating a deficiency of visual-motor performance, over other comparable mentally retarded, and increasingly so as the motor complexity of the tasks increases. An alternate conclusion would be that the RT difference is due to a hypotonic musculature, and to the accumulating effects of secondary neuropathology in older DS subjects.

The extent of the influence of hypotonia on RT was shown by O'Connor and Berkson (1963) who manipulated direction of attention and eye movement. They anticipated that fluctuation in attention (based on eye movement indices) might vary with intelligence level, complexity of stimuli and across aetiological class. Lateral eye movements to static and changing visual displays were recorded for DS adults, non-DS controls (mean IQ 32 points) and normals. The DS subjects made more eye movements under all conditions. Among the explanations offered was that 'hypotonus might prevent more controlled movements of the eyes' and therefore contribute to faulty attention and slower RTs. O'Connor and Hermelin (1961) had previously suggested that stereognostic and galvanic skin response (GSR) differences, between DS and other retardates, could also be attributed to hypotonus. Cerebellar damage or arrest and faulty circulatory system functioning were seen as underlying the hypotonia. Hermelin (1964) later compared a brighter DS sample (mean IQ 42 points) with MR controls matched for CA and IQ. The RT tasks engaged two modalities (vision and hearing). The results were of faster RTs for DS on the visual signals and when the warning signal was of a different modality than the RT signal. Otherwise, findings were for a slower overall RT for the syndrome; an indication that direction of findings are bound up with the receptive–expressive channels and by the nature of the stimulus conditions.

Astrup, Sersen and Wortis (1967) applied factor and multiple regression analysis to a variety of motor reflexive items. They found DS subjects to have higher loadings for motor retardation than did the undifferentiated and encephalopathic MR groups. Further analysis (using MA-matched controls) produced no significant RT differences, emphasizing again the need to separate the effects of hypotonia from the more complex input–output variables associated with reaction time. High weightings for DS were related to poor verbal facility and to a 'poor concentration of excitatory and inhibitory process' (p. 310) with resulting poor motor reflexes. Astrup et al. were of the opinion that larger samples would have shown DS to have longer RTs than other mentally retarded.

Clausen's (1968) study of RT to visual displays, for DS and controls, imputes mental age differences as relevant to outcomes. A representative task was the naming of familiar objects exposed tachistoscopically for 2 seconds. These tasks combined elements of perceptual and verbal speed and sensory function. Clausen considered the RT distribution to be a function of IQ, aetiology, and CA. These data, together with other auditory and perceptual speed findings, led Clausen to conclude that cross-aetiological comparisons might prove DS to be more impaired for some combinations of sensory function and perceptual speed than non-DS retarded. However, 'It is possible that we are dealing with a basic visual impairment which may be peripheral in nature.' Reaction time differences between aetiological classes of MR dissipated when samples were matched for age.

Hermelin and Venables (1964) tested RT for normals, DS and non-DS mentally retarded as part of an examination of the activation theory tenet that RT is faster if subjects are pre-alerted. Mean RTs, across six forewarning intervals, were approximately 700 milliseconds for DS and 400 milliseconds for non-DS controls. Since the longest RTs were achieved by DS subjects, in combination with maximal sensory activity (evident in alpha blocking), the authors concluded that a tardy task-related 'development of motor set' could be responsible. The mixing of modalities for forewarning (visual), and the RT task signals (auditory), could also be a factor if there is merit in the previous suggestion that DS exhibits a special disability of auditory-motor circuiting. However, the slower RTs for DS might be entirely a function of the five point mean IQ advantage of the non-DS controls and of the small sample ($N = 6$) employed. The O'Connor and Hermelin (1963) interpretation, in favour of simple motor speed differences, is of interest. They cite evidence that lowered muscular tension is associated with longer RTs and that hypotonia in DS would result in poor muscle tension and correspondingly slower reactivity. Their proposed connection between quality of motor skill and muscle tone for DS is not new (Cassell, 1949; Pertego, 1950; Kirman, 1951). Crome, Cowie and Slater (1966) subsequently related poor muscle tone to cerebellum involvement in DS, a phenomenon not particularly evident for other forms of mental retardation.

Knights, Atkinson and Hyman (1967) isolated the components of reactivity as comprehension of instructions, conceptualization, and basic motor functioning during tasks. DS subjects and non-DS controls were required to perform on a variety of size, texture, weight, kinaesthetic, and visual-motor discrimination problems. Many more DS than non-DS subjects failed to complete the requirements, despite careful IQ and CA matching. Those who did complete were older and brighter. Down's subjects who reached task criteria performed as well as non-DS subjects, there being little evidence of inordinate motor inferiority in either group. Knights et al. reported that a discrimination demanding the manipulation of concepts, such as 'rougher than' or 'bigger than', were more often beyond the intellectual grasp of DS subjects than MA matched controls. An interesting tactic (introduced during the second part of their study) involved excision of the conceptual-discriminative aspects of the tasks, exposing just the motor component. The motor performance requirements included maze coordination, hand steadiness, dynamometer performance, pegboard, tapping and RT tasks. Statistical findings were for no significant differences between DS subjects and controls on isolated motor skill performance and for no evidence of the special effects of hypotonia. The direction of the RT results, while not significant, supported Berkson's (1960) finding that DS is slower for RT than are other MR subjects at similar developmental levels. Their DS group performed less effectively on steadiness and dynamometer tests, than on the pegboard tests, indicating a possible drive component which might differ across aetiological classifications.

Wallace and Fehr (1970) identified slower RTs for DS (under baseline and distraction conditions and against normal controls), using measures related to motor-impulsivity and general skeletal-motor functioning. These differences can also be understood in terms of the auditory stimulus used insofar as Down's is claimed to have a particular auditory sequencing handicap. The significantly longer RT latency period for DS, under both baseline and distraction conditions, reinforces a mechanical or peripheral explanation for the findings. Straumanis, Shagass and Overton (1973) have offered support for a conduction pathway deficiency explanation for slow RT in the syndrome which would be more parsimonious than an exteroceptive model involving attention and distraction. The low IQ level of some DS subjects (as low as 5 points) poses the additional difficulty that purely reflexive activity is being measured, much of which would be incidental to the autonomic system lability hypothesis under consideration.

The major investigations have, in the main, agreed that reactivity is usually slower for DS than for other retardates but differ on interpretation. Berkson (1960), O'Connor and Berkson (1963), Astrup et al. (1967), and Hermelin and Venables (1964) make a case for cerebellar originated hypotonia as specific to prolonged latency of response for the syndrome. Despite the generally known connection between motor skill and muscle tone, Knights et al. (1967) found no special deficiency of motor function for DS, arguing instead for the role of conceptual handicap. Peripheral physiological explanations were offered by Berkson (1960), Hermelin (1964), Hermelin and Venables (1964), and Clausen (1968). These writers proposed that sensory and perceptual handicap or auditory-motor circuiting difficulty is more evident for DS than for other forms of mental retardation. Hermelin and Venables (1964), Knights et al. (1967) and Wallace and Fehr (1970) offered that arousal thresholds, the development of motor set, drive potentials and motor impulsivity differences contribute to variability of RT both within DS and between clinical conditions. To establish slower reactivity as a reliable, syndrome-specific phenomenon will require a better understanding of the various cognitive properties (attention and discrimination), drive potential (impulsivity, distraction and arousal phenomena) and intake–output circuitry of the syndrome. The latter would include the role of imbalanced sensory thresholds by modality, the effects of hypotonus, the influence of lability of peripheral physiology and a number of purely mechanical considerations. The task is doubly difficult because each of these classes of mediational events covary with maturation. The objective of future research would be to (i) chart characteristic reaction times developmentally and to isolate and manipulate the dozen or so suggested antecedents under various stimulus conditions and (ii) to determine if the modification of precursor and signal conditions leads to improvement of reactivity for the disorder.

Attention and distraction

The most venturesome pre-experimental opinion belongs to Brousseau and Brainerd (1928). They proposed that attention disorder is a 'noticeable peculiarity' of DS and that the more severely retarded among them lack even the non-voluntary or spontaneous types of attention; while showing no defect of the sensory organs. For the brighter and more mature, attention was said to be of short duration. Attention failure was most evident on psychometric subtests where sustained effort was not elicited, even by novelty or surprise. One exception was that musical sounds proved capable of sustaining greater attention. Retention and recall were 'noticeably deficient' as well. Brousseau collected psychometric data for 53 cases over 5 years of age. Of these, 38 failed on the year III Binet memory tests and three only passed the memory items at year IV. The normal child at 3 or 4 years compared favourably with DS at 9 or 10 years of age. The discrepancy for memory function was attributed to defective perception which could be traced to attention deficit. Alternative psychometric hypotheses are that limited comprehension and the adequacy of peripheral input–output capacities, are related to the quality of attention. Penrose and Smith (1966), considering Brousseau's memory defect hypothesis, proposed that DS subjects cannot make discriminations between weights of similar size and shape merely because they do not comprehend instructions. It might be that simple.

A high frequency of distractability and impulsivity, for DS, especially as age increases, is widely accepted. Yet Belmont (1971), evaluating the experimental literature, found that attention span deficit is among the most intensely debated of the behavioural artifacts of DS. He interpreted McCord's (1956) findings that 45% of DS subjects could not be hypnotized, because of presumed impulse control (attention) problems, as suggestive. Uncooperativeness, hyperactivity and negativism, all seen in formal task situations and expressed as attention disorder, have been observed in between 25 and 85% of DS cases; depending on IQ level, CA, care situation, medical history and sex status. Recent investigations have centred, in particular, on attention related to discrimination performance.

Girardeau (1959) tested discrimination differences between Down's and MA-matched normal children and found, not surprisingly, that normals performed significantly better. The DS children were less attentive to the task and more frequently distracted. A quite dissimilar task situation, involving interest generalization, led Martin and Blum (1961) also to assign their cross-aetiology differences to an attention disorder particular to the DS sample. Berkson, Hermelin and O'Connor (1961) pursued an excitation explanation of the differences. They tested the physiological responses of DS and other retardates to repeated stimuli by requiring experienced care staff to rate subjects for 'excitability' as a possible correlate of distractibility. The resulting scores did not differentiate the two older groups statistically, although the tendency was toward lower mean excitability scores for the DS cases (72 versus 81 points). Age differences across samples and the various ways distraction is defined for experimental purposes might tend to explain uncertain findings.

A provocative test of a number of distractibility parameters for DS and other imbeciles was undertaken by Brown and Clarke (1963). They employed adults at barely trainable IQ levels (27 points plus or minus 7.7 points for 14 DS subjects and 28.9 points plus or minus 6.1 points for 14 TMR controls). Their study was prompted by a pilot project which had indicated that distractibility differences, among the retarded, might be aetiologically specific. The task comprised the naming of serially displayed common objects. The distraction, when applied, was presented through a head set (uncoordinated naming of 'meaningful' task objects and non-meaningful nonsense syllables) while the task was performed. The DS group made significantly fewer errors under meaningful distraction than other imbeciles and performed, in fact, within the range of the much brighter 'subnormal' group. The DS sample, however, took longer to complete the task than the brighter group and in this respect were like the non-DS imbeciles. These findings generally run counter to those of other investigations that have contended for a particular auditory-motor deficiency in DS manifest as distractibility and attention disorder. Zekulin, Gibson, Mosley and Brown (1974) reported a greater susceptibility of the auditory modality to distraction in DS subjects compared with non-DS retardates. Miezejesk (1974) found that white noise distraction (a visual reaction time task) was more pronounced for DS subjects than familials. Belmont (1971) faulted the Brown and Clarke findings for inappropriate design, recommending instead a mixed analysis of variance for repeated measures. Brown (1976) has replied that:

While noting that we found differences in terms of errors under meaningful auditory stimulation (labelled distraction in the experiment), Belmont goes on to suggest that our analysis of variance is inappropriate. He also suggests that most of our subjects made zero errors or one error out of a possible twenty. In actual fact the meaningful distraction scores of the mongoloid group for three trials lay between five and seven scores. It is true that the mongoloid group and the subnormal group of rather high intelligence made mean error scores lying between one and three, and therefore the majority of subjects made more than one error. It is also true that distributions were highly skewed. Although a correction was made, some authorities would argue that non-parametric statistics would have been advisable to the techniques we employed. Had we employed other techniques (and in particular non-parametric statistics) the results would have been quite similar to those obtained. It is admitted that we were surprised at the difference obtained between mongoloid and non-mongoloid subjects of similar IQ. We would agree that a larger sample replication study is desirable. Further, Belmont compares our study with that of Fisher (1970) and seems to stand by Fisher's argument that there are no differences in distractibility between mongoloids and non-mongoloid subjects of similar intelligence levels. Although agreeing that further evidence is required in order to substantiate our hypothesis, a comparison with Fisher's experiment is absurd. There is no reason to suspect a common factor of distractibility within any particular population. Indeed, the available evidence suggests that a variety of variables, including the nature of the extraneous stimulation, the tasks being presented, the amount of previous learning, and the specific input–output difficulties of the subjects of concern are likely to influence the degree of distractibility. Fisher's experiment is fundamentally different from ours and indeed without questioning his results, differences of this type may be due to some or all of the foregoing variables.

Fisher (1970) examined attention deficit in brain-damaged children, including DS. The attention subtests selected included elements of impulse control, incidental learning, set change, contextual cue distraction, visual concentration and vigilance, and auditory vigilance demands. The sample comprised 31 DS subjects below IQ 50 points and 31 non-DS retarded (CA 8 years for both). The controls were almost 4 mean IQ points superior to the DS sample. The DS and non-DS subjects showed similar patterns of attention deficit. There was 'a trend toward fewer attention deficits with increasing IQ' (p. 507). The study is essentially a comparison of two causally distinct TMR groups against 'norms' rather than with each other, a procedure which might obscure cross-aetiological distinctions of a qualitative sort.

The foregoing studies support previous clinical opinion that DS subjects are about as distractible as other MR groups of similar IQ. Where there is disagreement, sample ages and the diagnostic composition of the control groups appear to be important. Distractibility among the mentally retarded has been associated with low IQ and age, personality status (impulse styles), conceptual limitations, the extent and type of neuropathology (progressive or not), training opportunities and physiological or psychological drive levels. To the extent that these differ among causally distinct groups of the mentally retarded then presumably so will distractibility levels under various circumstances. A more precise delimitation of the biological and stimulus components of distraction would need to be made in order to establish syndromic differences and appropriate remediation techniques.

Discrimination

The largest single body of behavioural research into DS is centred on problems of discrimination. These include the significance of modality, sensorimotor circuiting, stimulus differentiation and generalization, visual stimulus complexity and conditionability facility in respect to cognition. The burden of the discrimination research is on which input and output capacity differences, frequently noted in the psychometric studies, are real and if they originate principally in the CNS or the peripheral systems. The relevant studies will be considered in the light of their limitations and compatibility.

Gordon (1944) was first to contend that DS differs from MA matched normals in the execution of tactile discrimination tasks. DS children appeared to be inferior for stereognostic discrimination but equal for visual discrimination. Belmont (1971), employing a mixed analysis of variance for repeated measures, found instead that DS was 'uniformly inferior' across size, form, patterning and texture-type tasks and that selected modality was not important. Girardeau (1959) presented a discrimination problem requiring the matching of two series of five wooden forms (with appropriate token rewards) for ten normals and ten DS subjects comparable for MA. Mean IQ scores were 39 and 116 points respectively. Measures were taken for trials required to reach criterion performance. Stimulus differences involved form, size and colour. The MA-matched normals performed significantly better, presumably because equivalent MA levels for the two samples represent different intellectual qualities. Girardeau had attributed inferior discrimination for DS to attention deficit which was linked to degree of mental defect rather than assuming any syndrome-specific cognitive deficit. Rudel (1960) proposed differences between DS and brain-damaged subjects for discrimination performance and generalization, but these results defy cross-aetiological interpretation in view of the reported mean IQ difference of 45 points between the DS subjects and controls. Gramza and Witt (1969) and Gramza *et al.* (1969) compared normal and pre-school DS children on response to coloured block presentations. The DS children were inferior to the normal children. Responses for DS subjects ranged from non-structured patterning (throwing and scattering) to simple linear and vertical stacking. There was no evidence of discrimination activity based on colour use. Conclusions for poorer comprehension, motor output or perceptual discrimination are not possible because the normal children were between 4 and 5 years of age while the Down's subjects averaged less than 3 years MA.

Other tests of syndrome-specificity for discrimination and generalization deficit in DS have employed non-DS retardates as controls, to better effect. Martin and Blum (1961) compared institutional DS and familial retardates with normals using an oddity learning task, followed by a choice task. Generalization could be anticipated from first to second session. The first series included three triangles, the oddity features being size, colour, form and spatial orientation. Significant performance differences between causal groups disappeared when adjusted for mean differences in MA; although performance success was not appropriate to MA for the DS sample. The generalization of learning set from tasks I to II was assessed by providing a choice of the middle size of three objects. The inferior performance of DS subjects was explained as an attention deficit in preference to postulating any unique learning deficiency. Failure to equate familial and DS retardates more closely for IQ level (30 versus 52 points), and for age, would account for the findings; a criticism which has been made by Prysiazniuk and Wicijowski (1964). The latter investigators used essentially the same oddity discrimination problem as had Martin and Blum, taking care to match DS subjects with undifferentiated TMR controls for CA, MA and IQ (30 and 33 points respectively). The initial learning trials did not distinguish the groups. Subsequent tests of learning provided no evidence of spread of discrimination achievement, to criterion, or of differences between aetiological groups. Possibly, the MA levels were too low to demonstrate discrimination generalization ability in either sample.

Sersen, Astrup, Floistad and Wortis (1970) conducted a somewhat similar study within a Luria–Pevzner framework using DS subjects of good mean IQ (47 points) and optimal pre-deteriorative CA (4–13 years). Motor coordination and word association procedures were used for DS, encephalopathic and undifferentiated MR groups and normals. Conditioned responses were keyed to red and yellow lights, as negative and positive reflex conditions, and then reversed. The word association task (verbal functioning) was a test of the 'second-signal system'. While the degree of support for the Russian view is limited, the syndromic effects are of interest. No group-by-MA interactions were significant for the motor conditioning task. The largest number of significant performance differences appeared for the DS-normal comparisons. DS subjects differed from the encephalopathic group for RTs in some conditions, a phenomenon attributed to deficits of internal inhibition. Both the DS and encephalopathic subjects showed increased RTs to the stimulus which was initially positive while the DS subjects exhibited a delay in response to the stimulus which had been reversed in valence. Word association performance differences were not distributed syndromically, there being only a decline of primitive reponses with MA across groups; a kind of verbal facility index unrelated to motor conditionability or ease of adaptation to conditioned reversals.

The inhibitory deficit hypothesis was further examined by Zekulin, Gibson, Mosley and Brown (1974) using a peg placement task interspersed with auditory and visual distraction, both patterned and unpatterned. There was some support for a greater susceptibility of the auditory modality to distraction (either patterned or non-patterned) in that performance under the auditory non-patterned condition, relative to the no extraneous stimulation conditions, was significantly depressed. Such was not the case for the non-DS retarded and non-retarded control groups. Perhaps the DS subjects were slower to habituate to the auditory non-patterned extraneous stimulation (white noise at 80 dB) and, therefore, attended more to a distracting stimulus to the detriment of the motor task. Differences in pattern of performance between groups is shown in Fig. 7. Alternatively, DS subjects might have a higher initial arousal level and be more susceptible to conflicting stimulus conditions (Miezejeski, 1974). Whatever the source, the speed at which reactive inhibition builds and dissipates is apparently different for DS over other MR samples. McDonald and MacKay (1974) examined the effects of proximal and distal proactive interference on recall with DS, epileptics and undifferentiated MR subjects. A signal, preceding a digit message for recall, was varied by position, tone and loudness. The DS subjects were more vulnerable under all conditions.

O'Connor and Hermelin (1961) favoured Gordon's contention that DS exhibits particular discrimination strengths and weaknesses depending on the modality channel or input–output circuit chosen. Institutionalized DS and non-DS TMR were matched for mean IQ (38 points) and CA (24 years). Normal child and adult samples were engaged for comparison. Discrimination tasks included the presentation of five previously familiarized shapes, followed by five new shapes, randomly interspersed. Subjects were required to identify the new shapes from among the collage and within the experi-

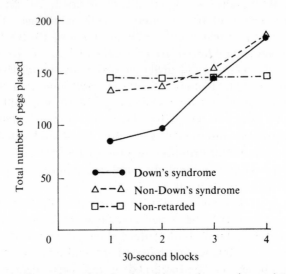

Fig. 7. The total number of pegs placed by each experimental group for each 30-second block across all experimental conditions. (From X. Y. Zekulin, D. Gibson, J. L. Mosley and R. I. Brown (1964). *American Journal of Mental Deficiency*, **78**, 575.)

mental context of either the visual or stereognostic (shape and tactile qualities) modality. Non-DS subjects were superior for tactile-shape recognition and DS subjects for visual-shape recognition. The authors cautioned that 'Whether peripheral insensitivity, faulty nerve conduction, or central impairment are responsible for such observations and findings will have to be determined by further research' (p. 65). They speculated, in part from animal studies, that ablation of the posterior parietal lobule (areas 5 and 7) could deplete stereognosis, and that a major anatomical factor in DS is the small cerebellum; which is implicated, in turn, with the organization of movement and is perhaps a main contributor to the hypotonia said to be characteristic of the condition. They challenged programme specialists to determine if muscle tone and stereognostic facility could be improved by training.

Elaboration of O'Connor and Hermelin's interpretation has been offered by O'Connor and Berkson (1963) who used a visual discrimination display involving a variety of tasks differing for complexity and monitored for eye movement. The argument that inferior discrimination performance in DS, over comparable non-DS subjects, might be assigned to attention deficit, was supported in the sense that DS evidenced more lateral eye movement under all conditions. They claimed that 'hypotonus might prevent more controlled movements of the eyes' thereby obscuring the distinction between visual discrimination and motor variables. O'Connor and Hermelin (1960) had previously affirmed that the shape-tactile disadvantage for DS subjects, compared with other imbeciles, can be attributed to inhibition and hypotonia rather than to differences in cognitive style or capacity to comprehend. Corroboration, in part, is offered by Kennedy and Sheridan (1973). They compared DS, brain-damaged and normal subjects of similar CA on a shape matching task using a visual and tactile channel. The DS group performed at chance difference levels for all conditions except the visual-to-visual matching where mean achievement was 97%. Sidman, Cresson and Willson-Morris (1974) sought practical application for the apparent visual processing advantage in DS. They required subjects to match through mediated transfer, using one auditory (A) and two visual (B and C) sets. Although the B–A and C–B matching was taught, visual to auditory matching was acquired without being taught directly. Their study suggests that elementary reading (instructed by matching via mediated transfer) should be programmed consistent with the modality strengths and weaknesses of the syndrome. It is undecided though if visual feedback capacity at a practical learning level, is superior to other classes of MR. Jackson (1974) presented three-letter words orally to DS and other retarded children, requiring them to match with the printed word. The DS subjects did no better in making this discriminate association than the others. Sample age and the storage requirements of the task are critical factors. Dalton, Crapper and Schlotterer (1974) tested short term visual retention on a delayed matching task with results indicating that older DS subjects make more errors than younger DS and other MR controls. Memory erosion, associated eventually with Alzheimer's disease, appears early for the syndrome and provides a confound of some consequence when testing discrimination and sensorimotor processing hypotheses. Another major confound was noted by Walthi, Salvisber and Auf der Maur (1973) who, while reporting poorer auditory memory for DS over other MR subjects, employed a task which required vocal response.

More careful scrutiny of the tactile discrimination facility, claimed to be comparatively poor for DS subjects over other categories of MR, was undertaken by Knights and his colleagues (Knights, Hyman and Wozny, 1965; Knights, Atkinson and Hyman, 1967). The first of the two studies avoided the issue of capacity and threshold difference (a problem faced by Prysiazniuk and Wicijowski) by pre-selecting only subjects who could correctly place eight blocks on a time-limited formboard task. Subjects were blindfolded and required to perform with the dominant and non-dominant hand. Comparison groups included 18 DS subjects (IQ 40 points, CA 12 years), nine brain-injured subjects (IQ 58 points, CA 14 years), and nine cultural–familial subjects (IQ 59 points, CA 11 years). Of the 18 DS individuals, only four could work to criterion. While the authors did not pursue these results statistically, they concluded that within the IQ range of 40 to 59 points DS appears to have a tactile discrimination deficit larger than can be reasonably expected on the basis of IQ alone. The DS sample also experienced particular difficulty interpreting their tactual-kinaesthetic sensations.

In the interest of clarification, Knights et al. (1969) developed a two-step test of tactual and kinaesthetic discrimination capacity for DS against a cultural–familial control sample. The first step engaged texture, size, weight, kinaesthetic and visual–tactile discrimination skills. The second step removed the conceptual-discrimination component of these demands leaving a battery of simple motor tasks. Their intention was to separate the effects of comprehension from those related to hypotonia (i.e., as indicated by level of motor proficiency). On the discrimination tasks, many more DS than non-DS subjects failed to complete and those who did were both older and brighter. Indications were that, despite MA matching to control samples, DS does not have equivalent comprehension or conceptual reach. The psychometric scatter evidence evaluated earlier tends also to indicate that DS subjects score relatively better for concrete demands, manipulative tasks, self-care sub-tests and on some repetitive and memory items, than they do for conceptual and verbal content. While qualitative disparities, inherent in MA-matching across MR causal categories, are common enough, Knights et al. are nevertheless impressed by the slight tendency for visual–tactual discrimination to be better for DS. Similar observations had been made by Gordon (1944) and Nakamura (1965). The strictly motor-based tasks, employed by Knights et al. (using DS and non-DS retardates with a mean CA of 14 years) yielded maze coordination, hand steadiness, pegboard, tapping, reaction time and dynamometer scores. No differences were statistically significant, although the direction of results favoured lower DS ratings for steadiness and dynamometer performance. Muscle strength, when coordination skill was not involved, seemed comparatively good. There is little suggestion here that hypotonia in DS is accounting for discrimination performance differences between DS subjects and controls.

Separating the motor component from conceptual tasks is a complex problem. Frith and Frith (1974) set DS, normal and severely subnormal subjects a simple pursuit rotor and finger tapping task. The DS subjects showed no improvement after a 5-minute rest whereas the two comparison groups made significant gains. Since mental development and initial task criterion were identical for all groups, some form of feedback or cumulative motor circuiting difficulty appears to be involved. An undifferentiated motor output hypothesis is apparently inadequate to explain discrimination performance differences across groups. An interesting implication of the Frith and Frith report is that because DS children have motor difficulty, as a result of an inability to evoke or express motor sequences, they compensate by dependence on immediate visual and kinaesthetic feedback. An additional suggestion is that the visual-motor loop superiority for DS is partly learned and could be further promoted by employing a training regime based on exaggerated feedback. Otherwise, comparative motor status for DS in any given study appears to depend on the composition of the control group.

The importance of control sample make-up, for data interpretation, is more precisely illustrated by Sackett (1967). He engaged DS, post-encephalitics, grossly brain damaged, and cultural–familial (C–F) children in a visual complexity discrimination experiment. Subjects were required to adapt to three initial complexity levels, followed by exposure to five complexity levels. DS and C–F subjects showed a preference for visual complexity levels superior to their adaptation level indicators. The post-encephalitics and brain damaged samples chose stimulus cards below complexity adaptation levels. Sackett interpreted these results as possibly indicating that DS individuals enjoy a greater potential for visual exploration than do exogenous mentally retarded subjects. Komiya (1973), comparing DS and other MR children on simple figure copying to time limits, found no differences. Although his DS sample was somewhat brighter than average, the suspicion remains that a visual discrimination advantage for DS subjects, over other discrete causal groups of MR, might be masked by the motor report requirement or by delayed kinaesthetic feedback when time is a task criterion.

Claims for the superiority of DS subjects for visual over tactual or auditory modalities, in discrimination performance situations, are further weakened by the failure to separate the stimulus and response components of traditional experimental tasks. Scheffelin (1968 a, b) studied the effectiveness of four stimulus–response (S–R) channels for combinations of visual, auditory, vocal and motor discrimination exercises (using paired-associate learning). The DS sample comprised 24 day-school children with a mean IQ of 42.8 points. The stimulus pairs consisted of a series of common objects in various presentation modes and counterbalanced for visual or auditory modality. Verbal or motor responses were possible and errors per condition were calculated following pre-training. While errors for the auditory-vocal condition were almost double each of the other S–R channels, statistical analysis showed neither stimulus modality nor response mode, alone, as important in influencing rate of error. Significant effects were detected for the combination of auditory stimulus and vocal response. Difficulty in associating pairs of spoken words may be experienced by all children at early mental ages, although O'Connor and Hermelin (1963) contended that DS subjects have particular difficulty because of specific language (central) and speech (mechanical) lag. Then, too, special problems of auditory-vocal sequencing in the syndrome could be a by-product of some peculiarity of attention, sounds and words having less alerting impact than visual cues. Scheffelin offered that poor tactual-kinaesthetic feedback might inhibit the proper development of articulation facility, or that hypotonia corrupts the development of speech muscles, or that DS suffers a unique disorder of auditory feedback.

Block, Sersen and Wortis (1970) implicate attention in their exploration of the ease of reversal of conditioned discrimination for DS subjects and controls. The controls were made up of encephalopathic mentally retarded subjects and normal siblings. The DS subjects did not distinguish themselves on classically conditioned cardiac discrimination reversal, whereas the encephalopathic group's susceptibility to conditioning was 'related dichotomously to the presence or absence of brain deficit rather than to mental age' (p. 784). One explanation would be for reduced attention in cases having obvious brain damage so that DS individuals might perform poorly, or not, on discrimination tasks depending upon the status of their age-related neuropathology. Compatability of findings among studies would, therefore, depend on the age and IQ level of the DS sample and on the precise nature of the control groups.

Support for a hierarchy of stimulus and response modes, exclusive to DS, is also equivocal. One sees that DS individuals compare favourably with non-DS retardates for visual–tactual and visual-motor sequencing. Central process deficit, sensory deficit, motor-expressive difficulty, attention disorder and cerebellar-related hypotonia have been proposed in a mediational role. However, tasks requirements have often extended beyond the general intellectual capacity of DS and, sometimes, of the controls. Control groups have been unrefined aetiologically or have differed across studies. Other workers have compared DS subjects with themselves in order to isolate an internal hierarchy of performance modes; but usually to task criteria which capture only the few brighter cases not characteristic of the syndrome as a whole. Age of samples has ranged from early childhood through to adolescence and adulthood, with little concern for the impact of developmental variables on performance within and across conditions. The problem is seen most clearly in the matching of DS subjects and controls for mental age; where global mental age scores are arranged to be equivalent across groups but represent quite divergent maturational configurations. Ability differences, subsequently tested experimentally, are guaranteed by the nature of the matching procedure.

What provisional consensus is there? A scorekeeper's view of the experimental literature indicates that DS is inferior to other mentally retarded for stereognostic, kinaesthetic, and tactile-shape discrimination and possibly for auditory-vocal channelling. DS samples are claimed to be equal or superior to other mentally retarded for visual-stereognostic, visual–tactual discrimination and for visual exploration potential. O'Connor and Hermelin (1961) proposed three explanations – effects due to peripheral insensitivity, to faulty nerve conduction, and to central impairment. The evidence emerging from the newer laboratory findings is not so neatly categorized. The observation that attention deficit acts to depress discrimination performance cannot be exclusively pinned to peripheral physiology, or shown to be clearly unique for the syndrome. More reasonable is the position that these deficits are the final product of a causal chain beginning with cerebellar immaturity expressed sequentially as hypotonia, motor speed slowing, reaction time lag and attention disorder. A major competing hypothesis favours syndrome-related conceptual limitations, but this position is weakened by a failure to control for peripheral and structural differences between aetiological groups. A case in point is the Scroth (1975) study which employed 40 DS and 40 non-DS retarded subjects on an oddity learning task. The more rapid learning of the non-DS retarded subjects was presumed to indicate that DS subjects tend more to level I ability (rote learning and memory) than level II ability (conceptual) than other classes of MR. Explanations of supposed cognitive strengths are harder to come by. Positive intellectual attributes might be compensatory in origin or else merely apparent in comparison with more severely brain-damaged types of mental retardation. Seriously damaged retardates display perceptual-integrative and impulse patterning disorders against which younger DS subjects compare favourably. The 'uniqueness' would be with the control subjects. A third route to establishing cognitive uniqueness for DS is through its drive properties.

Drive states

Brown and Clarke (1963) claimed that the drive characteristics of a stimulus influence level of performance differentially between causal groups of MR. Wesner (1972) reasoned that DS individuals in particular cannot sustain arousal states – and attention – without special environmental inducements

Subjects (32 DS equated for MA with normal kindergarten children) were invited to learn words by sight under 65 dB of intermittent noise. A significant increase in verbal learning was evident under the manipulated arousal condition. Discrimination facility, in tandem with motivation, has also been explored. Byck (1968) reported that concept-switching facility for DS, and other imbeciles, depended on reward conditions. Classical conditioning rates, when comparing DS with others, had been traced previously by Birch and Demb (1959) to variation in general activity level across causal groups and rather less to general level of mental defect. The importance of external motivational factors, for performance quality in DS, has been noted by Butterfield (1961) in a single case study of over-achievement and by Buddenhagen and Sickler (1969) using operant procedures. The valence of reinforcement, too, is relevant. Talkington, Altman and Grinnell (1971) engaged a DS sample in a marble dropping task. Negative verbal feedback for errors was more enhancing to performance than positive feedback for correct responses. The findings were interpreted as failure-avoidance in DS subjects and is consistent with personality constructs which hold that DS children are heavily dependent on their affectional environment and retain the capacity to monitor changes within it; a capacity which is possibly more intact than their general mental level would suggest. However, the numerically most important area of motivational research for DS has concerned physiological states of activation, a major objective being to identify the relation of arousal conditions to quality of cognitive output and the extent to which activation properties can be usefully manipulated.

Electrocortical evidence

Fehr (1976) claimed that there is general scientific support for a relation between rates of cerebral metabolism, including cerebral blood flow and cerebral oxygenation rates, and EEG reponses. Given the well documented circulatory system anomalies of DS individuals, it would not be surprising to find electroencephalographic correlates of performance particular to the syndrome. The study of neural activation levels for DS dates from Kreezer (1939). He detected a positive correlation of alpha frequency to Binet scores. Gunnarson (1945) reported slower alpha rhythm for DS compared with non-DS mentally retarded samples. Godinova (1963) noted excessively slow EEG activity for 50% of his sample of DS individuals. Hirai and Izawa (1964) examined 40 DS subjects who did not suffer from seizures and concluded in favour of neural immaturity. There was also evidence of atypical 'fast' activity, suggestive of 'damage' in some instances. Rinaldi et al. (1972) found spontaneous cerebral electro-activity faster than 14 CPS in DS but didn't consider it representative for the syndrome.

The extent to which depressed neural activation is characteristic of 'non-damaged' DS, as distinct from other TMR, has been tested by Berkson, Hermelin and O'Connor (1961). Alpha was calculated for percentage of time present during three 10 second periods. There was no significant difference between the DS (82% alpha) and other retardates (76% alpha). A second test was conducted for length (seconds) of alpha block to a light flash. Return to alpha was defined as a burst of at least five alpha waves, averaged over two independent judgements. These MR groups did not differ for habituation rate, or for their positioning on a behavioural excitability scale *vis a vis* magnitude of resting or responding alpha scores. While Berkson and colleagues took care to eliminate obvious neuropathology, known to distort alpha frequency, little concern was shown for the possible influence of different sensory threshold and response delivery capacities across aetiological groups.

Response time, in relation to alpha blocking, has been investigated since by Hermelin and Venables (1964) comparing six DS and six non-DS retardates. The assumption was that, for pre-alerted subjects (alpha blocked), reaction time should be faster than when an activating signal or stimulus was presented in a non-alerted (alpha status) condition. Since longest RTs were achieved for DS subjects, coupled with maximal neural activity, the authors suggested that development of motor set might be delayed for the syndrome; or that the mixed modalities engaged in the procedure have exposed a particular difficulty of auditory-motor circuiting. Alternatively, the five IQ point difference favouring the non-DS group and the meagre sample size, could have influenced the results. No conclusion was reached for a distinct neural arousal status for DS even though DS subjects, free of specific neuropathology, did appear to have slower alpha than would be expected using normal age-graded criteria. Whether such slowing would indicate neural immaturity for Down's, along with depressed activation levels, is not clear. Nor is there persuasive evidence that other lower-level retardates vary for basal or reactivity rates from DS; or of the extent to which aetiologically distinct sensory capacity, motor set and response mechanisms, have contributed to the observed variability of neural activation. Sackett (1967) found, for instance, that DS patients preferred visual complexity levels superior to previously demonstrated adaptation levels, a discrepancy not evident in CA and IQ matched post-encephalitics and brain-damaged subjects. Greater control of sensory and expressive factors, developmentally adjusted, will be required when examining neural activation hypotheses with defined causal groups of mental retardation.

The sensory intake parameters of activation in DS, examined by Brousseau and Brainerd (1928), have been discussed. Bilovsky and Share (1965) have since advanced the idea of a specific impairment of auditory channelling and Clausen (1968) has remarked on the reduced speed of perception evident for DS. Experimental studies of response artifacts, important in interpretation of physiological activation data, have centred on eye movement and related fluctuations of attention. O'Connor and Berkson (1963) monitored lateral eye movement for DS and non-DS retardates, assigning the greater eye movement of DS subjects to peripheral hypotonus inhibiting smooth control of eye muscles. Increased eye movement contributed, presumably, to fluctuation of attention and to depressed maintenance of activation states. Astrup, Sersen and Wortis (1967) also assigned response deficiency in DS to a retardation of motor function. Eyelid conditioning in DS was explored by Ross (1967). He reported that older DS subjects conditioned more readily but proposed that sample bias, as a function of selective institutionalization and the effects of age-graded mortality, could influence all such findings.

A major difficulty then is to effectively isolate the experimentally relevant central, sensory and expressive properties of the syndrome. Those who work with evoked-response amplitudes have claimed a centralist position, i.e., that such amplitudes might be larger for DS subjects than other types of mental retardation and that DS subjects will show, therefore, a particular deficit in central inhibitory processes (Barnet and Lodge, 1967; Barnet, Ohlrich and Shanks, 1971; Bigum, Dustman and Beck, 1970; Gliddon, Busk and Galbraith, 1975). These effects have been observed for visual, somatosensory and auditory stimulation. Gliddon, Galbraith and Busk (1975) say further that 'the usual balance between excitation and inhibition is presumably disturbed, and sensory stimulation thereby results in larger (uninhibited) evoked brain activity' (p. 186). Neural deficits in the processing of sensory information were especially characteristic of DS individuals, over MR controls, at higher levels of stimulus intensity and duration. Gliddon et al. (1975) employed DS subjects who were 23.8 ($\pm$ 7.0) years of age with a mean Binet IQ of 29.5 points. These figures indicate a sample well within the range of secondary deteriorative process so the conclusions would not necessarily be valid for the younger DS cases which comprise the majority of the syndrome. Evidence reviewed in the chapters on Development and Management suggests that increased intensity and duration of stimulus conditions tend to elicit better quality responses to the extent that an immature sensory apparatus obscures sensory intake. Further study will be required to determine if and why the equilibrium of excitation and inhibition for the syndrome is any more disturbed than for other discrete forms of MR and if the phenomenon is anything more than an artifact of progressive central process erosion.

Autonomic nervous system evidence

Other approaches to physiological activation in DS have focussed on autonomic nervous system (ANS) function, particularly the cardiovascular system (CVS) and galvanic skin response (GSR). Resting skin resistance measures are taken as indices of alertness or arousal, the expectation being that mental defectives will show either higher or lower resting levels than normals. Failure to predict direction of differences, for MR subjects in general, is understandable because high anxiety levels are characteristic of the exogenous and low anxiety levels of certain of the clinical and endogenous categories of MR. Research with DS subjects is more consistent, showing them to have higher skin resistance than other subtypes of retardation (O'Connor and Hermelin, 1963). Coarseness of skin has been offered as an explanation but is not entirely supported by the stimulus manipulation literature which tests reaction to buzzers, light flashes, verbal demands, etc. Birch and Demb (1959) assessed number of trials to GSR conditioning, between DS and brain-damaged retardates, the latter subdivided for hyperactive and non-hyperactive disposition. Achieving a classically conditioned GSR proved to be a more formidable process for DS than for non-hyperactive damaged subjects but about equal in difficulty to the hyperactive subgroup. Number of trials to acquisition was greater for the hyperactive than for either the non-hyperactive damaged or for the DS subjects. Differences of mean IQ level between samples, along with subject loss during the course of the experiment, prevented an adequate separation of activation levels from intellectual and other biologically important variables.

Berkson, Hermelin and O'Connor (1961) analysed resting heart rate and skin conductance for DS and non-DS retardates. Heart rate (beats per second) did not separate the two groups, either initially or following response to a stimulus series (light flashes). Skin resistance findings proved non-DS retardates to have significantly higher conductance than DS subjects. The two MR groups did not differ for the various psychophysiological indices in response either to the initial light flash or to a series of such flashes. The single difference of lower skin conductance for DS is attributed by Berkson et al. (1961) to the effects of peripheral masking. Supporting this is the finding by J. H. Clark that skin conductance in DS is lower than for other IQ-matched samples (reported by Berkson, 1960). O'Connor and Hermelin (1960) ascribed GSR differences, among causal groups of TMR, predominantly to hypotonus and cerebellar immaturity in the DS group. On the other hand, Clausen, Lidsky and Sersen (1975) interpreted their resting SR finding as indicating a higher arousal potential for DS than for familial MR.

Therefore, higher than normal (compared with other TMRs) physiological resting levels are not clearly established for the syndrome; possibly because it is not known how different sensory threshold patterns, across MR causal categories, serve the traditional activation-performance equation. It is proposed in Karrer's (1975) collection that performance deficit in the mental retardations can be understood in terms of an inverted-U arousal hypothesis and that DS subjects display a supranormal arousal potential such that distraction is more frequent. These findings would need to be elaborated for various input–output combinations if they are to be compatible with the modality literature. Wallace and Fehr (1970) found heart rate fluctuations for DS to be uncorrelated with performance (reaction time), and skin resistance to be negatively correlated. Motor impulsivity and general skeletal-motor function were implicated in their interpretation. It is the Lacey and Lacey (1958) position that spontaneous ANS activity is associated with these two factors and that autonomic processes serve as 'energizers' of cortical potentials. Moreover, the greater the cortical activity, the more active, as a rule, will be the motor system. Autonomically labile subjects should therefore display faster reaction times than less labile subjects. Another possibility is that the significantly longer latency of RT for DS subjects, over matched controls, reflects an auditory intake disorder or a slowing of auditory-motor circuiting as a function of hypotonus.

Despite the uncertain nature of the research literature, activation postulates provide an attractive adjunct to the purely cognitive process hypotheses. The approach of Block, Sersen and Wortis (1970) illustrates this promise. Block *et al.* proposed that deficient performance is tied to poor ANS potentials and that distinct ANS patterns might exist across different types of mental retardation. The task criterion for the study was ease of reversal of conditioned discriminations and subjects were age-graded to test developmental trends of ANS function associated with discrimination outputs. Basal heart rates did not differ between retardation groups. Important evidence was noted of decline in heart rate as age increased, presumably as a function of general maturation. Cardiac maturation co-varied with mental rather than physical age, suggesting a common developmental process affecting both circulatory system and CNS status. Cardiac-discrimination functions, too, varied with MA rather than with CA. Similar studies range from no difference in resting heart rate for DS over normal subjects (Berkson *et al.* 1961; Karrer and Clausen, 1964) to evidence for higher pre-stimulus heart rate for DS subjects (Block, Sersen and Wortis, 1970). Otherwise, DS individuals are less reactive than normals in response to stimulation of pulse rate (Vogel, 1961), vascular responses (Razran, 1961), HR variability (Karrer and Clausen, 1964), heart period variability (Block *et al.* 1970), blood pressure and finger volume measures (Vogel, 1961). These results are not unexpected given the circulatory system deficiencies of the syndrome. Whether certain activation indices are unique for DS, compared with other forms of MR, or consistent across stages of growth and decline, is unknown.

The particularity of motivation, drive, or activation states for DS is an ongoing issue. While Kreezer (1939), Gunnarson (1945) and Godinova (1963) demonstrated comparatively slow alpha in DS, due they say to neural immaturity rather than to neural upset, Berkson *et al.* (1961) were unable to confirm these findings. Appearances are for (i) depressed resting psycho-physiological and neural indices, compared with normal populations, but not necessarily differing from those of other retardates; (ii) a connection between physiological drive states and IQ level, regardless of aetiology; (iii) a poor concordance between resting and aroused physiological states and con-comitant behavioural sets; and (iv) depressed GSR measures in DS subjects compared with MR controls. Some of these differences may have peripheral explanations, including the sensory and motor inadequacies peculiar to the syndrome. Other differences depend on the nature of the control group, e.g., brain-damaged TMRs can display a magnitude of drive disorder and physiological over-vigilance against which DS, or even a normal child, might appear under-reactive.

Movement away from a cognitive model towards an arousal-motivational concept for MR performance is well advanced (Karrer, 1966; Zigler, 1966). Declining dependence on exclusively centralist explanations followed the realization that direction and magnitude of behaviours in mental retardation related rather imprecisely to mental test indices and only generally to the neuropathological particulars of any given aetiology or individual within the boundaries of mental retardation.

Evaluation

Like Thursday's child, the experimental enterprise, surrounding learning and arousal in DS, has far to go. The two most promising lines of enquiry have depended on the concepts of circuitry and activation. Of the first, Belmont (1971) has said: 'It is firmly concluded that mongoloids are deficient in auditory-vocal processing both to their own alternative channels and to the auditory-vocal processing of other retardates. There is, moreover, an indication that their visuomotor system is their strongest, and it may be stronger than that of other retardates' (p. 75). These are confident words considering the contradictions and poor comparability of the various studies. Johnson and Olley (1971) in their summary give preference to the role of depressed arousal states and lowered muscle tension in respect to reaction time, GSR, attention and tactile discrimination performance for DS subjects. Here too, the evidence is ambiguous.

A concern for how the DS subject learns began essentially with the use of mental measurement techniques. Binet test findings suggested comparative strength for the identification and naming functions and particular weaknesses for sequencing and relating activities. Language lag was more evident for DS than for other retardates at similar mental age levels. Psychometric indications of more serious symbol deficiency for DS, than for other MR, were inconclusive except for evidence of poor sense of numbers. Auditory-perceptual patterning disorder, attention deficit, and poor activation potential were offered as explanations. Eye–hand coordination, psychomotor ability and self-help skills appeared to be appropriate to, or slightly in advance of, overall mental age for DS children but less obviously so as physical age increased. The uneven expression of neuropathological processes, over time, has reduced the consistency of the foregoing behavioural picture. The growth and recession of finer visual-motor skills is claimed to match the emergence of self-help (social) skills and their subsequent decline in the total behavioural matrix. Otherwise, whether or not DS surpasses other retardates for any performance dimension is contingent upon sample ages and the aetiological composition of the comparison groups.

Recent evidence for a distinctive quality of cognition for the syndrome has implicated sensorimotor and activation constructs, primarily. Input–output circuiting appears weakest for the auditory-vocal and strongest for the visual-motor channels (Bilovsky and Share, 1965). Clausen (1968) found speed of perception to be deficient. He favoured an arousal over a sensory or cerebral deficiency explanation. Since perceptual speed is a function of response delivery capacity, perhaps motor deficiency (including speech muscle sequencing) should bear the responsibility. Cowie (1970) tied sensorimotor circuiting, DMQ and DIQ scores to the neurological and reflexive apparatus at birth, including hypotonia and the placing reaction. Jebsen *et al.* (1961) considered infantile muscular hypotonia to originate in the CNS. The poorly nurtured and enervated muscle system of DS also warrants mention. Many centralist studies of the syndrome have seriously undervalued differences in peripheral or sensory system physiology, probably because Brousseau and Brainerd thought these unimportant. Straumanis, Shagass and

Overton (1973 a) calculated somatosensory evoked response (SER) to demonstrate that (i) for a given conduction pathway length, latency of the initial SER peak was longer for DS than for normals or idiopathic MR subjects, and (ii) the expected high correlation between conduction pathway length and initial latency was abnormally low for the DS sample. Depressed arousal, reactivity, or discrimination facility for DS might, therefore, represent a failure of the sensory network. Age effects, however, are difficult to assess. The second Straumanis, Shagass and Overton study (1973 b) stimulated DS, idiopathic MR and college student subjects by auditory clicks of 105 dB at 2 second intervals. First peak amplitude for the DS subjects was significantly greater than controls. Mean latency of the first peak was longer in DS than in idiopathic MR subjects, indicating that the conduction system for DS is only initially faulty. A similar study using visual cues would be useful. Pending further research, the most obvious conclusion favours an attention-inhibition deficit somehow associated with the auditory circuiting function.

Exclusively centralist hypotheses are at present unsatisfactory if cognitive outputs for DS are corrupted by depressed muscle tone, activation lability, conduction latency, coordination skill, or modality strength. Limiting explanations to the peripheral system is equally hazardous. Thompson (1963), among others, has remarked on the comparative delay DS children exhibit in establishing cerebral dominance. If lateralization, an essentially CNS phenomenon, is poorly established then a number of coordination, perceptual, speech and circuitry problems will follow. Whatever the starting point, it is plausible that central, peripheral and mechanical factors contribute to learning and arousal patterns in a complex reciprocal manner. Much of the experimental research reviewed here has ignored these interactions.

It is not yet clear if DS individuals exhibit shorter attention span or slower reaction time than do comparable groups of MR subjects; and if so, under what circumstances. Rollin (1946) described DS as relatively alert, outgoing, impetuous and briskly reactive, but not necessarily attentive. It appears that the search for novelty and change by DS individuals is not matched by sustained interest. Maintenance of a single interest is more often evident when motor discharge is continuously engaged, as in dancing or mimicry. Whatever the conclusion, attention in DS has not been adequately tested across a range of stimulus types and intensities. Most studies, arguing for an attention or reactivity lag, have appealed to motor speed defect, auditory-motor circuiting difficulty, verbal deficiency, low arousal potential, sight limitation, retarded motor set or simple failure to meet task criteria (i.e., to comprehend). The general hypotonia and other structural peculiarities of the syndrome also have interpretative value. Once more, the need is to incorporate physiological events as independent variables in behavioural research with DS subjects.

The twin postulates of behavioural uniqueness and bio-behavioural specificity for DS are, in the final analysis, dependent upon the nature of the control groups used. Conclusions reached appear to depend on the selection of either familial, exogenous or normal controls (Girardeau, 1959); on the age level and psychometric comparability of DS and controls (Martin and Blum, 1961); on the motivational propensities of different aetiological categories (Brown and Clarke, 1963); and on the quality and level of IQ regardless of aetiology (Fisher, 1970). Down's is a progressive and regressive syndrome both physiologically and behaviourally. Mental age matching of DS subjects with controls, however meticulous, is a self-fulfilling process insofar as behavioural-aetiological differences can be built in. For example, a DS child may earn a 2 year Binet mental age, largely because of relatively good early indicators for habit training, whereas MA-matched non-DS control subjects often earn age-graded points for speech or retention facility. These qualitative distinctions, between causal groups, shift in turn with increasing CA. Furthermore, discrimination differences, between DS and other retardates, are obscured because of a failure to identify the parameters of attention, sensory input, and expressive abilities. The discrimination performance of DS subjects is variable depending on task attention demand, conceptual requirement, and whether or not tactile, stereognostic, visual inputs, or motor and verbal expressive outputs (or some combination), are prerequisites. Consistency of findings is not remarkable and no study permitted a clear statement about discrimination capacity for DS or the relative constraints of peripheral insensitivity, faulty nerve conduction, or central impairment.

The newer concerns for drive states, arousal potential, and motivational conditions in mental retardation, as these influence learning and thinking, contribute to the disarray. Behavioural asymmetry of all kinds, within DS and between types of MR, has been related to reward condition (Byck, 1968) and to physiological activation states (Birch and Demb, 1959; Clausen, 1968; Kreezer, 1939). Berkson et al. (1961) and Hermelin and Venables (1964) found no characteristic activation status for DS. Other workers have assigned differences to skeletal-motor status, auditory channelling deficiency (Sackett, 1967), a variety of response artifacts (Brousseau and Brainerd, 1928; Bilovsky and Share, 1965; Clausen, 1968; O'Connor and Berkson, 1963, Astrup et al. 1967), chronological or mental age, and sampling effects (Ross, 1967). There is only tentative evidence for a special activation status for the syndrome and no assurance that motivational research has controlled for irregularities of cognitive, sensory and expressive processes. Wallace and

Fehr (1970), and Block *et al.* (1970) bypass such issues by linking heart rate to the energizing of cortical mechanisms. Reaction time and quality of attention, as these influence comprehension, discrimination and generalization facility, would be seen as centred in peripheral physiology. Moreover, cardiac maturation covaries with mental age and with general development such that ANS function would differ reliably across aetiological groups if the maturational timetable for each differs. Wallace and Fehr (1970) admit, nevertheless, that longer reaction time latency, for DS, is also some function of motor capacity and auditory-motor circuiting lag.

The experimental study of special behavioural deficits or assets, for DS, must therefore be understood in terms of (i) the selection of comparison groups, (ii) chronological age at time of sampling, (iii) extent of circulatory disorder, (iv) degree of hypotonus and related cerebellar immaturity, and (v) the vagaries of developmental schedules in respect to establishing physiological arousal parameters and conceptual status with DS samples. O'Connor and Hermelin were the first to promote an inclusive explanation for the behavioural configuration claimed for DS. The underlying mechanism, they say, centres on the immaturity of the cerebellum and correspondingly poor muscle tone, as compared with other mentally retarded. One could expect slow motor speed, poor stereognostic and tactile discrimination, slower than usual (mental age related) speech growth, etc. They invoked the Davis (1940) finding that the 'greater the tension level in the responding muscle system, the shorter the reaction time'. Freeman and Simpson (1938) had demonstrated a decrease in skin resistance under increased muscle tension. O'Connor and Hermelin further claimed 'that hypotonia would minimize kinaesthetic feedback and thus impaired stereognosis seems plausible' (p. 101). Concerning arousal thresholds, they argued that a low arousal state could indicate merely a lack of muscle tone. Despite the dynamic symmetry of their postulates, purely mechanical explanations are available. These include the suspected influence of circulatory difficulty on the proper nutrition of muscles, nervous system and cutaneous tissues related to the quality of physiological activation; the effects on psychomotor abilities of the shortened distal bones of the limbs; the effects of ear structure and proper ear hygiene on audition; the role of various peripheral visual defects (reported often for the syndrome) on perceptual integration; and the role played by hyperflexibility in DS for lay impressions of dance, rhythm and melody skill as 'inborn'. These factors are overlooked as sources of 'unique' behaviours, probably because nervous system explanations are more prestigious.

A final source of understanding is found in the development process itself. Unlike the aetiologically capricious 'damage' categories of MR, DS is karyotypically programmed for relatively good early development, progressing through less accelerative growth periods, to subsequent deterioration at adolescence and young adulthood for many. Much of the psychological profile has been identified as emergent or magnified at various points on the maturational continuum; imperfectly, but reasonably consistently in terms of what is known about the underlying biological and neurological strata of DS. The prominent sources of explanation – centrally mediated hypotonus, cytogenetically programmed curves of maturation, arousal status, sensorimotor factors and the structural peculiarities which make up the classical somatic configuration of the syndrome – are not mutually exclusive. Taken together, they support a reasonable claim for a degree of behavioural uniqueness for DS.

9

Speech and language

The stereotype

The 'mongols' examined by Langdon Down (1866) were 'usually able to speak; but the speech is thick and indistinct'. Beyond agreement on the clinically obvious, there was little early concern for the extent and type of speech disorders or for the staging of language growth for DS children. Contributors to the later descriptive literature neglected to define what they mean by defective speech in particular samples. The role of age, the contribution of secondary handicap and sample selection biases (e.g., hospital versus home) have each added confusion to the various speech disorder estimates. Thus, Benda and Durling (1952) could claim that 4% of older institutional DS subjects are 'not using words'; Engler (1949), that past 5 years of age 19% are incapable of speech; and Gottsleben (1955), that of 39 Vineland training school cases 8% show 'a complete lack of speech'. Schlanger and Gottsleben (1957) found 95% of their speaking DS group to have articulation problems, a figure well in excess of any other clinically discrete class of mental retardates. Buddenhagen (1971) asserted that after 5 years of age 10% were fundamentally mute and Johnston and Abelson (1969) that 81% were unable to communicate with others understandably. All that could be concluded is that many or most have communication problems and that certain of these difficulties might be more characteristic, frequent, or severe than for other intellectually similar forms of mental retardation. But even that is not certain. Wing (1975) argues that seriously retarded children, with clearcut organic pathology, experience greater problems of language development than do DS children. Reviewing the recent literature, Villiger and Mathis (1972) proposed that DS is linguistically inferior to other mental retardates but has less hearing loss. Agreement on extent of voice deviation was limited. Linguistic ability seemed to them to depend on degree of retardation, yet comprehension was found to be superior to verbal expression. The contradictions are partly a function of the consid-

233

erable variability of language and conceptual development within the syndrome (Evans & Hampson, 1969).

Some frequency claims have been hedged developmentally. Brousseau and Brainerd (1928) implied that DS children talked rather later than might be expected of imbeciles at their mental age but talk they did. Engler (1949) claimed that timing of onset of speech was comparatively late, and McNeill (1955) and Thompson (1963) that speech in DS is proportionately slower to appear, than are the other common developmental indices. Lenneberg et al. (1964), Fishler et al. (1964) and O'Connor and Hermelin (1963) attempted to show that DS speech is both characteristically delayed and defective. Most growth studies have found DS speech to develop relatively later than the traditional motor, intellectual and social indices; within the syndrome and when compared with normal children and other retardates.

Transcending the debate about consistency of stereotype for speech lag in DS is the question of quality of defect. Schlanger and Gottsleben (1957) were among the first to detail kinds of speech disorder for DS, organic, familial and undifferentiated mental retardates. Down's subjects were outstanding for percentage of articulation defect (95%), stuttering (45%) and general voice disorder. Many more voice disorders were found in DS than in the other aetiological groups. A later survey (Blanchard, 1964) produced similar results across aetiological groups of MR. Spontaneous articulatory ability did not pace other abilities and was comparable with those retarded groups originating in mechanical injury at birth or from pre-natal infections. More normal communication patterns were observed in the post-natal injury and cultural–familial groups. Dodd (1975) added that articulation difficulty (number and type of errors) varies by mental age for DS subjects but not for the non-DS retarded. Castellan-Paour and Paour (1971) find DS subjects below other retarded subjects for quality of speech rhythm and syntax in addition to quality of articulation.

While it is commonly claimed that DS children make comparatively more errors in articulation, at all ages (Smith, 1975), the reasons are not clear. Degree of mental defect and structural pathology are most often mentioned. Lenneberg, Nichols and Rosenberger (1962) were not convinced that there was any connection between clarity of articulation and the major structural insufficiencies of the syndrome. Dodd (1975) speculates that spontaneous articulation disorder might be due to deficits in auditory processing and storage or to a disability in the motor sequencing of the speech act. She tested these alternatives, using real and nonsense words, to find superior performance for the DS sample on word recognition and a relative deficit on word reproduction after delay. The ability to store and retrieve auditory information in short-term memory did not appear to be impaired relative to the non-DS retardates. Dodd concluded that 'The poor articulatory performance of the Down's syndrome group would seem, then, to be at least partly due either to an inability to use learned sequences of articulatory movements or to an incomplete learning of sequences. This deficit is probably a symptom of the general motor disability associated with Down's syndrome' (p. 311).

Accordingly, our understanding of the dimensions of DS speech and its structural, peripheral and cognitive correlates is inhibited by a literature which seldom controls for syndromic or maturational effects. What follows is an evaluation of the speech, voice and language stereotype for the syndrome in a developmental context; including the infant responses, early speech acquisition in the face of various mechanical–structural limitations, and problems of communication in relation to ability profiles. The exercise is a necessary step to examining the several mediational and more numerous management positions and to supporting or not the authenticity of distinctive voice and linguistic traits for the syndrome.

Infant responses

The study of babbling and the cry response is moved by the assumptions that the development of speech sounds is related to later vocal proficiency and/or to degree of intelligence. If these early signals are precursors to later articulation disorder, or are linked to degree of mental defect for DS, an argument can be made for remedial intervention beginning in the first months of life.

Brousseau and Brainerd (1928) first mentioned the peculiarity of the DS infant's voice (crying). Experimental studies since have largely confirmed this. Karelitz et al. (1959) characterized the infant's cry as high pitched. Fisichelli et al. (1963, 1966 a, b) described the pain cry response as less active, of shorter duration, and as requiring more stimulation to elicit than that of the normal infant. Goueffic et al. (1967) examined the voices of ten 19-year-old DS individuals and reported the 'fundamental frequency lowered' from comparable normals. Others studies of abnormally low pitch for DS children (Michel & Carney, 1964; Hollien & Copeland, 1965) have not been entirely supportive. Lind et al. (1970) have criticized some of these investigations on methodological and theoretical grounds, attempting instead a wide ranging examination of a variety of cry components with a trisomy-21 sample ($N = 30$) and normal controls. The cry latency for DS was greater, the duration was greater, the minimum pitch cps mean was less and the maximum CPS mean was less. Nasality, stuttering voice, and flat melody forms all exceeded the normal means significantly. Five clinically equivocal cases of DS displayed a normal cry. Later chromosome analysis confirmed that these five cases were not Down's. The authors point out that the low pitch is not entirely pathognomonic, being seen also in congenital hypothyroidism and perhaps cretinism. Other findings were of a declining cry reaction to pain with increasing age and a special quality of tension in the pain cry. They say; 'the pain cry in Down's syndrome is also tense, but the tension often has a special 'stuttering characteristic' caused by rapid rhythmical variations in glottal pressure. The tenseness of the cry is in striking contrasts to the general hypotonia of the musculature' (p. 483).

Lind *et al.* (1970) then moved to the somewhat speculative position that experts could isolate the DS cry from that of others and that phonatory dysfunction analysis might be useful for the initial clinical diagnosis of the syndrome. This hope can be contrasted with their other findings of wide individual differences for DS voice quality, e.g., the stuttering variety of cry phonation appearing in only 16 of the 30 DS cases examined. They proposed that phonatory dysfunction might vary by chromosome subtype. The prospects are dim. While Reisman, Shipe and Williams (1966) observed good speech in an unusual form of mosaicism DS, Gibson and Pozsonyi (1965) found no difference in age of talking between the standard trisomy and the translocation subtypes. Speech distinctions across chromosomal categories are possibly artifacts of differences in temperament, intelligence and age of institutionalization. Less clear results emerge from the comparison of babbling patterns for normal and DS infants. Dodd (1972) compared spontaneous vocalization for frequency, length and type of utterance but found no differences between the two groups. Babbling does not appear to be related to mental or motor indices in the early months of life and gives no indication of later articulation skill.

At this point there is tentative agreement that many DS infants exhibit a cry response which has a prolonged latency and is high-pitched, tense or stuttered. The most palpable explanations are to be found in the respiratory, sensory transmission, muscle tone and arousal deficits of the syndrome. Later vocal proficiency might prove to be a correlate of infant vocalization but only to the extent that the foregoing somatic limitations continue to be extant.

Mechanical factors

An enumeration of the structural factors involved in the speech stereotype for Down's syndrome is required in order to balance current thinking that speech disorders in DS are the product of biased or impoverished linguistic environments or stem from stereotypic projection. The latter point can be disposed of now. Montague and Hollien (1973, 1974) charted voice quality deviations (breathiness, roughness, etc.) and resonance disability (nasality) in 20 DS children and 20 normals (mean ages 10.4 years). Matched verbal samples were played backwards to four evaluation groups (naive listeners, speech pathologists, etc.). The DS sample exhibited significantly more breathiness, roughness and nasality than normals regardless of the composition of the evaluation group. The vocal deficits are similar to those identified by West *et al.* (1947), Strazzulla (1953) and Jones (1963).

Brousseau and Brainerd (1928), Benda (1949) and Buddenhagen (1971) have detailed many of the peripheral pathological factors claimed to be associated with delayed and defective speech in DS. A number of these appear peculiar to the syndrome, by type and frequency, including pharyngealization (exhibited in a raspy, gravel voiced articulation), a buccal cavity too small for the tongue and a protruding tongue which might therefore swell. The shortened buccal cavity also distorts vocal tract configuration, from lips to pharynx. Benda found the larynx to be high in the neck and with a thickening of fibrotic mucosa. Myxoedema of the pharynx was thought by him to be associated with the guttural voice of the DS child and adult. The edematous tongue doesn't groove properly for the distinction between *sh* and *s* and is impaired in its motility. Buddenhagen says 'Not only does the motion of the tongue alter the buccal cavity but the pharyngeal cavity is altered as well since, as Lieberman (1968) explained, the root or dorsum of the tongue forms a moveable anterior wall for the pharynx' (p. 180). Oster (1953) recorded that 57% of his regional sample had noticeably enlarged tongues. It has been suggested that the large tongue is an illusion based on small mouth and oral cavity, although Oster found the mouths in his series to be of normal size.

Other anomalies included 29% with broad lips and 40% with lips irregular in shape, including lateral inversions of the lower lip. Oster's opinion is that while these anomalies are common, wide individual differences exist. A universality of structural features, coupled with speech lag or deficit in DS individuals, is difficult to support. In addition, frequency of structural anomaly is age dependent. Oster reported a husky voice for 156 of his 453 cases with little evidence in subjects under 4 years and increasing frequencies to age 14 when the voice quality becomes more stabilized. Palate anomalies are (otherwise) said to include a short 'steeple' palate (Spitzer *et al.*, 1961) which creates problems of sound production not heard in a normal linguopalatal relationship. Blanchard (1964) mentioned the fissured tongue as among the structural anomalies affecting speech. Strazzulla (1953) connected speech difficulty to numerous peripheral factors including hearing problems, aphasia, excessive salivation, poor oral closure, flabbiness of tongue and a too small jaw. Sibilant sounds give most trouble, especially *s* which requires the finer coordination of tongue, lips, jaw, and breathing muscles. The result is a lisp which is quite common in young normal children as well. Other difficulties of mechanical origin include the production of the affricatives (*ch*, *j*), the fricatives (*f*, *v*, *th*), the plosives (*b*, *d*, *k*) and especially the back sounds (*g*) the nasal sounds (*m*, *n*, *ng*) and the vowels and diphthongs. The last two categories pose fewer problems for the DS individual, it is said, because there are fewer lingual adjustments to be made.

Engler (1949) attributed speech problems in DS to defective teeth, muscular hypotonia of tongue and lips and an imperfect palate, so that sounds are produced explosively and incoherently. Benda (1960) found the mucous membranes to be often quite dry and thickened, but argued that these were basically physiological rather than structural defects. Kraus *et al.* (1968) reported dentition for DS to be the poorest of all the syndromes examined within the mental retardations. Down's subjects displayed 29 times the number of crown abnormalities as did the the normal subjects. Of these findings Buddenhagen (1971) says 'while abnormalities in crown morphology can have little effect upon the articulation of phonetic behaviour, the absence (either from extraction or delayed eruption) and irregular alignment of teeth certainly do. And if the incidence of such flaws parallels that of crown abnormalities, the expectation for a normal development of speech would be seriously challenged' (p. 181). He gives an appropriate illustration: 'The absence of incisors for example, renders, by definition, all labiodental, interdental and apicondental articulations impossible, and greatly distorts the qualities of sibilant sounds: (*f*, *v*, *d*, *o*), dialectal versions of (*t*) and (*d*) and (*s*), respectively' (p. 181). Strazulla (1953) made a similar report of sound production related to structural peculiarities. Most difficult for his cases were the sibilant sounds which required finer coordination of tongue, lips, jaws and breathing muscles. One result is the lisp already mentioned.

A possible sequence of events from structure to function might be as follows: from shortened cavity to protruding tongue, moistened and distended lips, cracked and bleeding lips, inhibited labial articulation and thus faulty articulation of sounds associated with lip rounding and lip mobility. The flattened nose, too is associated with the underdevelopment of the sinuses and nasal passages, the frontal sinus sometimes being absent (Spitzer *et al.*, 1961). Brousseau and Brainerd mentioned enlarged tonsils and adenoids in particular as contributing to speech defect. Articulation difficulty is further heightened by the consequences of respiratory infection, so common in DS, where inflammation of the pharynx, laryngitis and bronchitis produce coughing, hoarseness, aphonia and reduced breathing capacity. An unattractive side effect is the frequent presence of purulent nasal discharge which discourages both the DS individual and the onlooker from useful interaction, verbally or otherwise.

Other structural features influencing communication include auditory and visual defects. Rigrodsky *et al.* (1961) surveyed hearing loss across types of mental retardation. They found hearing loss in DS subjects to be much greater than for normal children and appreciable for all MR categories. Hearing impairment affected 60% of the DS sample. The loss was chiefly in the slight to moderately impaired range. Hearing loss for DS subjects (included in a sample of retardates of unknown prenatal origin) was among the three highest of eight categories surveyed and showed 11% 'perceptive' loss, 12% 'mixed' loss and no conductive loss. The mixed loss was defined as a depression of both the low and the high frequencies. Clausen (1968), comparing DS and matched non-DS subjects, found that when audiometric measures were better controlled, the DS subjects exhibited a depressed threshold of hearing for speech, the lack not being especially dependent on IQ level. Colton (1973), however, noted pure tone thresholds and intelligence to be superior for community resident over institutionalized DS subjects suggesting a somatic and intellectual deficit selection bias at work. Nor is it established that hearing deficit is a critical ingredient of quality of speech difficulty for DS. Thorum (1974) compared DS and hearing impaired subjects for extent of vocabulary development, use of syntax and ability to imitate sentences. The two groups differed systematically in their language deviations. Less obvious as causative factors are the peculiarities of brain morphology in frontal lobes and cerebellum influencing conceptualization and voluntary motor movement (Penrose, 1963). Lenneberg (1967) implicates arousal (motivation) status, at least in relation to articulation disorder.

Ocular defects in DS are well known and are important to the learning of communication skills in the sense that visual attention is involved. These defects include strabismus, myopia, cataracts, nystagmus and lens opacities. All impede sustained visual focus (MacGillivray, 1968). Watering and crusted eyes, conjunctivitis, and respiratory infections reduce visual efficiency appreciably. These disorders are more evident in institutionalized DS groups. Preventing colds and teaching the DS child to attend to the discharges from mouth and throat, nasal passages, eyes and ears, is obviously vital to the acquisition of language.

A small amount of somewhat uncertain literature exists on the speaking fundamental frequency (SFF) of DS subjects as against normals and other retardates. The SFF is an index of rate of vibration of vocal cords in cycles per second, essentially pitch. Michel and Carney (1964) and Hollien and Copeland (1965) reported SFF levels to be the same as for normal children of the same chronological age. Weinberg and Zlatin (1970) found significantly higher SFF levels for the pre-school DS children of the trisomy-21 variety. Differences in findings could be function of 'purity' of karyotype across samples but are more likely to be understood in terms of the nature of the verbal task (standardized reading versus spontaneous speech) and the closeness of subject matching. Montague, Brown and Hollien (1974), exercising care in both of the foregoing respects, report no difference for SFF between normal and DS children and no correlation between SFF and IQ. Greater variability of SFF was noted for DS over normals and a possible tendency for SFF measures to approach the norm as age increases. Montague *et al.* speculate that disparity of findings, over time, could be a result of sample age and sex differences and of the improvement of medical care (for respiratory and thyroid disorders in particular) in recent years. Otherwise, they say, speaking defects in DS individuals might relate more closely to resonance parameters, breathiness, hoarseness and nasality than to SFF. An examination of these affiliated variables, along a developmental continuum, is needed.

Those who believe that the voice qualities of DS children are distinctive and founded in syndromic processes, are supported by evidence from the structural and peripheral systems. The importance of these qualities for the language characteristics of the disorder will be considered now.

Language characteristics

Muir (1903) claimed that the development of language in DS is essentially like that of normal children: 'first 'mamma', 'tata', 'papa', then the names of persons, then the names of things and next a few verbs. My most accomplished mongol got no further than this' (p. 167). Brousseau and Brainerd's analysis is consistent with that of Muir, except for a 'disinclination' to use sentences. Canbanas (1954) found speech blocks and other cluttering symptoms in language use, but no active stuttering in a sample of 50 DS children. Preus (1972), on the other hand, reported stuttering in 34% of his sample ($N = 47$) on at least 5% of the words tested and excluding whole word repetitions. Secondary symptoms were observed in 30% while 32% had a tendency to clutter. No correlation was found between the stuttering and cluttering. Lubman's (1955) group of severely retarded children contained 12 severe stutters of whom 10 were DS. Benda (1963) found stuttering more common in the brighter DS children, presumably as the result of the stress of greater performance expectation. Lind *et al.* (1970) reported the stuttering cry to be very common among DS infants when subjected to threshold pain stimuli. Biogenic and psychogenic factors possibly operate interdependently.

Lyle (1960a) tested the language and verbal aspects of DS subjects including proficiency for word naming (50 common objects and actions), word comprehension, word definition (by use), speech sounds, sentence complexity, speech clarity and speech frequency. The DS cases were observed to develop at a slower pace and to a lower achievement level (for language) than otherwise comparable non-DS imbeciles. Lyle claimed, 'they suffer a particular difficulty in discriminating and reproducing speech sounds' (p. 6). A number of regression equations were worked in order to apportion the variance associated with a composite verbal score. Being diagnosed as DS contributed significantly. The disadvantage of the DS subjects was maintained across home, institutional and 'experimental' environments and was not noticeably related to IQ level. Lenneberg *et al.* (1962) also failed to discover a relation between language proficiency and IQ level although there was evidently some connection with chronological age.

Semmell and Dolley (1971) attacked the cognitive aspect of language growth and facility in DS. Responses were elicited using four pairs of pictures depicting, for example, boy kicking girl and girl kicking boy (as one pictorial pair). For each pair of pictures, declarative, negative, passive and negative–passive sentences were presented to the subjects. Comprehension scores varied significantly with sentence types but not with CA or IQ. The DS cases responded best to simple declarative sentences, and weakly to negative declarative and passive sentences. These researchers viewed the difficulty pattern of DS individuals as related to attention disorder, to decoding strategy peculiarities or perhaps to short-term retention deficit. Yet, imitative language facility was associated with IQ level. To conclude in favour of syndrome-specific language characteristics which are independent of degree of IQ deficit would have required the use of comparison groups.

Mein (1961) undertook a grammatical analysis using 11 pairs of DS and non-DS retardates. They were aged 20 years on the average and had a mean mental age of between 4 and 5 years. Word counts were done over nine interviews based on general conversation and on picture description proficiency. The experiment was founded on the assumption that the typical developmental sequence is from noun content, to verbs, to prepositions, to pronouns, and finally to adjectives and adverbs. A comparatively large noun percentage in a developing vocabulary is said to signify cognitive immaturity. While both groups had about the same vocabulary, quantitatively, the DS subjects employed a higher percentage of nouns in picture description and in conversation whereas the non-DS subjects used more articles. Down's subjects appear, therefore, to have a distinctive language lag not attributable only to mental age level or to environmental opportunity. Lyle (1959), using the Minnesota pre-school scale of intelligence to separate verbal and non-verbal scores, found that the hospitalized DS subjects were significantly less adept with the verbal component of the test than was the hospitalized non-DS group. The mean discrepancy was equivalent to 9 months of verbal mental age. Since the retarded groups were the same for non-verbal MA, verbal mental age differences must be associated with parameters other than general intelligence. Lyle favoured an environmental explanation coupled with the proposition that DS might be more susceptible to the external inhibition of speech development than would other MR in the moderate to severe range.

A novel approach to language analysis for the syndrome engaged the Flesch (1949) method in the counting of verbal outputs for a comparatively bright DS individual over the period of his childhood and early adulthood (Seagoe, 1965). The material was in the form of personal diaries. These were analysed for readability, verb–adjective ratios, word counts, pronoun use, sentence structure and so on. The most important of Seagoe's observations about language structure included (i) a tendency, despite intensive training, for the DS subject to remain at the descriptive verbal level and (ii) an indication of some growth of verbal output to age 19 years but with obvious deterioration by age 33 years. Both Blount (1968) and Spreen (1965) were of the opinion that DS individuals, on the whole, display a greater concreteness of language use than would be expected on the basis of age equivalent norms; but that language complexity (sentence length and total vocabulary) were otherwise correlated with mental age level. The problem of cognitive concreteness in DS has been mentioned by Kolstoe (1958). He cautioned that they are able to produce grammatically complex word combinations and build an adequate vocabulary, but that genuine word comprehension and the management of conceptually complex word combination does not keep pace. Thompson (1963) observed that word output for DS consisted mainly of initial sounds. Short sentences were characteristic of them as was a tendency to run words together as compound words. There appeared to be a deficit in whole–part appreciation. Binet items grouped for mental age level, including non-verbal and verbal direction and response items, showed DS to lag verbally. The lag could not be assigned to mental age gradations, exclusively or importantly.

Smith (1975) confirms the tendency of DS subjects to perseveration and cognitive rigidity in language use. He displayed pictures of familiar items to DS and MA matched normals requiring that they identify the picture content verbally and subsequently imitate the experimenters verbal identification. The DS sample was less able to recognize and subsequently respond verbally but had little trouble modelling the appropriate identification when made for them. Errors included perseveration, gross reduction of words to vowel sounds and inconsistencies of response. Beyond these limitations, they used the same phonological rules as the normal children. Share (1975) confirms the presence of conceptual problems in relation to language use. His sample had particular difficulty with words denoting spatial relationships, e.g., the prepositions, in, on, under, over, etc. The DS population is possibly unique for language and speech use in relation to normal children but not necessarily among the mental retardations.

A cross-aetiological study of speech disorder was conducted by Blanchard (1964). She compared DS with other MR groups (of congenital, metabolic, infectious and mechanical origins) for articulation growth patterns. All were hospitalized. Articulation staging was measured by recording errors on an object naming task. Misarticulations included sound omissions, substitutions or variants of these. The findings are reproduced in Table 13. Mental capacity was not the dominant influence in early consonant development, certain consonants being a product of the same structures and actions as infant sucking and other sounds. These are designated as vegetative consonants. The DS subjects advanced little beyond early consonant sounds, if compared with other intellectually comparable subgroups of mental retardation. Verbal communication status was poorest for the groups suffering from Down's, mechanical birth injury and pre-natal infection. Functional retardation, post-natal brain injury and post-natal infections were the least deviant categories. Language disorder in the mental retardations appears then to be associated as much with clinical category as with general physical and mental growth measures.

The DS group is evidently different from normal children and other categories of MR in respect to language use. Among the differences are a preference for certain parts of speech over others, a better verbal understanding than word use, a tendency to emphasise the first consonant and vowel sounds of words and a propensity to communicate with a minimum verbal complexity. Except for the ability to imitate speech and word naming,

Table 13. *Patterns of articulation*

Condition or cause of mental retardation	Measurable articulation								Not measurable			All patients		
	Stages (ages in months) of normal patterns of articulation						Deviant articulation	Deviant language	Total deviant	Conditions that may accompany any foregoing				
	30	42	54	66	Nearly adult	Total				unusual voice	physical anomaly	Total	M	F
Functional retardation	33	48	29	9	17	136	73	14	87	27	6	150	106	44
Mongolism	28	8	—	—	1	37	50	13	63	29	9	50	32	18
Congenital cerebral defects	17	17	9	5	8	56	30	9	39	19	23	65	38	27
Metabolic disorders	3	2	1	—	—	6	4	1	5	—	—	7	5	2
Postnatal brain injury	3	3	—	1	4	11	6	1	7	3	3	12	9	3
Asphyxia at birth	1	3	5	—	2	11	5	5	10	7	15	16	9	7
Mechanical birth injury	11	3	3	1	—	18	20	4	24	19	27	22	11	11
Rh incompatibility	3	1	—	—	—	4	3	2	5	5	5	6	4	2
Pre-natal infections	—	1	1	—	—	2	2	4	6	5	8	6	1	5
Post-natal infections	2	9	2	1	2	16	7	—	7	4	3	16	7	9
Totals	101	95	50	17	34	297	200	53	253	118	99	350	222	128
Male 222	63	53	33	13	27	189	121	33	154	54	46	222		
Female 128	38	42	17	4	7	108	79	20	99	64	53	128		

none of these is exclusively associated with mental age level or with the structural defects mentioned earlier. The foregoing generalities are offered with full knowledge that the evidence is incomplete. Notwithstanding, many of the reports include speculation about the antecedents of language disorder for the syndrome; tending specifically to favour cognitive explanations. Among these are peculiarities in decoding strategies, attention and retention disorder, whole-part perceptual problems, perseveration and cognitive rigidity and aberration of spatial sensing. Since the tactics of remediation will depend on the assumptions we make about mediational processes, the latter will be considered now.

Mediation hypotheses

Langdon Down offered that DS speech could be improved 'very greatly' by a simple scheme of 'tongue gymnastics'. Others have proclaimed that degree of gross retardation is the primary basis for the speech prospects of DS children, structural factors aside. West, Ansberry and Carr (1957), pronouncing on the speech habilitation potential for DS, offered that the 'possible result will be meagre and in proportion to the patient's level of intelligence'. A few have suggested that the brain mechanisms for language are particularly arrested (e.g., Brousseau & Brainerd). Brain pathology explanations date from Benda (1949) but these do not tell us (according to Buddenhagen) why some DS subjects are better verbalizers than others. Once again, the competing issues are shaped more by expectation than evidence. Neuropathological studies have identified impressive individual differences within the syndrome such that the existence of particular brain–speech links for DS and whether or not they are primary (neuro-maturational) or secondary (neuropathological), will be difficult to settle. Equally trying are the exclusively environmental explanations of how speech and language patterns are originated and sustained for the syndrome. The recent literature has avoided the distortions of oversimplified or extreme mediational positions (pure mechanics, IQ levels, injury or nurture) in favour of more inclusive cognitive process and peripheral system process explanations.

Speech and cognition

Debate on the relation of cognition and language can start from either of two assumptions; language as cause and language as effect. O'Connor and Hermelin (1963) allowed that retarded speech and language in the moderately retarded, including DS, restricts cognitive growth. Attenuated vocabulary is in turn associated with limited life experience. Rhodes *et al.* (1969) contended that language enhancement is the key to both intellectual and social growth. They say that intellectual gains are multiplicative and that 'the acquisition of structures or schemata make possible the acquisition of still other and more complex structures' (p. 75). The argument has problems of logic insofar as the deaf–dumb child, with no intellectual deficit, exhibits cognitive ability patterning much like that of the general population (Vernon, 1972). There is little doubt, however, that speech revives traces of past experience and enhances ongoing verbal performance (Luria, 1963). An alternative position is that neurophysiological processes, including their alteration by pathological events, are paramount to shaping rate of language acquisition and type or extent of language handicap. Gibson *et al.* (1959) tested academic success with core school subjects across three aetiological classes of mental retardation and reported IQ scores to be predictive of performance for only certain school subjects, regardless of IQ levels. Of seven primary school subjects tested, language and arithmetic appeared to be more closely bound to aetiological class than to gradations of mental retardation.

Engler adopted a two-headed centralist view. He acknowledged the contribution of anatomical limitation to the expressive facility of the DS individual but assumed that severity and quality of mental defect was equally important. Speech growth and styles, he contended, will certainly reflect primary imbecility, apart from aetiological considerations, but will also reflect the distinctive cerebral, other anatomical and peripheral-structural pathology of any given causal group. Benda (1960) conceded that 'comprehension is usually superior to expressive language for mongolism' (p. 70) whereas Spreen (1965 *a*, *b*) found that mental age attainment is the single most reliable correlate of communication disorder in the mental retardations. Thompson (1938) found receptive language better than expressive language for his single case study of DS, but claimed a similar developmental phenomenon for normal children and presumably for other classes of MR. Most textbooks on expressive ability in MR draw no distinctions among the aetiological categories in respect to the antecedents, mediation or remediation of speech and language. The recent literature does attempt to set DS apart by demonstrating how the apparently unique cognitive and peripheral characteristics of the syndrome impinge on speech and language facility.

The cross-aetiological comparisons of patterns and deviations, including the DS child, date from Blanchard (1964). Her approach, however, does not stratify for mental age and cannot support a clear separation of general cognitive deficiency from syndromic effects, whether central or secondary in nature. The Bilovsky and Share (1965) treatment of characteristic styles of psycholinguistic abilities for DS does control for age and cognitive specificity. Twenty-four non-hospitalized DS individuals were administered the Illinois test of psycholinguistic ability (ITPA). It was believed that: (i) subjects of similar mental age, across the mental retardations, would display dissimilar cognitive (i.e., language and symbol related) patterns, and (ii) declining IQ for DS would not be substantially due to a diminution of general cognitive potency, but represent instead a failure to respond to the intensification of psycholinguistic demands with increasing age. The nine subtests used included a decoding group (receptive language ability equated with understanding) and an encoding group (expressive ability). The subject groups ranged from 6 to 23 years of age with IQs between 31 and 86 points and a mean of 46.6 points. Internally compared subtest scatter showed visual decoding (understanding pictures and low verbal content) and motor encoding (expressing thoughts by gestures) as most advanced. Auditory-vocal sequencing (digit span) behaviours ranked lowest. Bilovsky and Share concluded that DS is possibly unique psycholinguistically; being poor for auditory channelling (encoding or decoding) and strongest for visual decoding and motor encoding. There was good intra-sample agreement. Other indications were for a special deficiency in the use of abstract symbols and a possible strength for the handling of representational types of material.

McCarthy (1965), also using the ITPA, questions some of the foregoing findings. While DS subjects were more homogeneous for pattern of psycholinguistic development, than controls, the major qualitative difference was a superiority of manual expression. Differences noted by Bilovsky and Share could, therefore, be an artifact of motor potential. Rempel (1974) has replicated the McCarthy study using older and more severely retarded DS subjects. His results show that DS individuals are indeed superior to comparable non-DS retardates for manual expression and visual memory, but inferior for auditory association, grammatic closure and auditory memory. The greater homogeneity of psycholinguistic pattern, recorded by McCarthy for the syndrome, was shown by Rempel to relate to visual reception, grammatic closure and auditory memory. In general, the visual components of the input and association processes were superior to the auditory equivalents.

A test of the relation of language potential and more basic conceptual capacity has been undertaken by Cornwell (1974) for five mental age levels, using Binet verbal and numerical test items. The differences between recognition and designation capacity, while equivocal, tended to recede with increasing age. Cornwell interprets the evidence for number concept lag in the syndrome as supporting a centralist viewpoint for language lag as against an auditory receptor deficit. He says, 'Apparently the impairment we observed in some aspects of verbal capacity was due not only to deficiencies in oral skills, but may also be attributed to abnormalities in cerebral integrative activity which are manifested as maturationally more primitive verbal behaviour' (p. 187). To what extent the results of these three ITPA studies are exclusive to DS and whether or not the 'circuiting' distinctions are central, peripheral or structural in origin is difficult to assess.

Other investigations, reviewed earlier, have touched on the question of circuiting and channelling patterns for DS using laboratory manipulations. Some have involved a communication component, e.g., O'Connor and Hermelin (1961), Knights *et al.* (1965, 1967), Clausen (1968) and Scheffelin (1968 a, b). A few merit second mention in the context of language anomaly. Gordon (1944) had been among the first to guess that DS individuals might display cognitive variability tied to modality channel or input–output circuit. O'Connor and Hermelin (1961) used a discrimination task for DS and other retarded subjects, varying the modality. DS subjects were superior for visual-shape recognition and other imbeciles for tactile-shape recognition. They, like Gordon, hesitated to speculate about the relative importance of peripheral (sensory) or central impairment in the equation. A CNS hypothesis was favoured, i.e., hypotonic inhibition tied to cerebellar damage or insufficiency would have important modality-related implications for both receptive and expressive functioning. Knights *et al.* (1965, 1967) attempted to separate motor-expressive factors from central events and reported a tendency to better visual-tactual discrimination for DS over other retardates. This observation was shared by Sackett (1967) in his cross-aetiological study of visual complexity discrimination.

A major problem with the foregoing studies has been a neglect of the possibly separate roles of input and output potential in assessing the precursors to communication efficiency. Scheffelin (1968 a, b) employed four stimulus response channels for combinations of auditory, vocal, visual and motor tasks in a paired-associate learning situation. Error rates for the auditory-vocal condition were almost double each of the other S–R channel combinations, although statistical analysis failed to show that stimulus modality or response mode alone were disproportionately influencing error rate. What seemed amiss was the channelling process itself which could involve central process failure peculiar to the syndrome. Further, Scheffelin suggested that poor tactual-kinaesthetic feedback can inhibit the easy development of articulation and that DS subjects might suffer a specific disorder of auditory feedback. Coupled with the postulate of centrally mediated hypotonia, which is maximal at the most vulnerable period of speech development, the soundest present conclusion would be that mechanical, sensorimotor and central anomalies act in collaboration to shape communication patterns. The mixture of factors, rather than the components as such, is probably critical. The tragedy is that as the hypotonia recedes and as sensory efficiency improves in later years of maturation, central neuropathological processes are accelerating. Accordingly, while the puissance of the antecedents shift, their interaction continues to disadvantage the speech and language status of DS individuals over their life span.

Artifactual considerations

Although structural limitations, input–output circuitry patterns and general intellectual defect are central to the development of speech and language for DS, other factors are germane. Circulatory defect and skeletal anomalies contribute to slow or defective psychomotor growth. Associated with these is the timetabling of cerebral dominance and lateralization. Van Riper (1954), among others, considers proper motor maturation important to the unfolding of speech readiness and to such related functions as directionality, spatial orientation, and auditory-perceptual patterning. With respect to DS, it has long been suspected that lateralization is particularly delayed (Thompson, 1963) and that muscular control lags disproportionately (Berry & Eisenson, 1956; Spreen, 1965a; Strazzulla, 1953). It can be fairly contended that lateralization and motor control delay are related to delayed speech (Share, 1975), whether the subject is Down's or not. Any procedure which would hasten motor coordination, such as patterned exercise, might advance the establishment of cerebral dominance and therefore of speech readiness. These possibilities have not been adequately explored for the DS child.

A number of investigators have identified slow reaction time as characteristic of DS (Berkson, 1960; O'Connor & Berkson, 1963; Hermelin, 1964; Astrup et al., 1967; Clausen, 1968; Hermelin & Venables, 1964). Other researchers have claimed that depressed arousal potential (Wallace & Fehr, 1970) and the reduced attention span are especially inhibitory to learning efficiency in DS subjects, including language learning. Kolstoe (1958) and Buddenhagen and Sickler (1969) found that attention training does enhance language growth and that attention span deficit is a by-product of hyperkinesis in many DS subjects. Buddenhagen and Sickler assumed, incidently, that hyperactivity in DS is largely learned and that as attention improves with training, speech skills too will advance. The biological predispositions of the DS individual to considerable impulsivity and to reduced attention is documented in an earlier chapter. Adverse environmental conditions no doubt aggravate these tendencies.

Impulsivity and temperament as components of general performance for DS has been discussed in the context of personality status (Chapter 6). Strazzulla (1953) identified personality factors as important to communication effectiveness in DS. Pototzky and Grigg (1942) were more specific. They observed that when DS subjects are 'angered they often seek solitude and review the disturbed situation aloud' (p. 508). What is implied is that the supposed stubbornness of DS inhibits speech use in a social context. Wunsch (1957) claimed that the 'phlegmatic, self-sufficient tendencies might disincline them to communicate with others'. A similar adumbration is made by Johnson and Abelson (1969 b). Lyle (1960 b) did note that, concomitant with speech improvement in DS, was a growth of affectional relationships with staff and of social participation generally. It is difficult to decide which is chicken and which is egg.

Finally, a wide selection of compensatory factors have been offered to account for speech problems in the syndrome. The proposed pantomime and motor encoding talents of DS individuals (e.g. McCarthy, 1965) are said to incline them to gestural rather than to verbal communication. There are others who consider the communication problem to be in the eye of the beholder. The reasoning goes that DS, as a clinical stereotype, invites a low verbal expectation and that the verbal environment is thus depleted. Possibly there was an element of this in the older institutional settings (Lyle, 1960 b). The expectation hypothesis has been examined more directly by Buium, Rynders and Turnure (1974) using six DS children and five normal children (CA 24 months) in home settings. Analyses included sentence use, length of utterances, word rate per minute, presence of negatives, and use of personal pronouns, all taken from recordings of language interaction between mother and child. Findings were that DS children are exposed to (i) a higher number of utterances but a lower mean length of utterances, (ii) a higher number of sentences and a lower mean length of sentences and (iii) a higher frequency of grammatically incomplete sentences, imperative sentences and single word responses. The authors conclude that the linguistic environment of DS children is different from normal children and that language acquisition in DS is somehow a function of that difference, biological determinants (Lenneberg, 1967) aside. The study proves only that, since the DS children were about half the mental age of controls, mothers provide a semantic releasor system appropriate to the readiness of the child. An investigation of DS and normal children matched for mental age might be instructive, nevertheless.

Management

Adaptations of traditional approaches

The popular approaches to speech management for the DS child share the assumption that a suitably diluted training regime will adequately serve, whether it be an adaptation of procedures used by parents and teachers for normal children (Brinkworth & Collins, 1969) or of those employed by specialists for the mentally retarded in general (Schiefelbusch, Copeland & Smith, 1967; McLean, Yoder & Schiefelbusch, 1972). Even conceding that there is considerable technology in these approaches which is applicable to DS children, the outcomes have not been impressive. The intent of the present section is to inspect those treatment studies which have something to say about the particular potential and limitations of the syndrome in regard to speech development and correction.

Those who have been impressed with the structural idiosyncracies surrounding speech problems in DS children have tended to be most optimistic about remediation. Brousseau and Brainerd (1928) echoed Shuttleworths' prescription that breathing exercises and lip–tongue drill would enhance communication effectiveness. 'To improve the power of closing the lips he (Shuttleworth) advises an ordinary pen holder-stick on a bone ring which may be held by the child between his lips for a few minutes at a time.' Further, 'blowing a whistle, puffing into motion a pellet of paper or a flake of cotton-wool helps in the power of pursing the lips necessary for labial sounds'. Finally, 'Opening and closing the mouth, so as to bring the teeth together, putting out the tongue and moving it to the right and to the left, and touching with it the teeth of the upper and lower jaw respectively are forms of exercise that Shuttleworth recommends as useful in overcoming many defects in articulation.' The foregoing quotes are from p. 171 of Brousseau and Brainerd (1928). These procedures represent an extension of Down's initial observations about treatment.

Benda (1949) linked speech and voice problems with poor nutrition, thyroid deficiency, myxoedema (associated with the raucous voice) and the failure of the DS individual to achieve motor proficiency. He recommended thyroid treatment to reduce the drying and thickening of the mucous membranes connected with voice quality and other hormonal combinations to improve general growth. Strazzulla (1953) tested thyroid therapy but with modest results. Of 16 cases receiving thyroid medication (specific to the hoarse, deep voice quality), five returned to normative levels appropriate to age and sex. None of the 23 non-treated DS subjects displayed similar gains in voice quality over the life of the experiment. Further study is required of optimal dose and age of maximum susceptibility. Other prescriptions have included the removal of adenoids and pharyngeal tonsils, etc. (Ardran, Harker & Kemp, 1972) laterality strengthening (Iida, 1973), directionality training (Share, 1975), and the exploitation of imitation (Voelker, 1936). It is Share's notion that directionality training might advance the use of words denoting spatial relationships. This conjecture could be easily tested, as could the suggestion that since brighter DS children employ gestures with some effectiveness that the encouragement of gesticular communication might provide a firmer conceptual base for later language training. Many of the programmes to be mentioned have tended to discourage non-verbal communication to force vocabulary development. Voelke found that an enriched language and social environment and the dramatization of semantic situations benefits DS children. The intention is to capture the emotional interest of the child and to exploit his supposed imitative facility. The echoic reproduction of sounds by DS subjects is possibly superior to other forms of mental retardation (Smith, 1975) but does not guarantee the acquisition of meaningful speech.

An imitation of modelling strategy has been tested by MacDonald et al. (1974). A five months programme was conducted using three DS children subjected to 2 months of language training by professionals in collaboration with mothers. Three months of additional home training was undertaken by the mothers. Three control children received no special programme. The imitation–conversation technique resulted in an improvement of length of speech and of grammatical complexity for the experimental subjects comparable to the expected rate of growth for normal children over a 3 month period. The results do not permit the separation of transitory echoic speech gains from more substantive or lasting language advance. Nor is it possible to determine if the major forerunners of these advances are primarily of a modelling or affective nature. A combination of techniques which exploit the relatively undamaged affect and suggestibility of the DS child, at appropriate ages, have been useful for other areas of habit training. Additional problems of interpretation are introduced by Tawney (1974) who gave ten DS children up to 1 year of daily interaction in a speech enriched environment which included the use of demonstration, imitation and appropriate reinforcement. The institutional setting provided total contingency management but no control group was used against which to calculate maturational effects over one year. All teachers and aids rewarded, for example, two word chains and then three word chains. As well, children were kept clean and encouraged to exhibit acceptable general behaviour so as to attract satisfactory verbal exchange. Findings were for an increase in intelligible responses but no significant increase in mean length of response. Disorders of articulation would be expected to recede over one year, especially under improved overall living conditions.

Those who have paired speech proficiency with general intelligence have been less optimistic about treatment outcomes. Mathews (seen in West, Kennedy and Carr, 1947) concluded that 'the true mongoloid is particularly unresponsive of speech rehabilitation and it is particularly useless to attempt such training'. Engler (1949) admitted that his speech training regime for institutional DS children was unsuccessful. He says, 'While I was able to obtain satisfying results in other respects, such as housework, gardening, easy handicrafts under patient supervision, I had no success whatever in improving their speech' (p. 84). While excepting the few mildly retarded cases and formes frustes, Engler says that families who have 'spared neither money nor other sacrifices...have had no better success than he' (p. 84). Others recommend a compensatory approach to speech remediation. Taking advantage of what Benda (1960) considers a relatively good memory, O'Connor and Hermelin (1963) proposed that an enlargement of the naming facility by intensive training would lead to improvement of the associative capacity and eventually to more complex speech. Barthel (1952), exploiting the child's affect needs, advised that an active relationship between DS child and mother can reduce speech handicap. Both suggestions have value in theory but are untested against control groups.

A number of studies have exercised proper controls while testing the efficacy of traditional treatment methods. Strazzulla (1953) undertook speech and language training with 17 DS subjects (IQ 25–60) and controls for up to 1 year. A parent managed regime was designed to stimulate speech play at home. Only one member of the treated group made no progress. Two showed excellent gains, ten good gains, and four fair gains. Seven of the fifteen controls displayed no gains, six showed fair progress and two good progress. Strazzulla concluded that relatively unspecialized speech management is profitable but that progress is dependent on the subject's status regarding orientation, socialization, academic readiness and gross muscle control. Given no serious structural defects, speech was seen to develop in DS at about the same rate as for other comparable retardates.

Lubman (1955) takes the position that the treatment possibilities are, in fact, greater for DS children than for other forms of retardation. Programming 150 retarded children, 48 of whom were DS, she found the DS child to demonstrate' more rapid and permanent improvement than the brain-damaged child with a comparable intelligence. Being generally more placid (the mongoloid) it was not so difficult to retain his attention during the lessons' (p. 299). Therapy was 15 minutes per child, per week, and included instructing teachers on classroom procedures to be used between visits. Parent counselling was geared to home supplementation of the classroom procedures. Lubman enumerated four principles of speech management for any mentally retarded person under IQ 50 points. The DS subjects were not differentiated specifically. A major guideline is that the therapist recognize and exploit, the 'eye-mindedness' of the severely retarded. Eye contact was maintained, although the use of a mirror for this purpose sometimes acted as a distraction. Phasing of the treatment sessions were altered *ad hoc* to renew patient interest and to maintain attention. Bribery, appeal to pride, stress on accomplishment (goals), all proved less effective as rewards than simple praise. The therapist preferred to initiate sessions with familiar tasks (sounds). 'This method served not only as a means of offering the child praise for a job well done, but also introduced the method of instruction. By this process the child was given a sense of achievement which encouraged him to greater effort when more difficult lessons were introduced' (p. 300). Practical and limited goals were pursued which recognized the restricted conceptual ability of the DS subjects. Satisfactory outcomes favour the younger children.

A test of speech remediation for institutionalized DS children was undertaken by Kolstoe (1958) making use of the principles enunciated by Lubman. The sample ranged from 5½ to 14½ years of chronological age with a mean IQ of 24.53 points for the experimental group and 23.07 points for the control group. Matching for the 15 pairs was based on IQ, CA, MA and age at admission to institution. Comparison measures included the Kuhlmann, the Illinois language test, and an observational rating scale. Three teachers gave instruction to five students for 45 minutes daily for 5 days per week. Treatment lasted for just over 5 months. The goals of the programme were to increase attention span and to introduce verbal symbols in play situations where the context of the verbal presentation could be varied. Reward (approval–praise) followed any successful word use. One goal was to achieve a state of overlearning. Materials employed for verbal discussion included picture books depicting home events, animals and trains. Scrap books were built by each child and depicted familiar events. Flashcards, dolls, household articles and so on were introduced to stimulate re-enactment play. Phonograph records, silent movies and field trips supplemented the programme. Results showed a 2.87 point IQ drop for the control group and a 1.2 point IQ drop for the experimental group. The differential retention of IQ, based on extent of language learning, is a questionable finding in view of an initial

IQ difference of 1.2 IQ points favouring the treatment group. A test of outcome for labelling and association training clearly advantaged the treatment group, nevertheless. Observational ratings of how the child subsequently used words and sentences in free play were disappointing insofar as the formal gains of the treatment sample did not seem to extend beyond the experimental situation. Most provocative was a finding that where the treated of the pair exceeded the matched control for formal language growth, relatively good initial mental age was evident for both. The results support the evident futility of intensive individual speech therapy for low IQ patients, the failure of gains to generalize for everyday use, and the uncertainty about optimal duration of therapy. Other problems are whether or not institutional and community placed DS subjects are clinically comparable with regard to speech potential, and the differential effectiveness of treatment approach (formal or permissive, group or individual). Tizard (1966), observing DS children in an open play nursery programme (institutional) cautioned that too much unstructured stimulation is counter-productive for speech training purposes.

The Brookland experiment in language enrichment by Lyle (1960) shares some of the problems seen in the Kolstoe study. Institutional and experimental DS samples were matched for CA and non-verbal IQ. They were part of a larger group including other varieties of imbecility. Over the period of study, DS subjects developed verbally at a slower rate than the other imbeciles, a discrepancy which was not altered by placement in the enriched environment. Thus, the DS cases appear to have some special disadvantages, related to developing communication skills, which are not exclusively a function of degree of mental defect. The finding is in accord with that of Mein (1961) and of Mein and O'Connor (1960), i.e., that severely subnormal patients differ with respect to language development depending upon aetiological class. Again, durability of gains and the generalizing of verbal improvements to non-laboratory situations have not been adequately examined. With respect to retention of gains, the evidence is discouraging. Harvey et al. (1966), using trainable mentally retarded children in a well-defined school programme, recorded the expected language improvement at the end of the school year and a notable loss over the summer months. Only the growth of social competence seems to have endured.

Syndromic approaches

Language treatment programmes for DS children, considered thus far, have not insisted on distinctive remediation procedures for the syndrome despite the clues they provide that such separation might be of value. Because outcomes have not been impressive, the more recent literature has attempted to capitalize on those aspects of communication deficiency which are specific to DS children (Rhodes *et al.* 1969; Talkington and Hall, 1970; Buddenhagen, 1971; Glovsky, 1972).

Rhodes and her group established a language stimulation and reading programme for the severely retarded DS child. Subjects, aged from 1 month to 4½ months, were admitted to an experimental unit of a state hospital designed to offer intensive individualized stimulation. A group of home-care DS infants were identified as controls. The language environment of the experimental group was stratified according to mental growth stages. Articulation training was also given, although the emphasis was more on directing the use of generous praise or enthusiasm for attempts at receptive or expressive language. Articulation correction was delayed until there was evidence of 'conceptual pegs on which to hang the appropriate sounds' (p. 24). Reading training was initiated at a more advanced point. The programme was graduated in easy steps from words to phrases to sentences, each step reflecting the child's progress. Stress was placed on reading as a vehicle for conceptual development, word concepts being acted out or made concrete in various ways, e.g., fast, push, pull, here versus there, etc.

Following 2½ years of language stimulation, the mean IQ of the experimental group had moved from 31 to 42 points, the percentage of spontaneous work combinations had increased, and articulation errors (substitutions, distortions and omissions) had decreased. The programme illustrates the possible benefits of (i) an early start to long-term training, (ii) communication training as a foundation for intellectual and social growth, (iii) the value of enthusiasm and intimacy in programming and (iv) the need to train ward personnel (or parents) in the mechanics of language stimulation. Speech, they say, does not magically emerge even in so-called good environments, especially if the verbal content is thin and if gestural communication is permitted. It is not evident, from the data presented, what improvements were observed in the home controls or what progress would have been made by equivalent DS children in the regular programme of the host institution. The approach is of interest because it recognizes a number of the intellectual, motor and affective properties of the syndrome.

Two other recent language training studies of DS have stressed speech remediation as a promoter of conceptualization (Talkington & Hall, 1970; Buddenhagen, 1971). Talkington and Hall employed Gotkin's (1967) matrix language programme for 30 DS subjects with an average IQ of 40.7 points and an average CA of 24.2 years. Twenty control subjects were given music activity classes with a quantitatively similar involvement opportunity. Their mean IQ was 39.1 points and mean CA, 24.5 years. The matrix games, purporting to develop receptive and expressive language, comprise a series of pictures and shapes. The child was instructed to 'place a red circle on the boy wearing a hat', and was then required to say what he did. Subjects were given ten daily trials over 20 days. Tapes of performance were evaluated for language and concept usage, particularly in respect to the increasing appreciation of prepositions, articles, sentences, colours, shapes, plurals, similarities, differences, missing parts and number analogies. Total language use and total conceptual performance were also assessed. Testing was conducted 'before and after' for all 40 subjects. The experimental group experienced significant gains for sentence and total language use and for four of the five areas of concept formation. While the immediate gains were convincing, the impact was short-lived, raising once again the questions of long-term retention of language learning and its transferability to non-laboratory situations.

Intensive remedial procedures for limited gains is best illustrated by Buddenhagen (1971). His therapy is based on Sapon's (1968) procedures. Paraphrased, these include (i) the phonetic analysis of initial behaviours to determine which component of the subject's extant repertoire could serve as a remediation base-line and lead most rapidly to viable speech, (ii) ensuring effective social and material reinforcement for successful responses, and (iii) providing a context which would make the subject's responses appropriate in terms of meaning or content. That is, when the child had been taught 'Iwanna' he was offered a toy animal to elicit the 'Iwanna' (horse) response and was then given the horse. This device was said to promote the target response and to provide the reinforcement 'which was made contingent upon successful responding'.

Buddenhagen's four non-talking DS subjects were notably aggressive and had IQ scores of 'less than 10'. These scores are probably underestimated insofar as all four had learned self-feeding and dressing, were toilet trained, and were able to perform simple cottage routines. Treatment consisted of a two-part programme of 22 and 10 hours of individual instruction over 11 and 15 weeks respectively. Subjects did learn a few words but these were evidently not used outside of the experimental setting. No attempt was made to assess the permanence of gains either at the verbal or conceptual level.

No controls were established for maturational events over the course of the study, these being thought unnecessary. The notable advances appear to have been non-verbal in nature, subjects achieving some improvement in general behaviour. Buddenhagen concluded that speech, in severely retarded DS individuals, can be initiated or improved providing there are no serious structural disorders; an unrealistic expectation. He identified the institutional environment as a 'most serious impediment to the acquisition of vocal, verbal repertoires by mongoloid children' (p. 162). Among his other findings, relevant to DS individuals, are (i) the need to work with attention disorder, (ii) the remedial value of social reinforcement when combined with material reinforcement and (iii) the particular suitability of an imitative approach for communication training. While these observations might each hold true (more or less) for all severely retarded children, they suggest an overall philosophy of language therapy which is consistent with what is known about the socialization and arousal status of DS children.

What Buddenhagen will demonstrate for many readers is that intensive effort can be modestly effective for speech improvement, in the short run, but that the secondary gains provide the major pay-off. A more tractable and less distractable DS child is a worthwhile goal, even though communication continues to be substantially postural, gestural and guttural. Glovsky (1972) is among the few who promote a flexible combination of voice and language therapies for the syndrome. He maintains that the symptom picture shifts with age and that language difficulties are shaped by the sensory and perceptual peculiarities of the condition at different maturational stages.

A number of less programmatic remedial studies of DS speech problems have been conducted (Castellan-Paour & Paour, 1971; Mansfield, 1972; Sidman & Cresson, 1973; Jeffree et al. 1973; Tawney, 1974), two of which are relevant here (Mansfield and Jeffree et al.). Mansfield conditioned abstract motor responses to prepositional speech for 24 DS subjects ranging in age from 8 to 36 years. Subjects used a small object and container so as to learn the prepositions, 'in', 'under', 'beside' and so on. Food, praise and patting were the rewards and new objects were introduced to ensure conceptual spread. The findings support the proposition that 'spatial-contextual' training hastens language acquisition for the syndrome. Curiously, good and poor performers did not differ for mental or physical age. An analogous approach is taken by Jeffree, Wheldall and Mittler who argue that the language difficulty of DS children is more acute for the construction of sentences than the mere learning of words. Subjects were two DS boys, at CA 4 years and MA up to 2 years, who had achieved single words. A pivot-open practice instrument (POP-IN) was devised which is a large posting box into which familiar articles can be dropped and retrieved by use of a lever if a pivotal word is used, e.g., gone. Teaching was undertaken in a play setting with social reinforcement employed throughout. The key measure of success was whether the two-word sentences, so acquired, would generalize outside the experimental situation and whether pivotal words would be attached to other open class words (gone dinner, gone potty, etc.). The two subjects showed short-term gains under both controlled and real-life situations but only one retained these gains. The approach recognizes the conceptualization and directionality difficulty of the DS child and the relevance of these skills for language growth beyond simple word naming.

In a nutshell, the management of speech in DS children has had limited success compared with other areas of functioning and with other categories of mental retardation. The blame is two-fold; the assumption that remediation practices need not differ from those used for other classes of MR and the belief that environmental manipulation provides the most powerful or sole treatment approach. Where environmental methods have been relatively effective there has been an emphasis on the syndromic aspects of motor function, temperament, modelling, memory, etc. However, where strong initial gains have been shown, follow-up has been negligible.

Evaluation

Enquiry of any kind can yield impoverished results for two reasons; because the question is poor and because the answering data are badly generated. The area of verbal and voice disorder research for Down's syndrome suffers in both ways. Most investigators have worked from academic and professional assumptions based on research with normal children or on unrefined MR samples. One extreme argues that the improvement of verbal facility, by intensive training appropriately timed, enhances cognitive facility. The other extreme counsels that the correction of the structural defects associated with speech will (at best) uncover whatever native intellectual ability is available for language promotion. The first approach ignores the somatic features of the syndrome and the second under-estimates their complexity. Zisk and Bialer (1967) in their study of the symbolization, articulation rhythm and phonation qualities of DS, concluded that more appropriate management techniques will emerge as our appreciation of the biological bases of speech and language for the condition improves. Language remediation without regard to the mechanical, sensorimotor, circuitry, arousal and cognitive peculiarities of the DS child is likely to fail. Many of these qualities can be manipulated as part of treatment.

Articulation and other expressive limitations have been attributed to auditory processing and storage difficulty, and to limitations of kinaesthetic feedback and inhibition process. The impulsiveness, short attention span and motivational attributes of the syndrome are also important considerations when designing treatment. A number of workers have suggested that a general cerebral integrative fault exists for DS in addition to any specific cognitive anomalies; although it is a moot point considering that comprehension is often in advance of expression. Language training and treatment would proceed on a broad front, begin very early and be closely allied with continuing medical and behavioural programming. For example, bilateral motor system strengthening would be followed by laterality and directionality training. Sensory training would be extended to grouping and classing exercises to improve conceptualization. The demand and capacity of the DS child for affectional bonding can be exploited through the use of imprinting, modelling and play situations as a background for language experience. Social reinforcement is especially useful for the DS child, as is spatial-conceptual training. The visual-motor system would be favoured for language training as would any regime which capitalizes on rote memory and the perseveration tendency. Exclusive dependency on the latter, however, would fail because simple word naming drills do not necessarily lead to more complex or abstract language.

In short, the chances of successful speech and language training for DS children is dependent on the overall remedial approach. Even so, speech and language gains might continue to be fewer than for other areas of development. We could reject the need for intensive language training, pleading that semantic behaviours have an artificially high priority in modern society, were it not that the acceptance of DS individuals in society is a matter of transactional skill and that it is the intention of policy-makers to expand the community integration of all MR.

10

Behaviour management:
I. Decision and reaction

What happens to the DS infant, child and adult is dependent on the quality of our helping technology and on contemporary social attitudes as expressed by parents, professionals and the community. The two sets of conditions, management practices and server or receiver group attitudes, are never easy to separate. For instance, the decision in the 1950s that institutional care be abandoned rather than improved was as much culturally as empirically founded. The emerging demand for preventive public health measures in the form of compulsory amniocentesis, while scientifically motivated, is difficult to reconcile with existing public policy and individual beliefs. Accordingly, an evaluation of current support technology for the syndrome will first require a consideration of the literature on disclosure of diagnosis, reactions to disclosure, and the responsibilities and rights of the child, the family and society.

Much has been said and written by the experts on what to do with a retarded child. The advice comes in two parts; making the initial decision for or against maintenance in the family unit and shaping the decisions about care style and procedure, whatever the domicile. Advice varies subject to whether the child is of custodial, trainable or educable calibre but, beyond that, all retarded individuals are treated as more or less similar for purposes of psychological handling. Manuals of instruction are readily available on problems of habit training, socialization and habilitation for the retarded as a class. There is much less material on management problems particular to Down's syndrome because parents often contend that their DS child needs no more than the love and consideration due any child and because many professionals tailor remedial regimes to degree of mental defect only and to the availability of local resources.

The purpose of the present chapter is to identify those factors which

261

influence the overall management decision for DS; including the effects on family and community and the nature of counselling services. The chapter to follow will deal with techniques of management as these distinguish the needs of the DS individual from those with other forms of mental retardation.

The decision for management

DS is different

Yates and Lederer (1961) commented that parent reactions are not only those of having a retarded child but also of having a 'mongoloid' child. The impact of parents is syndromic at the outset, at least in respect to images. The reasonably consistent physical features are evident at birth thereby reducing diagnostic equivocation, or self-deception about prognosis, so telescoping the usual family adjustment period between suspicion and decision. A span of hospital nursery care, commonly enforced while the paediatrician and others test and debate the condition, is usually unnecessary for the DS infant. As a result, there is unmitigated shock, shame and guilt which can colour parent willingness to cope with the child. Unlike many other categories of MR, the immediate temptation is to place the infant for nursing care until old enough to be institutionalized (Stone & Parnicky, 1965).

Where the temptation to care for the child at home does persist, it is muted by the stereotype. The still used term 'mongolian idiot' carries an aura of monstrosity and of potential danger to siblings and community. Friends, relatives and neighbours reflect these fears, however subtly, offering less sympathy and support than they might have for a blind or damaged baby (Parmelee, 1956, Hormuth, 1953). Nor is there any hope of spontaneous arrest or significant expectation for corrective neuro-surgery, maturational catch-up, diet or drug treatment. The placement decision and management processes are distorted accordingly; a problem of diagnosogenesis (Hormuth, 1953). Tizard and Grad (1961) report that the most asked questions by parent of DS infants are whether or not maturity will bring violent behaviour or psychosexual difficulties. It is not surprising that institutional requests in the pre-school years disproportionately favour DS individuals, even though they are paediatrically less difficult than other custodial or trainable levels of mental retardation. (Giannini and Goodman, 1963).

The parents too are different. Saenger (1960) traced mental retardation across all socio-economic levels and ethnic groups, recording a tendency towards higher frequencies in the less culturally and biologically advantaged strata of society. The DS child, however, represented a higher family socio-economical level, was a product of better established families (Giannini

& Goodman, 1963) and had older (more experienced) parents. The families were more often northern European in extraction, demonstrated upward mobility in the social and economic system hierarchy, were nuclear rather than extended, tended to be self-sufficient and were more sensitive to exhibition of shortcomings. Their reactions took the form of anxiety about community opinions, fear that the child will fail to achieve prescribed goals, and concern about 'bad seed' in family lines. The DS child can become the focus for these concerns as well as provide a pivot for whatever other family stresses are associated with middle-class striving. The result is an inclination to early institutionalization, often encouraged by the family physician who shares their cultural values. If the DS infant and child is retained in the home, without external aid, the conflict heightens. The mother soon discovers that the DS infant is not so difficult and begins to form emotional attachments. The reaction is either to hasten a disposal decision or to over-compensate through care (Katz, 1972). If extended home care is undertaken, the mother eventually discovers that the first evidence of benign reactivity does not promise well for later motor, cognitive or communication growth (Share, Koch, Webb & Graliker, 1964; Lyle, 1959). Her disappointment can be doubly bitter, because the investment has been highly personal and the expectations centered around middle class achievement values. It is not surprising that the debate about home versus institutional care for Down's syndrome has been both vigorous and unscientific.

Changing approaches

The management decision for DS is usually faced just following birth and in an atmosphere of diagnostic or prognostic shock. In the fourth and fifth decade of this century it was fashionable to recommend that the child be placed on an institutional waiting list while receiving early care in a private nursing home until eligible for public care. The primary concern was for the psychological and social welfare of the family. Styles have changed during the past and present decade to favour home care supported by a network of community facilities. The concern is obstensibly for the physical and psychological well-being of the DS infant and child. The shift was prompted by a number of factors having little to do with the merits of the various care alternatives. North American and European society had become more child-oriented and relatively affluent. At the same time, the large public institutions had failed to recover from the decline of standards, budgets and quality of staffing suffered during the depression and war years. The pressure was squarely on parents to undertake extended home training and to participate in the building of community support services. Institutions were vilified, being viewed as a terminal resource likely to be considered only by the unfeeling or the desperate. The body of corroborative research which appeared was consistent with the cultural and sentimental swing to home care and with the more respectable animal and infant research on the effect of extreme deprivation. The analogy was an improper one for many group care facilities but did apply to a number of especially derelict institutions.

The major home versus institution studies have been reviewed in the chapters on development and intelligence. They demonstrate that at-home DS children enjoy a better physical and behavioural status than DS children in institutions. The conclusions was that institutions, of any kind, were unhealthy and home care was universally preferable. Physicians and other professionals were advised to counsel accordingly, the only exception being for severe multiple handicap or genuine family incapacity. Foster home placement was recommended as the preferred alternative in the latter case. What about the evidence? The most common sampling tactic has been to compare age-matched DS children who had been institutionalized with those still at home but on the waiting list for admission. The early intake is presumably from among the more medically and psychologically difficult or represents families in difficulty. The two sets of circumstances are not independent. Otherwise, there is no convincing research concerning nurtural effects on DS children randomly assigned to clearly different care situation. The major problems have been to match properly for physical, psychological and family status prior to taking a care decision (home versus hospital) and to assess development rates reliably across types of group care or across different traditions of family care. The influence of home care for the DS child, on other family members, is even less well understood.

Among the more satisfactory comparative examinations of management outcomes is the work of Stedman and Eichorn (1964). They reason (i) that if type of early environment (home, foster-home, hospital, etc.) is not linked differentially to growth rates for the DS child then placement decisions could be centered on overall family well being, and (ii) that if quality of care regime only is significant we should identify the components so that effective nurture can be practised across various settings. Ten of their cases were admitted to institutions in infancy while ten others continued in home environments. The home-reared showed superior social and mental maturity. Little difference was detected for motor growth between care regimes. MacNeil (1955) reported a similar finding. One exception in the Stedman and Eichorn sample was a length and weight difference favouring the home care group. There was no important disparity at age of walking to explain the length difference. Looking at the Centerwall and Centerwall (1960) data, Stedman and Eichorn extracted only those DS children from the home and hospital samples who had walked at equivalent ages. When motor status was held constant, IQ and SQ differences largely disappeared. The evidence suggests that comparison samples are seldom matched for initial neuro-maturational status, and therefore, any general conclusion about the origins of other behavioural distinctions between care groups are suspect. A second part of the study was experimental. It included an intensively staffed hospital nursery situation with many of the nurtural features of the home. The results showed that the major shortcomings of traditional institutional training is in the verbal area and in finer motor coordination. The provision of small play objects and the use of older patients in the language environment significantly reduced the lag between the home and hospital samples for both performance areas. Francis (1970) had found his institutional sample to be less object-orientated and to display more self-orientation and diffuse movement than the home-reared sample. Lyle (1959) also singled out traditional hospital programmes as being less efficient for communication skill training. More opportunity for social contact and response-provoking programmes were recommended. The problem would seem, therefore, to lie with the content rather than with the geography of the care programme. Location in or out of home is probably less relevant than the provision of appropriate releasor systems for growth. Spcecial group programmes are being designed to achieve goals similar to good family care and with the additional advantage of technically expert staffing.

Family care varies by style, quality and outcome in much the same way as across types of group care. Carr (1970) tested motor and mental growth for at-home, fostered and institutional DS babies. The home samples were further stratified for social class (manual and non-manual family employment). Examination at regular intervals disclosed better progress for the at-home infants on the average and a spread of developmental indices favouring infants of the non-manual family group, although the latter finding is not consistent with a second study (Carr, 1975). Noteworthy is that motor growth favoured the at-home over the fostered sample from the outset, a finding which illustrates the difficulty of sample matching. Similar results, across family socio-economic strata, have been reported by Kostrzewski (1965) and by Gibson (1967). Very capable or well-provisioned parents appear able to provide sufficient stimulus intensity to surmount the depressed sensory thresholds of DS infants and to encourage early motor growth in the face of muscle and reflex system immaturity. They probably also provide superior nutrition, give suitable attention to the respiratory and circulatory risks, and take advantage of the relatively unimpaired affective potential of the DS child in order to guarantee a strong mother–infant interaction leading to effective social learning. Less inspired parents, working mothers and families close to the poverty line – the majority – might not be able or willing to meet these priorities without direction and assistance. In short, a specialized technology now exists for the care of the DS infant and child but must be applied very early in his life span. A large number of families do not adjust to the calamity of a DS child soon enough to seek specialized management or can not cope with an arduous training regime for other reasons. Group care, located within the community and begun in infancy, can involve parents to elicit the combined effects of professional and family care. Two problems yet to be faced are cost and countering the view that routine family care is magical, whatever its quality and whatever the alternatives.

Striking a balance between the rights of the DS child and those of his family and community involves many imponderables. Parents have been known to institutionalize the DS child when quite young only because of family guilt or fear. Other parents institutionalize, sooner or later, because of severe behavioural difficulty and compounding physical disorders requiring intensive care of the DS child, major emotional effects on the mother, social and psychological damage to siblings, economic hardship or imminent marriage break-up. A few families sense the need to give a period of residential training to a DS child whose future in the family unit is limited. Lyle (1959) found that 59% of his sample were admitted because of parent inadequacy while only 8% of admissions were attributed principally to the difficult behaviour of the child. Menolascino (1965, 1967) reported that 13% of his outpatient DS sample were psychiatrically disturbed whereas DS children being admitted to hospital showed a 36% frequency of psychiatric disturbance. The statistics of custody choice (Saenger, 1960) are difficult to evaluate given the tendency of parents, seeking admission for their child into crowded institutions, to create the impression of child or family inadequacy. That they would do so is evidence of inadequacy of sorts.

Negative effects on the mother, of rearing a DS child, are not well appreciated. Aldrich (1947) observed that the easy infant–mother attachment, during those first quiescent months, is of little prognostic value and can predispose to later family disappointment and rejection. Mothers also suffer the effects of removal from normal family and community activity. Fotheringham et al. (1971) documented evidence of more frequent family break-up for at-home DS children over those families who had institutionalized the child. They also reported that the two sets of children, one year following the hospital placement of one set, were developmentally similar. A longer follow-up period would be necessary before reaching conclusions about the differential effects of venue. It is conceivable that circumstances exist where the well-being of the parents and family take precedence over those of the DS child. In these cases, supervised foster homes can be employed at considerably less cost than intensive hospital nursery care. Foster care is not a popular option, however, because infant separation in our culture is tantamount to child abandonment whereas 'hospitalization' is socially sanctioned. Otherwise, families who hospitalize and those who do not come to see their decision as the best for all concerned. Caldwell and Guze (1960) found no ultimate difference in mothers and siblings for either alternative although he wondered if both groups might differ from families where no retarded child had been involved.

The influence on the normal siblings of home-bound DS children and youth is a separate issue to some extent. Hormuth (1953) claimed that the normal siblings are not harmed and that home management for DS is no different than for any other child. He offers a list of 'rights' for the DS child but does not relate these to human cost or to the rights of others. Schipper (1959) argued that most stable parents do adjust to the demands of home-care but was less sure about the adjustments of the normal siblings. Sibling problems were related by him to the effects of having two sets of child-rearing rules. Normal siblings viewed the double standard as discriminatory. Dittmann (1957) wondered if normal children are able to provide a suitable peer environment for the DS child or whether a more realistic care situation would include other DS children. Carr (1975) concluded that the presence of younger normal members tended to disadvantage the DS child. Various writers have mentioned the unfortunate effects on younger normal siblings who model the inadequate behaviour of the older DS brother or sister. The social isolation of the DS child in his neighbourhood, the decreasing mobility of DS families because of the fear of making unsatisfactory adjustment to a new neighbourhood or town and the anxiety or embarrassment of normal sisters at the dating age, are all documented in the literature. Good effects have been mentioned as well. Certain parents experience social awakening with the presence of a handicapped child which is translated into community leadership. Some normal siblings find a vocational interest from their home experience or else develop a tolerance and understanding well in advance of their years. On the whole, though, the evidence on sibling effects is not encouraging. Fotheringham et al. (1971) found the largest decrease of family stability to be in the 'areas of sibling functioning and the parents' adequacy of caring for their children' (p. 67). They also say that 'the decrease in sibling function would seem to be the result of the retarded child's continuing presence, when considered in the light of other studies (Farber, 1959; Farber & Rychmann, 1965), which indicate that the presence of some retarded children has a detrimental effect on their siblings'. (p. 67–8.)

These findings are in accord with those of Gath (1974) on the siblings of DS children living at home. Antisocial disorders among the school age sisters were especially obvious when compared with control families. Normal children most at risk were those with mothers over 40 years old at the birth of the DS member and those from large families in the lower socio-economic classes. Perhaps the adjustment of the normal siblings is some function of the demographic status of the family rather than of 'mongolism' as such.

What surfaces from a generally weak literature on the issues associated with the care decision is that much of the research has been designed to denigrate group care. There is no doubt that early and sustained home-care is effective and economical where the severity of the condition is not too great and where the family is willing and able. Many families are not especially strong and many DS individuals are not promising in terms of the ratio of care effort to prognosis. Professionals who fail to make balanced recommendations in the best interest of the DS child, the family and the community are negligent because they are moved by prejudice, one way or the other.

In summary, it is now evident that properly designed group care can replicate good family care and that the unique assets and deficits of the syndrome might require some form of grouping for remedial purposes. It is also obvious that specialized community care for DS individuals will require a considerable network of support services and that the population of DS adults, as it increases in absolute number, will lead to demands for quasi-institutional residential services. It is unfortunate that the institutional model was not revised soon enough in the form of community-living modules with strong professional services and easy family access. While the de-institutionalization and de-professionalization of services for the mentally handicapped has provided mixed results, the exposure of the damaged child to society has been useful. Now that routine 'disposal' is discouraged and the retarded are visibly among us, social attitudes about genetic counselling, therapeutic abortion and the ethics of withdrawal of treatment are changing. So, hopefully, is our insensitivity about adequate research support for early detection and prevention and our reluctance to experiment with legislative guidelines to family planning and integrated management systems, The future of these issues is dependent on reaction and decision at the parent level.

Rights and responsibilities: the child and family

The White House Conference on Children and Youth has drawn a Bill of
Rights to be applied regardless of race, creed or handicap (American
Association on Mental Deficiency, 1973). The particulars include such rights
as understanding parents, a decent home, adequate shelter, religious guidance, maximum opportunity for development, life in a community where
the welfare of the child is of primary importance, appropriate and non-
injurious employment commensurate with ability and prompt diagnosis and
treatment. The DS child had not enjoyed most of these advantages. Parents
would feed and cloth them, physicians label them mongoloids and recommend institutionalization, psychologists test them and pronounces imbecility,
social workers counsel adjustment to inevitable separation, and educators
declare them uneducable. (Hormuth, 1953). Much has changed, especially
the understanding of parents and the advances in diagnosis and treatment.
However, parents and siblings, neighbourhood and society, also have rights
as well as responsibilities. The rights of the DS child will sometimes be in
conflict with the rights of others and compromises will be sought. The
assumptions about children's 'rights' too, are tenuous. Some societies prac-
tise surrogate family care, teach ethics and morality on a non-religious basis,
and apportion limited community resources such that the child's needs are
important but not primary. Some even question the necessity of everyone
having a job, i.e., that the handicapped continue to do the least interesting and
most tedious tasks when a machine technology could well afford them the
opportunity of self-fulfilment in non-vocational ways.

Given such wide disparities in working assumptions and codes of conduct,
between and within societies, it is not surprising that professional practices,
parent reactions and care decisions are so diverse. Aldrich (1947) identified
a fundamental incompatibility of family goals and nurtural effectiveness with
the DS child. He recommended immediate institutionalization and initiated
separation counselling at birth; including realistic disclosure about prognosis,
the description of institutional programmes and the anticipation of guilt which
accompanies the ultimate abrogation of the mother–child bond. Schipper
(1959) argued against early hospitalization because high infant mortality for
DS, coupled with immediate placement, are apt to produce lasting guilt
feelings in the parents. A number of medical counsellors have recommended
a pregnancy reasonably soon after the DS birth, to produce a normal infant
and to satisfy the expectation void. Gustafson (1973) tells us of a mother
who refused routine corrective surgery for her DS child's intestinal blockage
thereby hastening death. The mother had exercised a natural right to govern

the number and quality of her progeny, but in so doing, denied the right of the DS child to life. The issues are not so different from those surrounding the abortion debate. They are a matter of priority of rights and the dispersement of responsibility in given cases, religious and metaphysical considerations aside. Parsloe and Rose (1972) give an account of a 75-year-old mother looking back on her life of 33 years with a female DS offspring. She expressed bitterness and cynicism in regard to community reaction and to the professional treatment she received. Her expenditure on home care was not justified in personal retrospection. We do not yet understand the long-term effects of home care either on the child or on the family. Would most parents agree, 40 years later, that their initial decision for home or institutional care had been the best one? Would most agree that there had been no damage to parents or normal siblings or that the gains of intensive management had been worthwhile? Share *et al.* (1964) conceded the difficulty by recommending home care on a tentative basis until the assets of DS child and the coping ability of the family, became clearer. Most professionals today propound home-care on a long-term basis. They claim significant benefits for the child and at no enduring cost to family or community. They submit that the initial decision of many parents for separation is a matter of misunderstanding or social discomfort and that negative sibling and neighbourhood reactions are marks of immaturity and prejudice, to be ignored. A more guarded assessment is made by Edgerton (1975). He proposed that we know only that parent and community attitudes to DS vary considerably by region, class, religion and ethnic origin. All are honestly acquired beliefs which have survival and adjustment value for the individuals and groups represented. To influence them we need (i) to know more about the stratification of beliefs across society and (ii) to test the tolerance limits of the community to the Down's individuals who are increasingly among them. Edgerton recommends further research into the nature and limits of the interaction of DS individuals in various community settings and situations, including with parents, siblings, neighbours and teachers, and in various strata of the cultural hierarchy.

Disclosure styles and methods

Accounts of reaction to disclosure are either anecdotal or statistical. Wilks and Wilks (1974) provide one of many anecdotal treatments of the subject. These parents remember most clearly the subconscious nagging that idiots come from idiots, the fear that the other children would suffer and an apprehension about neighbourhood reaction. Each is a legitimate problem of pride and guilt, self-definition or fear for the future of child and family. Of the considerable and conflicting advice they received, some proved useful, e.g., having home help, mother maintaining her career interests, having another and healthy child as promptly as practical and realizing that clumsy or negative community reactions are symptoms of the uncertainty and embarrassment of others which time and familiarity usually soften. These buffers are not available to all families.

Tizard and Grad (1961) asked 80 mothers how they had been told and how they would have wished disclosure to be managed. Seven were informed at first suspicion, 11 when the diagnosis was medically confirmed and 28 somewhat later. Self-discovery was the route for 29 mothers. Data are lacking on five families. The preference of the mothers was in the order of immediate disclosure (89%), disclosure after diagnostic confirmation (17%) and self-discovery (3%). The realities and the ideals of disclosure are not well matched. Kramm (1963) studied 50 families including 20 who were advised that the child was normal (at birth) and eight who were told nothing for up to 2 years. Some of these valued not being told until a rapport had been established between mother and child. Other families appreciated the immediate and often blunt disclosure. There is evidently no formula for telling, timing or manner, which will fit all cases. A third of the parents appreciated either the blunt or the late disclosure whereas the majority wanted to know early and fully. The soft or evasive disclosure was prognostically confusing to some families because it created uncertainty and the false hopes that delayed their accepting the condition. Blunt disclosure and negative prognosis pleased other families because having the worst declared initially, they were subsequently pleased to find some assets and better than expected development for the child (Kramm, 1963). Perhaps there is a difference between forthright disclosure and clumsiness or insensitivity. One case of disclosure, in my experience, was made by the family physician and paediatrician who argued about the diagnosis in the nursery, to be overheard by all. Another is of a physician who telephoned the father at his office while he was distributing the festive cigars. He was told quickly and crudely. The father dissociated himself completely from the mother and baby and the mother underwent psychiatric care.

The question of whether disclosure should be immediate or withheld for a short period (weeks to months) is a difficult one. Confirmation of diagnosis by karyotyping takes a little time and is a justification for delayed disclosure in equivocal cases. In some instances, the mother has had a difficult pregnancy or delivery and prompt disclosure might slow her recovery (Drillien & Wilkinson, 1964). Others advise withholding diagnosis until the mother–

child relationship is strongly established. For the clinically obvious DS infant, the danger is that a neighbour or relative will make the diagnosis, thereby distressing both the parents and the physician. According to Drillien and Wilkinson (1964), over 50% of mothers had suspicions before formal disclosure. Parmelee (1956) advises immediate disclosure as a parents right, done tactfully, simply and with proper follow-up. Carr (1975) has confirmed the earlier findings of Berg, Gilderdale and Way (1969) that 60% of mothers were told in the first months and that while early disclosure is generally advisable, who does the telling is less critical than the manner of telling and the ability of the news-bearer to respond to questions about prognosis. In too many instances, the informant was not sympathetic and was not able to give accurate information about the syndrome. For the majority, therefore, disclosure should be prompt and professionally managed. There will be other occasions (e.g., uncertainty of diagnosis, maternal problems) where disclosure could be delayed or presented in stages.

Manner rather than timing of disclosure is possibly the nub of the problem because initial reaction to the medical opinion tends to influence later decisions for placement or home care and degree of parent commitment in either case. The physician, too, has his problems since he is as reluctant as anyone to be the giver of bad news and shares the middle-class aspirations of his patients. He might anticipate their disappointment in the form of reluctant or clumsy disclosure. Drillien and Wilkinson (1964) found physicians' disclosure to be especially delayed for the first born. Otherwise, disclosure timing did not relate to parent social class. In some instances, errors of disclosure are simply a lack of experience with a syndrome that is seen relatively seldom in community medical practice. In the final analysis, disclosure technique will be consistent with the professional style of the physician and guided by what he knows about the family. However well done, the reactions will be different and sometimes difficult.

Reaction and advice giving

The correspondence between poor quality of initial reaction to a DS birth and an unfortunate manner or timing of disclosure, while strong, is neither perfect nor irrevocable. Attitudes to the DS birth can be modified by counselling and information-giving processes for many parents. Others are unyielding. Kramm (1963) found that a minority of parents refused the diagnosis, however delivered. Seven of 50 families blamed the hospital or physician. Eight blamed family genetics (the other side of the family) and twelve identified the birth with God's punishment or test. Six families continued to deny any serious problem, holding to the belief that the child will catch up, needs special therapy, or has been a victim of unreliable IQ tests. Perhaps self-deception protects the affectional bond and should remain undisturbed, especially in those cases where acknowledgement of the disorder brings strong rejection or serious family upset. Another personal example involves an immigrant couple who had married late to produce one child, a DS female. They refused the diagnosis which was obvious, clinically and dermatogly-phically, because the physician had concluded that the first few months of development were essentially normal. Their affection for the child and gratitude at having produced any child was intense and not to be denied.

Lobo and Webb (1970) identified three distinctive reaction groups; those who rejected the child, accepted after initial shock or gave a degree of acceptance after the passage of time and experience. Of ten families, two rejected, five accepted and three eventually offered limited acceptance. These ratios are reasonably consistent throughout the literature and have led to a search for antecedents of reaction. Schachter (1960) favoured a social-class explanation. Parents of limited education and economic circumstances accepted the condition reasonably well and took professional direction easily. Families at the higher cultural and social levels were of two types, (i) those wanting placement away from the home and the district, either for status reasons or because of a fear of negative effects on the normal children, and (ii) those who accepted the challenge of home training, read professional journals, reached their own prognosis (usually optimistic) and ignored the physicians opinion about the future of the child if not in agreement with their own. Lobb and Webb (1970) had found the best acceptance correlates to be with families of stable wage earners. These families were not especially ambitious and not strongly religious; but they did tend to be emotionally secure, with satisfactory marriages and larger than average numbers of children. Rejection was associated with good parent education, self-employment, and social striving indices. Other rejecting parents showed marriage difficulty and emotional instability in the mother. Previous ex-perience of the family with the syndrome, as relative or neighbour, was a negative contributor to initial reaction. Presumably, these families had a more realistic view of prognosis or had experienced at close hand the community disavowal of handicapped persons. In the main, though, resisting parents are of two types; those who have family goals built around formal achievement and community place to which the DS child cannot aspire and those who cannot absorb the additional strain on the integrity of the home unit. Both sources are legitimate, or not, depending on how one views the priorities of family life.

Schipper (1959) associated negative initial reactions with self-renunciation and guilt about adequacy of pregnancy care. Projection of blame on the physician or the father and his family was evident for some mothers. Grandparent reactions were generally disruptive and the father's reaction was more often than not comprised of denial and an intellectualization of the problem. In large families, catholic families and immigrant families, the fathers reaction was more tolerant (Kramm, 1963). The initial impact on the parent relationship was the most dangerous effect. Ten of Kramm's 50 families reported marriage disruption and discussion of divorce. Nine parent sets decided on no further children and eleven sets delayed further children. The balance were older mothers who wanted no additional family. The influence of a DS birth on family planning is considerable but out of proportion to the genetic risks. Social activities were severely restricted for 12 families, somewhat restricted for 16 and unaffected for 22. Sixteen families diverted their social activities into community helping fields. Only 10% of the Kramm families admitted to a sustained negative reaction and 14% to having benefitted not at all from the experience. The balance (76%) claimed to have found maturity, spiritual growth or purpose. It is not certain whether these 'gains' have any practical value beyond the resolution of cognitive dissonance.

Reaction to disclosure is one thing and reaction to follow-up advice quite another. All of Kramm's families displayed a degree of tension and disruption for the 6- to 10-year span of the study. The weight of physical care required was most often the central factor. Over the period, 25 families of the home care group had essentially coped while 25 others had serious difficulty. Certain families strengthened their internal ties and developed stronger protective instincts both to the DS child and to each other: a response to real or imagined community rejection and to the initial tragedy. Yates and Lederer (1961) found some family strain to stem from uncertainty about growth expectations and the helping resources likely to be available to them as the child grows older. Many parents expressed anxiety about how to interpret their dilemma to relatives and neighbours. Stone and Parnicky (1965) discovered that family reactions differed depending on if a preliminary placement decision has been made, however tentative. Where a management decision had been taken there was less intense interest in the DS child and less sense of crisis. The result might be premature abandonment or neglect of the DS child in some instances and a useful objectivity to the problems of nurture in others. The placing of the child on a waiting list for institutional care appears to be an adaptive device insofar as expected failure to cope is hedged. Many waiting list DS children, are, in fact, not placed when their turn comes, despite continuing external pressures to place (Stone and Parnicky, 1965). A case can be made for waiting lists as their own reward.

Edgerton (1975) believes that the diversity of parent and community reactions to the handicapped child is natural and that an improved understanding of the motives behind different care decisions would be useful. Research of this kind is just beginning. Holroyd and McArthur (1976) compared parent stress as between a diagnosis of DS and childhood autism, noting that the nature of the handicap is an important determinant of direction of parent reaction. Fifteen scales, representing 285 true–false items, were applied to several dimensions of parent, family, and child problems. The canonical correlation analysis showed greater distress in the mothers of autistic children compared with DS children. The separation of syndromic effects (the nature of the handicap) from expectation level (higher socio-economic status for the parents of autistic children) is, however, not clearly made. The scales did reflect a greater concern by mothers of DS children for the developmental status of the child and, at the same time, a greater pessimism about outcomes. Effective parent guidance will need to be based on an appreciation of both the biological and value system variables which shape parent reactions and their subsequent care decisions. The Chigier (1972) cross-cultural study of DS children, in the family context, is an example of the latter concern.

The four concerns; child, parents, siblings and community

The placement decision (whether, when and where) has many sides which are shaped by family and community attitudes, social resources and professional practices. Immediate institutional placement is, in any event, difficult unless the family has the finances to afford private care or unless family breakup results in enforced custody or foster-home placement. The greater majority of parents are counselled by their physician, family agency, parent organization, or diagnostic screening clinic. The advice is almost always for home care, at least to whatever age is accepted regionally for institutional admission. Most professionals advise continuing home maintenance to adolescence but allow that a family can reverse that decision if serious difficulties develop. The parents are encouraged to enlist a wide range of facilities; community pre-school and clinic programmes, home visit teams, parent relief programmes, special schools for the retarded child, sheltered industry and community group homes. Parents follow this route, sometimes reluctantly, because hospital care for the very young is out of fashion and is decreasingly available at reasonable cost.

Despite growing community support capability and organized pressures for home care, parents still institutionalize or apply to do so. Some of the reasons have been mentioned. These include the social stigma of the term 'mongoloid idiot' or any of its euphemisms, the impact on the parent and siblings of long-term home care, neighbourhood prejudice and a concern for the welfare of the DS offspring, when the parents are too old to cope. The ingredients of the parent decision are therefore complex and made more so by the idiosyncracies of professional advice. Kramm (1963) found that 44 of his families ($N = 50$) had been advised to institutionalize and 32 at once. Others were told that death was imminent so that home care would be brief. Advice aside, fewer than half the parents applied to institutionalize their DS child and of these the action was perfunctory, the majority having never visited an institution. When asked, 15% of the families believed the institution to be a setting for special training, medical care, recreation and companionship. About 50% of the families viewed institutions as custodial and of use to them only when the parents could no longer sustain home care. The balance declared institutions as useless or had no opinion. Parents who sought hospital placement most vigorously tended to have a DS child who was the oldest in the family or found the growing DS child increasingly difficult to manage, i.e., fear of his strength or impulsiveness. The home-bound waiting list of DS children was otherwise indistinguishable from non-applicant families. As the DS child aged the family acceptance of institutional care increased, indicating that many of the reasons for placement are bound up in the changing nature of the condition with age. Other later sources of pressure to institutionalize were the welfare of the other children, the growing restriction on family activity and the social shame felt by the normal siblings concerning real or imagined constraints on courting. The older DS child or young adult on the waiting list displayed a lower social quotient and was more severely retarded than average for the syndrome. Kramm cites the problem of ageing DS individuals at home who now have no suitable comparisons and who suffer loneliness and boredom. Parents who opt for home care in the pre-adolescent years often find that the changing nature of the condition, coupled with changing family needs, favour an eventual move to group care.

It is evident that factors favouring early placement differ from events contributing to a similar decision for older DS individuals. The elements determining early placement include young parents planning further children, financial problems, inadequate disclosure, marriage instability, external pressure and the 'status maintaining norms and values' of the family (Farber, 1968). Lobo and Webb (1970) reported that the mother is the key to immediate acceptance and the father to the long term decision about continuing home care. The determination to place, sooner than later, was a function of the severity of primary handicap and secondary behavioural problems; determinants which influence in turn, family stability and extent of community acceptance. The influence of professional advice on the placement decision, was less than the clinical status of the DS child and the opinion of mate or relative respecting the welfare of the family as a whole.

Wolfensberger and Halliday (1970) consider many of the foregoing clinical and family factors, entering into the management decision process, to be moulded by social and subcultural pressures – i.e., the gross socio-ecological variables. They surveyed the state of Nebraska by county for any relation between rate of institutional placement and county population density, buying power, voting patterns, distance to hospital, etc. No single factor was significant, although all factors combined to represent 50% of the variance associated with a choice for institutional placement. Since the grouped factors co-varied with family and clinical variables no linear cause–effect inference was possible. The argument appears to be that if middle-class striving could be blunted, or if community concern for the quality of its members could be reduced, then all DS individuals would meet with a happy tolerance in home and neighbourhood. The vision has merit. Inevitably, however, the goals of any modern society and its nuclear unit, the family, assign a high priority to competence and productivity as a guarantee of its overall stability and survival. All else is secondary.

An interesting criticism made by Wolfensberger and Halliday of waiting-list studies bears repeating. It is that waiting-list families differ according to whether or not they eventually exercise the option. We would need to know more about the personal and cultural variables associated with families who use waiting lists for supportive purposes and those who firmly intend external placement at some suitable age. An equally interesting question is how the families of DS children, who have taken the option of early institutionalization, differ in value systems from socio-economically similar families who have not experienced a retarded member. The survival 'instinct' of many parents might well dictate expedious disposal of the DS child, if not otherwise restrained by professional advice or special interest group pressures. For other parents, the protective 'instinct' predominates whatever the cost or advice.

Varieties of psychological counselling

The counselling of parents of DS children, usually in groups, provides a clear example of difference in objectives among the various helping professions and between families. Yates and Lederer (1961) found parent concerns to be directed first to the practical problems of prognosis, immediate manage-ment and the interpretation of the disorder to relatives, friends and neigh-bours. Even late in the counselling process the expected cathartic reaction did not develop strongly, most parents continuing to be concerned with information seeking. Docile acceptance and adjustment to the seeming intractibility of the disorder was less satisfying to them than dealing with the pragmatics, either regarding home care or placement planning. Group counselling did result in some guilt reduction for the mother, over time, although the tendency of mothers to sustain their guilt or anxiety is possibly a key motivating force to problem solving. It is believed that a dispropor-tionate number of the prime movers in parent associations for the mentally retarded are parents of DS children. The condition is particularly anxiety provoking because it is clinically visible and because the parents of DS children are often themselves among the more visible members of the community.

Giannini and Goodman (1963) assessed the impact of a DS member on 'rejecting' families and the effects of special clinic and counselling services on the mutability of the placement decision. Their sample was the first 100 families to make contact with the clinic. Of the DS children 60% had been privately placed and 40% were in home care awaiting placement. The findings confirm previous research. The parents of the DS children were at higher socio-economic levels and were more generally 'adequate' than families representing other forms of MR. Still, the tendency to institutionalize the DS child was stronger and was attributed to greater middle-class striving and social-mobility needs. The negative community image of the 'mongolian idiot' also played a role. Giannini and Goodman recommended temporary placement as a device to give parents a 'before and after' ex-perience. Success of clinic counselling was measured by the reduction of the waiting list, although the favourable results might be a product of the popular but uncertain advice that parents should expect less development for the DS offspring while in group care.

In the same vein is an investigation by Stone and Parnicky (1965) involving 103 families of DS children. Institutional care of the child was applied for by 50 families. The eager placers were less affluent or had greater family difficulties than the non-eager. Among the most provocative aspects of the findings were that parents with the most knowledge about the syndrome were least willing to place. Tolerance to home-care declined, however, as the DS child grew older; especially if the child was male and if family integration problems became subsequently acute. The quality of parent life style was a vital component to a decision to retain the child in the family. Like other studies of this nature, the important counselling needs were for information rather than for catharsis, guilt reduction or other psychodynamic prescription. The success of counselling required the involvement of both parents, the counselling of the mother only leading to care decisions which were later vetoed by the father.

Parmelee (1956) was among the first to stress appropriateness of counselling content and tactics. His primary goal was to reduce the strangeness of the syndrome, chiefly by didactic means. Parents were told that the DS child is often happy and manageable in the early years. Other problems in counselling included countering the impression that the growing DS individual is dangerous to himself, family or neighbourhood and that an initial decision for home care prohibits a different later decision when the prognosis is better established. Murphy *et al.* (1973) have added that adequacy of counselling requires the professionals involved to be technically qualified with respect to the distinctive aspects of the syndrome and that more emphasis be given to the adjustment problem of the normal siblings. Many failures in home-care can be identified with the shifting attitude and needs of the normal brothers and sisters.

The label is one of the major barriers to family and community acceptance. Hormuth (1953) claimed that the initial family acceptance of the DS child is better before than after the diagnostic tab has been affixed. Many writers have recounted the prominence of the term 'mongolism' for the direction of parent reaction and decision. The public conception is more readily that of a creature or monster than for any other major category of mental retardation. Diagnosis is usually obvious at birth, is distributed across all classes of society and appears in families having no history of mental retardation. The temptation of the surprised family, relatives, and neighbourhood is to cast the event as an affliction, or as a punishment somehow deserved. Public education is likely to be more corrective in the long term than revising labels every decade or so.

Social and community prejudice has played a significant part in shaping parent decisions about care. Kramm (1963) reported that 27 of his 50 families had difficulty facing the neighbours and 16 avoided neighbours. These families reduced their mobility so as not to have to explain the syndrome again to new neighbours. In the end, however, 35 families made a satisfactory adjustment to their community. General social activities of the family were severely restricted for 16, somewhat restricted for 16 others and not at all restricted for the remaining. All recalled neighbourhood cruelty to child or family during the process of adjustment. Schipper (1959) found that a significant minority of his families were met by negative community reaction. A major feature of district acceptance was how open the parents were and how they appeared to accept the DS child in the family unit. The neighbours tended to govern their responses accordingly. It appears then that the more the parents understand and come to terms with the condition, the less is the overt resistance in the immediate community. Appropriate counselling can hasten that understanding.

Whereas parents deal with community prejudice by isolated self-sufficiency or by meeting it directly, the growing normal siblings face it in stages as their social sensitivity and vulnerability increase. The discovery crisis is repeated at different steps of the sibling's growth and social learning experience. Kramm's data is corroborative. Social distress in the normal siblings was reported by 18 of the families. These events were more common where the parents were also embarrassed either for the DS child or for the normal siblings. Among the particular sibling problems were unwillingness to entertain friends at home, the distortion of the dating behaviour of normal female siblings, and the difficulty of explaining the syndrome to essentially immature peer groups. Internal perplexities included resentment about the distribution of family resources, the distortion of attention appropriate to sibling ages and the restrictions on family social and recreation travel. The difference between sibling acceptance and non-acceptance of the condition appeared to depend on parent attitudes, whether or not the normal siblings were themselves well-adjusted, the place of the DS child in the sibling line (youngest is best), family economics, family life style and achievement strivings and the age-related social aspirations of the siblings. Early institutionalization raised different problems for the normal siblings, including guilt fantasy, genetic fears and the dread of discovery (Jolly, 1953). It is likely, then, that parents who have entered into long-term home care with only modest reservations and appropriate resources will trigger fewer frustrations among the normal children. The ultimate effects on normal siblings of the DS child institutionalized early, but firmly rooted in the family album, are unknown. Counselling has not extended very far beyond responding to disclosure reaction in parents; and, all to often, in only the mother.

The research on reaction to diagnosis and the initial decision for care supports the relevance of style and timing of disclosure, up to a point. Many families are immune to counselling efforts and many professionals or lay counsellors give advice based on some single belief system. Two extreme positions are that DS infant and child care can be delivered effectively only by the birth-parents or that a poor prognosis for DS does not merit the heavy commitment of family resources even in the short term. It is now known that most families can cope with the DS infant and pre-school child and that many can continue to manage into the later growth years, especially where family support and relief services are well developed. A significant minority of families cannot cope, however, and these require early placement opportunities for the child. The experimental literature indicates that we know enough about the special developmental needs of the syndrome to design such services, although the high cost is problematic. The future debate will be in the area of care styles for the DS adolescent and adult. Family configurations change with time and some of the less desirable features of the syndrome are emergent with age. If the custodial model is to be avoided, the community should evolve residential-training services which permit a gradual transition from family to group life in a community context. Tied to these services will need to be a programme of ongoing guidance so that parents can anticipate changing management needs as the DS child grows to adulthood and beyond.

Psychological aspects of genetic counselling

Jarvik, Falek and Pierson (1964), in their review of Down's syndrome for the psychologist, asserted that the 'Quotation of accurate facts and figures without consideration of their impact upon the individual seeking advice may have devastating consequences' (p. 395). Three aspects of genetic counselling having psychological implications are informing the general public, advising parents and siblings, and assisting the increasing number of DS adults in the community on matters of marriage and birth control.

Public health counselling

Recent evidence is that life expectancy for DS has risen from 12 to 16 years and continues to rise (Stein, 1975) as heart and respiratory disorders, accidents, leukaemia and childhood infections are better controlled. Stein refers to the growing imbalance between incidence and prevalence for the syndrome. While incidence is probably decreasing, prevalence and visibility are increasing. Most parents no longer seek institutional care because support services for home care are improving and institutional bed space is shrinking as a matter of public policy. These related events have contributed to a public awareness of the condition and a readiness to respond to public health measures and preventive screening procedures. Stein, Susser and Guterman (1973) have focussed on certain of the difficulties of such programmes. The information that mothers over the age of 40 contribute ten times their proportionate share of DS births, or that mothers over age 35 contribute five times their share, is frequently noted in the media and will likely result in a modification of these data for the future. There are problems, however. Women are being encouraged to establish and sustain careers, to remain longer in post-secondary education and to postpone childbearing. The creation of a good deal of public anxiety about childbearing, past 30 years of age, might reduce normal childbearing in a female group which is positively skewed for educational status. In order to protect this gene pool, a case could be made for tolerating the increased risk of DS births. The spreading use of amniocentesis, to detect chromosome anomalies during pregnancy, will reduce the dilemma considerably in the coming years.

Amniocentesis as a public health measure, on a compulsory basis, is another matter. Amniocentesis is the aspiration of amniotic fluid from the uterine cavity. The cellular content is cultured for identification of the karyotypes associated with DS and can lead to a recommendation for therapeutic abortion. Pre-natal diagnosis and selective abortion, if problem free, could mean total prevention. The caveats, as seen by Stein (1975), include accuracy of the process, risk to mother and a number of ethical considerations. Among the specific concerns is a success rate of culturing which is less than 100%, the possibility that a clinically anomalous mosaicism could be missed, that a mosaicism which is clinically normal could be aborted and the difficulty of pre-natal diagnosis for dissimilar twins. Other questions concern the effects of amniocentesis on the fertility of aborted younger women. The dangers of induced abortion are not apparently greater for older mothers than the problems associated with uninterrupted pregnancies. Possibly the greatest restraints to mass screening are cost and manpower. Stein speculates that the cost of universal pre-natal screening could exceed the cost of caring for the existing population of DS and that amniocentesis and karyotyping are delicate technical processes requiring considerable vigilance and training. Finally, the religious and cultural debate on compulsory screening and abortion, in an open society, would be a bitter one. Further research into better and easier screening techniques and the development of a compatible social ethic will be necessary steps to the prevention of DS and other handicapping disorders of genetic and pre-natal origin.

Family counselling

Interest in genetic counselling often follows the turmoil of disclosure and the period of family agonizing over competing strategies of care. Genetic counselling undertaken in that time frame should be sensitive to the guilt, fear, and ethical concerns of the parents. Family superstitions and the educational background of parents, relative to coping with technical information, are also important. Parents evaluate risk figures and other genetic data in terms of their beliefs, community and family pressures, social position, economic circumstances, age of mother and the number and ages of other children in the family. Antley, Ray and Hartlage (1973) testing the effects of genetic counselling on parent self-concept, noted the greatest improvement (employing before and after self-concept scales) in the mother. Genetic counselling should, moreover, be continually available because personal concerns and the readiness to explore technical material will differ within and among families as they adjust to the condition over months or years. Initially, the family is interested in assurances about the genetic status of the family line, past and future, and in relieving anxiety about pre-natal mismanagement. In the great majority of cases, the cytogenetic record permits the giving of these comforts and sets the stage, technically and emotionally, for more complicated counselling. That opportunity comes after a care decision has been made, however provisional. It might focus on a family plan to risk a further pregnancy, be a product of the interest of older normal siblings anticipating marriage, or reflect parent uneasiness about the eventual reproductive status of the DS offspring as physical maturity and the prospect of community habilitation approaches.

The primary tool for genetic counselling will be the result of careful karyotyping taken from tissue samples of the DS child, family members, or prospective mother. The client will need to know if the clinical condition is a non-hereditable standard trisomy – over 95% of all cases – or a potentially hereditable translocation form. Mosaicism carriers can be identified in terms of percentage of affected body and sex cells and the extent of genetic risk calculated for parents and normal siblings. These risk indices might vary by maternal age, region and ethnic origin. The availability and reliability of amniocentesis can be discussed if a further pregnancy is planned. Finally, the fertility prospects of the DS adult, along with the management of his sex education, will be important counselling concerns for the future. Much of the relevant information can be found in Penrose and Smith (1966) and Benda (1969). The chance of giving birth to a DS child, for any mother, varies from about 1 in 2500 at the age of 19 to 1 in 45 past the age of 45. The danger is especially accelerative beyond maternal age 35 years. Once a mother has a DS child, however, the general risk increases by over twice the population risk. Barring other complications a risk of 1 in 20 will be acceptable to many whereas 1 in 10, or less, will not be. The decision about what constitutes a tolerable risk is one best left to the informed client.

The 2–4% of all DS individuals who show other than the standard trisomy karyotype leads to a number of special psychological problems for genetic counselling. Clients with translocation DS children want to be told if sibling karyotypes are normal and the significance of the distinction between the D/D and D/G types. Fathers carrying the D/G translocation have a low risk of producing a DS child but can have up to 50% phenotypically normal carriers in their offspring. From pooled data, it is evident that mothers who carry the D/G translocation will have about equal proportions of normal children, (normal karyotype), phenotypically normal carriers and transloca-tion DS children. These ratios are for full-term births and do not include the significant frequency of spontaneous abortions (Reed, 1963). More com-plex still are the G/G translocations which can involve (i) the fusion of chromosome 21 and 22 to produce proportions of normal, carrier and DS offspring similar to that seen for the D/G translocations, or (ii) the fusion of two 21 chromosomes or the presence of an iso-chromosome 21 (combi-nation of the two long arms of 21). Repeated miscarriage might suggest the latter case. However, the distinction between chromosomes 21 and 22 of the G group is difficult to make: especially to determine if the two acrocentrics are both DS. Until the evidence is better elaborated, it is safe to assume that the genetic risk is high. Chromosomal analysis and expert counselling is especially indicated for young parents of a DS child, parents with more than one DS child and parents whose relatives have had DS children (Becker, 1966). Karyotyping and counselling of the normal siblings is also indicated. The ideal would be to screen all new born for chromosome disorders.

Another prospect for the future includes the extension of genetic coun-selling into behavioural prognosis. The classical stereotype for DS is possibly most representative of the majority standard trisomy-21 condition. A number of studies, reviewed earlier, point to (i) a separation of certain intellectual, motor and personality characteristics for trisomy and translocation subtypes of Down's, (ii) a possible graded quality of intellectual potential depending on percentage of cell mosaicism and (iii) an extension of somatic to beha-vioural consequences which might be specific to karyotype.

Advising DS youth

The genetic and psychosexual counselling of the DS adult will become necessary as more such individuals find places in the community. These could include, disproportionately, the mosaicism and translocation cases. A component of the popular movement to 'normalization' is that the mentally handicapped be allowed to marry and to enjoy a relatively unfettered life-style. Although fecundity and sexual responsiveness are apparently reduced in DS individuals, the possibility of fathering or bearing children is likely to be increased with improving health standards and relaxed supervision. Some jurisdictions have managed the problem by compulsory sterilization legislation, much of which has now been repealed (Gibson, 1974). What remains is voluntary sterilization or sex and marriage counselling. Many parents rebel at the notion of further biological assault on the DS youth or the use of coercion, however subtle, to gain consent for sterilization. The alternative, sex education, is not a convincing one because retention of consequences in the abstract is not a strength of the DS individual. It is likely, on balance, that parents and other advocates will be persuaded that sterilization is indicated in those cases where community integration is the preferred goal. While techniques for the prevention of Down's syndrome (by public health measures and by family counselling) are at hand, the problems of implementation are ethical, cultural and psychological.

Conclusions

The literature on disclosure, reaction and follow-up counselling does not support simple formulae for solution and does not convince the writer that current practices are especially influential. The major value of the research reviewed is in the complexities it exposes and the need to provide services which recognize different needs among communities, families and the DS population.

What we now suspect is that:

(1) Some families are so inadequate or unstable that prolonged home care will be to the detriment of DS child and family unit. Other parents are geared to intellectual achievement and are reluctant to expend resources on a member who will not enhance the status of the family in the community. These positions work against the DS child but have real or imagined survival value for the family as a whole. The happiest circumstance is the family of a DS child which is not organized exclusively around intellectual and social class achievement, where non-material considerations

are valued or those which support traditions characteristic of the extended family ideal.

(2) Life with a DS member proves, for certain families, to be rewarding. A useful study could be undertaken to determine if 20 or more years with a DS offspring or sibling has been, on balance, productive, and for whom. A better sense of care priorities might emerge. The impact of the DS child on the family is never negligible and we understand so little about benefits and losses, beyond the early years of care. Carr (1975) offered the encouraging data that most families were able to cope in the pre-school period. Mothers' health, holidays, discipline problems, and extent of fathers' participation in child rearing were not different from a control series of non-DS families. There was no promise of similarly favourable comparisons for the later years and dread of the future was identified as the main source of family stress.

(3) Family attitudes to care are governed importantly by the place of the DS child in the sibling line and by the age of the parents. The DS member, as last child to older parents, enjoyed the most willing acceptance. Family readiness to offer early home care was also influenced by the prospect, if not the fact, of external options should the parents be eventually unequal to the task.

(4) The medical and behavioural prognosis of the DS child is important to his acceptance in the family. The application of significant family resources to the nurture of the DS individual who shows less promise than usual for the syndrome or where prognosis has not been adequately reviewed, does not satisfy common-sense values.

(5) The needs of parents for early counselling, individual or group, is oriented to information about the syndrome for planning purposes. Most do not want professional intervention in their personal sorrow or cathartic release. Counselling for a management decision is also complicated by the fact that fathers, mothers, siblings and other relatives react in distinctive ways and base their decisions on different information.

(6) Normal siblings have less of a committment to the DS event than parents and, being less mature, are more subject to the longer term psychological consequences than are the parents. Too little research expenditure has been made in this area.

(7) The decision for home management or external placement, including the timing of placement, differs for DS children over other equally retarded children. The reasons, both sociological and syndromic, require further study.

(8) Factors contributing to the early placement of a DS child are not the

same as those bearing on the disposition of the older DS child or adult. The elements of early placement are much better understood than those contributing to a decision for later institutionalization.

(9) Community readiness to accept the DS individual, as child and adult, is tenuous. Families who have come to terms with home care appear to invite adequate community reactions. The evidence so far, though, is based on the DS child in society. Reactions to the DS adult in society, in any increased numbers, is unknown.

(10) Long-term home care can be successful if appropriate community support services are available. It is also evident, from recent pilot projects, that residential group care can achieve good standards of infant and child training and that parent involvement is useful if only to avoid the suggestion of child 'abandonment'.

II

Behaviour management:
II. Varieties of care

For the first 50 years following the identification of Down's syndrome the scientific and professional literature was largely descriptive. Little advice was given on management because, after all, life expectancy was short and hospitalization was socially sanctioned. When a formal treatment literature did emerge, its recommendations were built around degree rather than quality of handicap. Management distinctions among types of mental retardation were hardly necessary in custodial settings where gradation of mental handicap could be related to intensity of group care requirement. Parents were the first to believe that the condition exhibited peculiarities of growth and behaviour which might warrant more exclusive management practices. Researchers, notably in paediatrics, psychology and education, have followed that lead and produced a considerable body of information about the conditions under which DS children learn and grow. A current stage is the translation of research to practice in the form of demonstration projects, worldwide. When these projects have born suitably controlled longitudinal outcome data, we will be in a position to choose among the present experimental techniques to construct a syllabus of management specific to the syndrome.

The present chapter presents the unfolding of our thinking about remediation for the syndrome.

Varieties of early care

The conference reports

Among the first multidiscipline conference reports is *Mongolism – A symposium* (1953). The content includes sketches of the psychological, communication, family and educational needs of the DS child as these were viewed

288

a quarter century ago. The Yannet chapter on paediatric management and the Rosenzweig material on school training are especially conspicuous because distinctions are drawn between the needs of the DS child and the other forms of mental retardation. Yannet argues that, even given an MA of 5 years, the DS child is not necessarily a candidate for regular kindergarten because their frustration tolerance is too low and because the resulting resistance creates learning blocks. He favours a personal adjustment and life-skills approach to education. At home, the emphasis is placed on a closer than usual mother–child bond which is gradually reduced as external control is established through training. The nub of these pathfinding opinions is the admonition that we (i) intervene early in the maturational process, (ii) stress social skills and (iii) build on the relatively good effect or temperament of the DS child.

Rosenzweig noted a dearth of educational material prepared for the disorder: a product, he says, of the assumptions that its members are uneducable and not different from other moderately to severely retarded children in quality of learning capacity. The distorted or elongated growth schedule of DS children is mentioned as having educational significance. Benda (1969) agrees. He claims that we do not exploit the mental plasticity of DS individuals into the second decade of life. Thus training is terminated too early. There has been evidence since to question these observations. Of special interest in the Rosenzweig report is an early reference by Talbot (1937) that when sensory, structural and motor difficulties in DS are abated, general learning aptitude improves. Otherwise, Rosenzweig appeals to environmental constructs, e.g., 'the emotional and intellectual behaviour of the adolescent or adult mongoloid may be an artifact rather than of genetic origin' (p. 286). These positions were popular at a time when little was known about the biological basis of behavioural potential for the syndrome.

The Wisconsin Association for Retarded Children conference (1968), reported as *Mongoloid Conference Proceedings* (1969), demonstrates that the accretion of management research, specific to the disorder, is variable across disciplines. The contents range from a consideration of the common medical problems of DS infants and children to the residential and vocational needs of the more mature. One of the better remediation chapters is by Elisabeth Kaveggia. Congenital heart anomaly, bowel obstruction, hernia and the incomplete separation of toes and fingers are mentioned as correctable. Respiratory tract disorders are attributed to the small nose, very narrow nasal airway and enlarged tonsils. Hence the child is a mouth breather with an innordinate intake of unfiltered and unwarmed air. The heart anomaly permits a mixing of oxygenated and returned blood and, as a result, the heart must pump faster. Blueness, skin mottling, easy fatigue and low energy output are a few of the consequences. Coupled with a tendency to low sensory system acuity and overfeeding, the result can be a lethargic and overly placid infant or a child whose drive for experiencing is below his capacity to benefit. Circulatory problems also contribute to hypotonia, including the muscles involved in breathing. As well, the diaphragm is weak and the lungs are not properly ventilated. Contrived movement or handling, so as to improve air supply, serves to enhance arousal and motor potentials. Immunology procedures require particular attention because of an increased susceptibility of DS infants to infections. Special procedures include medical services for tonsils and adenoids, the use of infant seats to encourage sensory and postural growth and frequent position changes to develop more effective breathing patterns. By the age of 5 years, or so, muscles systems are maturing and the danger of infection is receding; a point when more strenuous training programmes can be implemented.

Kaveggia is particularly concerned with feeding problems as damaging to growth rate. The DS infant has difficulty adapting to milk because it causes phlegm, congestion and choking. Skim milk and the use of cereal and fruit are recommended. If protein intake from other sources is adequate, milk refusal should not be of great concern. Fresh fruit, vegetables or their fluids prevent constipation as well as providing alternative nutrition. Bowel movements should be recorded for the DS infant and child because, while bowel obstruction and peritonitis is readily signalled by the normal child, these might go unnoticed in the DS child. Skin dryness and lip cracking can be reduced by not bathing daily, by using soap sparingly and by careful rinsing. Hair should be shampooed only every few weeks. Humidifiers in the nursery and the use of skin creams on uncracked surfaces is recommended. The effects of these elementary precautions influence both health and behaviour.

From the same conference proceedings are several articles on education and training. Educational opinion (Contrucci) stresses discrimination training (colour and sound differentiation, finer motor control, etc.). Setting appropriate limits and providing consistency of handling are thought to be the routes to improving self-discipline. Formal education is not especially valued, classes for the DS child being seen as principally recreational for the pupil and respite-giving for the parents. The material shows little sensitivity to the research literature on the special learning handicaps of the syndrome. Allen talks about sheltered employment and promotes the view that DS adults are more or less like other mentally retarded with respect to programme requirements. Probstein discusses adult day centres built round the needs of the parents. These needs are not always those of their DS offspring and should not be allowed to distort training priorities. Townsend overviews the residential care choices to conclude against institutionalization unless forced by medical or behavioural crises. A shared programme, using community and institutional resource, is promoted for most. Thus, with the exception of the paediatric material, the emphasis of the conference proceedings is parent organization invested and 'human rights' directed. The reader is helped to understand the philosophy of the parent movement but is told little about specific remediation methods for DS beyond the suggestions for improving psychological status by close attention to health needs.

The parents' reports

The classical texts on Down's syndrome had a lot to say about aetiology, neuroanatomy, epidemiology and metabolic process but offered little on behavioural outcomes or their manipulation. The assumption was that early care would hardly differ from that required by any infant or child and that later care would follow established practices for the mentally retarded as a whole. It was the articulate DS parent who did most to broadcast the differences. The Wilks and Wilks (1974) account, for example, offers a chronology of the growth problems of the home-bound DS child. The Wilks' are a working professional family who could afford in-home help to spread the work and emotional load. They recommended several key principles at the outset: to have family aid, to extend compassion to the child and to oneself, *and* to stress firmness of training. The early difficulties were deceptively few. The infant slept through the night at 10 days of age and made limited demands. One result was slow weight gain and a susceptibility to illnesses such as mumps and measles. The respiratory and circulatory immaturity of DS also attracted infections of the lungs and alimentary canal, along with later catarrh, chilblains, and dental troubles. Feeding was messy and solids were rejected, especially the protein foods. A mixture of baby food with milk and mashed banana proved adequate when made attractive with a chocolate additive. Sausage meat was sliced into the mix as tolerance for solids increased. Motor development was equally slow despite the will (to sit up) which could not surmount the reduced muscle tone, without assistance. Improving feeding habits were complicated by the hypotonia, pudgy hands and clumsy fingers so that utensil handling was slower than might be expected on an IQ-equivalent basis. Food was stored in the mouth and swallowed reluctantly. The long tongue became a plate licker or a tool for feeding parallel with the table. These tendencies can be attributed to muscular hypotonia (postural), reduced or immature sensing and low arousal potentials. The Wilks' describe the latter as laziness. An objectively administered 'smack' at such times was effective in breaking through the sensory and motor barriers.

Dressing, too, was difficult and since the problems were architectural, so were the solutions. The child had a tendency to fiddle with buttons and to poke button holes out of shape. T-shirts and jumpers proved most resistant. Tendencies for the child to be chubby, to have short legs and no waist dictated the use of jump suits or pants with suspenders. Toilet training was managed using a 'wake-up' system. Overall, the early years were managed in a context of affection and acceptance accompanied by appropriate doses of discipline administered by guilt-free parents. Socially toned psychological problems emerged as the child aged. Visits to town, the stores and friends, were fraught with mischief. The choice of leaving the child house-bound was rejected in favour of suffering the public discomfort in the cause of learning by social modelling. Difficult behaviours included temper tantrums, speech frustration, and stubbornness, all stronger than in the normal siblings at similar ages. When such propensities reached the stage of aggressive punching and kicking, threat of affection withdrawal and a spanking were useful control devices. Denial of television privileges also proved an effective method.

Early schooling incorporated busy self-help activities, physical exercise (swimming and climbing), various visual, tactile and auditory experiencing opportunities and memory training (to bring something next day). Personal projects were encouraged (bird feeder) and modelling games were used to teach road signs, door signs, etc. There were community excursions and visits. A useful monitoring device was to chart progress frequently enough to expose gains at more finite levels than would ordinarily be necessary for the purpose of remotivating pupils, teachers and parents.

Talking was slow, a problem of articulation rather than comprehension. The child was encouraged to gesture and later to associate his private sounds with important objects (bet, ber-ber and ser were bread, butter and syrup). A major challenge at age 10–12 years was managing the end sounds in words. Formal speech therapy was employed but the child would frequently 'plateau' and fatigue so that treatment required suspension for several weeks. The therapist noted a growing inclination to stuttering and speech therapy was finally terminated. Other reasons for abandoning formal therapy included an inability to retain gains between sessions, short attention span and considerable difficulty in organizing a complex series of mouth movements. The structural and arousal properties of DS were probably the basis of failure.

As adulthood approached (age 17) a tendency to backslide continued and the easy affection of the boy began to take on a sexual tone.

The Wilks' have several observations in retrospect. These include the need for an ongoing guardianship plan and the necessity of group living experienced in childhood rather than in the late adolescent period when a degree of personal inflexibility becomes evident. As for long term adult care, they are not sure. The small community hostels are viewed as philosophically attractive but tend to lack resources and have a high turnover of staff. The larger institutions, if they improve to include suitable programmes, could provide a stimulating and varied community for the care of the older DS individual.

Brinkworth and Collins' *Improving mongol babies* (1969) is another parent account of the special problems of raising a DS child. It is a collaboration between parent and physician. The Penrose introduction stresses that the most vigorous growth periods are in the first months and years of life and should be judiciously managed in anticipation of later deterioration. The first problem faced by the authors is that the stigmatization or clinical visibility of the condition might inhibit 'mothering' at the critical infant stage. They offer the comforting dicta that stigmatization has no relation to mental development and that 'many family likelinesses of appearance, character and temperament' are evident. Little appeal is made to the research literature on these or other issues. Nevertheless, many useful points are made in respect to practical care, some of which are summarized now.

From birth to 2 years nutrition is a major challenge. The DS infant tends to slip into sleep while nursing, a victim of a shallow arousal and sensory incapacity. His feeding is seldom vigorous and provides little reward for mother. Metabolic characteristics of the syndrome are said to predispose to overweight – a combination of such factors as a particular liking for sugars, low energy output and poor circulation. Cane sugars are to be avoided, they say. Protein foods, fresh fruit and vitamin supplements are recommended. Skin care is another area of concern. Bathing and drying provide an opportunity to stimulate circulation and to improve the child's sense of balance. Creams and body massage are recommended for the dry skin of DS children and especially the use of lip salves. Ears and nose should be kept clear and colds taken seriously. The peripheral sensing apparatus of the DS infant is comparatively immature and he does not readily signal temperature changes.

The first 6–9 months are especially critical for motor and sensory system growth. A regime of frequently handling and rocking will enhance breathing and muscle tone, two major contributors to unfolding mental development.

The goal of exercise is to entice conscious movements of the body, e.g., pushing on the foot, stimulating the edge of the sole, passive exercise of arms, positioning of baby to encourage head and neck movements, even if uncomfortable, and drawing baby to a sitting position to achieve head balance which he will attempt to maintain. The problems of the first speech stages are attributed to structural, energy output and conceptual deficiencies. The DS infant is not actively aware of much of his stimulus environment such that normal language background should be intensified so as to establish receptive speech. Single important words (no, good, kiss) can be taught through play and gesture and should be suitably reinforced. Television provides a useful language and visual background which can be controlled for volume to break through the sensory mask peculiar to the syndrome. The strengthening of sensory and motor tracts (through exercise, play and stimulus enrichment) in the DS infant and young child are presumed to provide a foundation for more structured training. Later educational emphases are on social stimulation and word acquisition. Here the authors speculate about the interaction of language and cognition and the planting of neural traces as the foundation for abstract thought. Having raised the hope that language training benefits cognition, the authors hedge the bet by observing that abstract abilities are little used by most of us and over-rated as an educational goal for the majority who will enter non-intellectual vocations.

The balance of the Brinkworth and Collins' account builds on the premise that developmental slowing past 5 years of age is a result of passivity (arousal deficit) and a failure of early stimulation, especially the verbal variety. The extensive literature on secondary neuropathology is not acknowledged. A purpose of the book, however, is to reduce parent anxiety and promote hope. To this end, it takes an unabashed environmental viewpoint respecting remediation but one which fails to recognize the considerable spread of potential across individuals and the distinctive timetabling of development for the syndrome as a whole.

In addition to the conference reports and parent accounts, on raising the DS child, are the professional pamphlet writers who direct their advice to the new parent. Only two of these are examined here because most cover the same ground and none are supported by data. Following that is a more detailed consideration of the newer 'demonstration' studies which do permit critical evaluation.

Professional pamphleteering

The Pitt pamphlet (undated: see also Pitt, 1960) is among the best examples of the 'tips to parents' approach. The advice is essentially paediatric including guidance on nutrition and dealing with weak sucking, the dangers of overfeeding, the rudiments of physical care and the value of sensory and motor training. Baby should be nursed as upright as possible to prevent a tendency to inhale the milk and then placed on his or her side, rather than back, after feeding. Solids should be introduced only after swallowing is well established. Sensory training exercises include steadying the infant's head while moving objects slowly before the eyes. The infants hands can be placed around various objects to introduce tactile and spatial experiencing. Arms and legs can be manipulated in imitaton of creeping, etc. and later the limbs can be manoeuvered to encourage muscle tensing through reciprocal resistance. After 4 months or so the baby is pulled to the sitting position to exercise back and neck muscles. Propping baby with pillows provides a better visual field and improves movement potential. Physical care includes guarding against colds, the appropriate use of cod liver oil, vitamins, lotions and creams for skin and lip care and the use of antiseptic soaps (past babyhood). Ongoing training includes swimming, marching to music and trampoline exercises as contributing to motor growth and the strengthening of kinaesthetic feedback. Vision and hearing checks are recommended, as are strict safety measures about the house.

It is characteristic of most medical pamphlets that little is said about methods of training, behavour management or the special problems of the older DS child and adult. Smith and Wilson (1973) cope with some of these issues in addition to dispensing the usual medical advise and exploring a few of the links between chromosomal events and outcomes. The more demanding neurological and behavioural science literature is not referred to with the result that a number of stereotypes go unchallenged. For example, they consider poor muscle tone to be seldom problematic. Love of music and dance, general good humour and stubbornness are recited as reliable characteristics of the syndrome for management purposes. The physical disorders section mentions susceptibility to lung infection and intestinal disorders, the high frequency of stabismus (correctable) and that cataract disorders increase with age. They report that structural disorders of heart and intestinal tract can be corrected surgically but at some risk. These procedures are elective and pose an ethical dilemma for the parents and physician. Full and frank discussion between parent and physician is recommended in reaching a decision. The authors observe that the mortality rate has been 50% for young DS children but is now about 30% as medical skills improve.

Adjusting the family to the disorder is built around three recommendations: (i) parents should face their feelings realistically; (ii) the home care or placement decision must be made in view of the rights and needs of each member of the family; (iii) successful long-term management is more likely if a base of reciprocal affection is developed early. Parents are counselled to spend enough time with the DS child to appreciate his essential individuality and to form an emotional attachment. Membership in parent associations is advised for information and support purposes. Smith and Wilson do not push any one care option. Early home nurture is recommended not because group care is wicked but because early institutionalization demands an intensity of programme which is beyond the budget and staffing of most. When the DS child is 5 or 6 years old, the parent can seek day care facilities, special schools or group residential care in those areas where there are adequate resources. Several experimental institutional programmes are mentioned which exploit the enjoyment DS children draw from mutual association and which encourage home visits and parent involvement. Smith and Wilson caution that the ideal age for institutional training is between 6 and 15 years, out-of-home adjustment being more difficult later. The photography is extensive and excellent, designed to show DS individuals as more than clinical material.

The demonstration studies

R. B. Kugel is the author of *Combatting retardation in infants with Down's syndrome* (1970). In it he describes a pilot project at the University of Nebraska Mental Retardation Clinical Research Center. Six of seven DS children improved over a period of 18 months, although with no controls for maturational comparison or 'placebo' effect it is difficult to pinpoint the origins of the gains. The major programme ingredients were a home-like atmosphere, one-to-one staffing and a regime of sensory stimulation and physical strengthening. The equipment suggests the training programme – carpets for maximum tactile experience, mirrors at floor level, birds in cages and ample greenery. Training for balance was encouraged by the availability of rocking boats, rocking horses and tumble tub items. Other motor training devices included jolly jumpers, spring chairs, bolsters and tricycles. A good language environment was maintained by the staff and the frequent visitors to the center.

Programmes were constructed around one nurse or aide responsible for one child (admitted at between 4–17 months) with support from outside adjunctive therapists. Consistency of routine was stressed. Motor skills training was an important feature including exercises in head movement and neck control, creeping by the use of a toy skateboard and feet-pushing drills. Subjects were taught to rotate to a sitting position, a difficult manoeuvre for DS children with shortened extremities and poor muscle tone. Standing and walking were encouraged by the provision of objects at the correct height for the child to pull himself up. Shortened extremities and hypotonia made standing from an unsupported position especially difficult. Once standing, the child was encouraged to push wheeled but weighted wagons. Finer motor and relational skills were enhanced by putting balls into bottles, building blocks and fitting keys into locks.

By the end of the study most had achieved gross motor activity ratings appropriate to CA and were only somewhat depressed for finer motor controls. Parents were also more willing to take the child on home visits as improvement was demonstrated. All were later placed in foster-homes for follow-up training and study. The sensorimotor training emphasis during infancy appears to be the secret to improved general status, although we will need to know if these gains are maintained over time and if they provide a useful foundation for later development. A similar difficulty exists for the Fallstrom and Aronson (1972) experiment where a control sample was employed. The treatment and control groups were matched for initial status, the former receiving a course of sensory, habit and motor training. Intellectual stimulation included the use of puzzles and verbal games. The trained children showed a mean gain of 10.5 months of development against 3.5 months growth for the control children. Once more, the tenacity of the gains is unknown. Studies of pressured acceleration of sensorimotor development in normal children have been disappointing in respect to long-term effects, the 'untreated' child showing no later disadvantage by comparison. The analogy could be bogus, however, given the differences in neuromotor status between DS and normal neonates.

Coriat *et al.* (1967) believe that the DS infant, having a distinctive chromosome set, differs in quality of maturation from the normal baby and from those with other kinds of disorders. Among these deviations, initially, are the oral, postural, tonic neck straightening and walking reflexes. Oral reflexes, they say, 'are primitive traits whose responses gradually model the activity of organs in which basic human functions are established; taste, oral touch, language and kiss' (p. 378). Search and suction elements are especially disturbed for the DS infant and can lead to a too early weaning with the reduction of mother–child intimacy. The loss of sucking as a gratification is easily compensated by tongue and lip sucking, a result of the hypotonia of both. Tongue sucking can lead, in turn, to characteristic vocalizations and grimaces which shape the behavioural stereotype. Ocular fixation is also slow to appear such that the baby rolls his eyes in the manner of non-sighted infants. Coriat *et al.* observe that the stimulus needs to be sufficiently intense to engage these reflexes but not so demanding as to lead to retreat. The latter result is viewed as sheltering in autism and can be associated with rocking and other pointless rhythmic movements.

Tonic neck reflexes are especially reduced in the DS infant. These reflexes are associated with postural patterning and during the early months facilitate control of 'extero- and introceptive afferent impulses' separately to each half of the body. The division aids the 'primary integration of the body scheme' (see also Coriat, 1961). One result of the deficiency in DS infants is that head rotations are few and thus the hand is infrequently in front of the face for receptive purposes. In the normal infant, hand–face alignment facilitates incorporation of the mandibular limbs into the body schema and the integration of visual, touch and kinaesthetic perceptions. The feeble grasp reflex, in the absence of adequate tonic neck reflexes, leaves the hands free to engage each other rather than to explore the environment. Other consequences of the weak tonic neck reflex are inadequate head rolling and elevation which does not permit the infant to easily free his nostrils for breathing. Pelvic postures which inhibit crawling, are also more readily sustained. Straightening and walking reflexes are disturbed as well, being further distorted in expression by the poor muscular tonus. Added to this is a feeble palm grasping reflex which leads the child to reject mechanical support as an aid to postural growth. The main result is the often documented decline of DS infants on development schedules, noted by four months or so, and the appearance of stereotyped motor-autistic behaviours.

Treatments undertaken by Coriat and her colleagues during the first three months of life include: (i) stimulating the primitive reflexes to improve external contact, (ii) stimulating the senses and (iii) encouraging strong physical and affective contact with the care agent.

The anticipated result is a more rapid integration of the body schema and the avoidance of autistic habits. These goals are met by frequent patting, talking and embracing, the liberal use of a soother, regular head exercises and extending or positioning the arms to permit ocular fixation. Objects with auditory and visual appeal are employed to stimulate hand grasping. During the second quarter, primitive reflexes are prevented and maturation reflexes are stimulated. Mothers are instructed on holding and sitting the child, stimulating following movements of eye and head, creating a language environment, repeating the infants vocalization and providing more intense sensations of all kinds. Head and thorax elevation training is given during this period. The third quarter demands new exercises for supported sitting and standing, passing objects from hand to hand and feeding. The final quarter includes preparation for crawling and walking, digital pinching movements, the development of spatial appreciation, and the beginning of oral language. The techniques used here are similar to those described for other demonstration studies. In addition, the child is stimulated to greater motility and is encouraged to explore. Attractive objects are placed, like a carrot on a stick, to increase approach behaviour and objects are thrown to induce eye-following. Body-part naming games are initiated.

Results of the programme were tested against a control group stratified for age. The untreated (spontaneous evolution) had achieved developmental levels of 83 points at the outset but declining to 43 points by the tenth semester. The treated group achieved an IQ equivalent of 93 points at first semester and 61 points by the tenth semester. Personality gains are also noted. The findings are encouraging but difficult to evaluate because it is not clear how the control group differed from the treatment group initially and how to interpret the considerably greater loss of subjects in the control over the experimental sample. The major contribution might well be the cataloguing of the reflexive apparatus of DS infants from birth and the relating of these insufficiencies to beginning and later psychological development.

Marjorie Ann Buresch takes an anecdotal ' question and answer ' approach to management in *Mongoloid psychology* (1975). The preface states ' I could find no literature giving an understanding of the mental make-up of the mongoloid – or how to work with them.' And indeed no references to the extensive behavioural and treatment literature are offered. It is claimed that IQ tests are of doubtful value and that IQ and attention span are unrelated. The burden of the programme is that DS children mimic so that appropriate modelling opportunities are important. Stubbornness, on the other hand, is acquired through frustration and a relaxed atmosphere is encouraged so as to induce placid behaviours. On scientifically sounder ground is the programme tenet that affectional-dependency characteristics, seen in many DS children, are exploitable as reinforcement during training. Speech is induced by discouraging gestures in favour of word use. Overall, the recommendations are for generous praise and the encouragement of role playing.

What the DS individual supposedly cannot do is also critical to Buresch. Among these is that he cannot acquire or learn judgement, cannot aspire to competitive employment, and has difficulty when natural affection assumes a sexual connotation in the post-pubescent years. Buresch recommends that IQ levels of 50 points or more be separated for educational purposes and that attention span – inherently normal – be managed by improved teaching tactics. Terminal training is conceived of as a life-work situation including such mundane tasks as folding letters and filling envelopes. The plea that management be based on the unique characteristics of the syndrome is a good one; but apart from designating certain of the old behavioural stereotypes of DS as innate and others as learned, Buresch says little about 'mongoloid psychology'.

More comprehensive experimental programmes, focussed on early motor and sensory stimulation are now appearing. They have in common an appreciation that (i) the decelerative nature of growth in DS requires early and intensive stimulation of the peripheral systems and (ii) monitoring of outcomes is required in order to improve programme content choices. Zausmer, Pueschel and Shea (1972) applied sensorimotor stimulation to the young DS child with a resulting inhibition of the maturational decline rate. Bayley, Rhodes, Gooch and Marcus (1971) placed DS infants (prior to 4½ months) in a special institutional setting which duplicated home conditions but which was not explicitly tied to the unique qualities of the syndrome. A good patient to staff ratio, an enriched verbal environment and a formal pre-school programme were central to the plan. By the age of 8 years the experimental group was approximately equivalent in development to a home group. An IQ of about 40 was reached by both groups.

The programmes mentioned thus far are based on two characteristics of the syndrome: (i) that early social and emotional gains are within the capacity range of Down's and (ii) that intensive infant and child stimulation of motor and sensory systems provides some protection against later central process decline. The mechanisms of improvement are unclear but are probably related to the amelioration of circulatory system sluggishness, to the severity of the hypotonia and to the engaging of cortical process prior to the onset of irreversible neuropathological events evident by mid-childhood. What we don't know is whether or not promising short-term findings will survive to later years and what programme ingredients contribute most to real and compensatory growth relative to the non-treated.

An experimental programme of longer standing had been conducted from the University of Washington (Hayden & Dmitriev, 1975) and is better articulated than most. The goals of the centre are to improve motor, sensory and vocal development, to involve parents as treatment participants and eventually to integrate the DS child in the regular school system. Each child is assessed for motor, vocal and social skills or deficits at admission. The Denver developmental screening test is used subsequently as a programme monitor. Specific self-help training effects are charted daily (e.g., the toileting sequence) so that small gains will have reinforcement value for students, staff and parents. Other reinforcers include the generous use of social praise, the application of error free gradations of task complexity and fading techniques. For example, the DS child practices pouring with an empty jug, then with some water and finally with juice. These steps are manually guided by the teacher who 'fades' when the subsequent steps are likely to be successful without further help. Failure and frustration are thereby avoided.

The Washington programme is grouped around four age and competency levels. The infant learning programme ranges up to 18 months of age, children attending once a week for 30 minutes of individual instruction. Motor exercises such as head lifting, head turning, etc., are encouraged and the techniques demonstrated to parents for home use. The motor items chosen parallel those of the Denver and Gesell infant schedules, a procedure which will predispose at least to the appearance of progress psychometrically. The pre-school and kindergarten sections meet for two hours. Skills are taught in small steps with verbal command and physical guidance used in the first stages of training (e.g., removing clothing, hand washing, toilet training). Gross motor control and reduction of the wide gait is encouraged by such tactics as board walking, stepping over obstacles and crawling up inclines. Finer motor development requires class and home use of crayons, paste blocks, peg boards and dolls. Marching, placing, pointing and attending tasks are integral parts of the concept learning schedule. All programme steps are offered in units small enough to ensure success. Hand washing is a ten-step sequence, e.g. standing on a stool, touching the faucet, turning the faucet, etc. Communication skills development is also staged and can be chained to other skill programmes; so that requesting different food items (crackers, juice) succeeds when accompanied by a distinctive sound, spontaneously presented and reinforced through imitation. Imitation facility is further exploited in rhythm groups where clapping, stamping and swaying are elicited to the beat of sticks, bells, drums and xylophones.

The objectives of the programme are similar to the others described. These involve motor enhancement, increasing the impact level and variety of sensory events, improving arousal, drive and attention, initiating communication, and encouraging self-definition, relational and self-help skills. The management philosophy is (i) to make an early beginning, even by 5 weeks, (ii) to introduce appropriate schedules of reinforcement so that small gains are visible and motivationally important to student, teacher and parent and (iii) to exploit modelling procedures. Motor and self-help gains are claimed to be between 85–100% of age norms. Language and concept development competencies are described as between 39–100% of age norms. Gross motor development was the area of greatest advance while language and conceptual advances proved more difficult. In the advanced pre-school programme, all the children met the recognition target of 30 words after 1 year. Children completing this level showed a developmental lag of only 5.6 months versus new admissions who showed a 21 month lag. Over 1 year, treated children showed IQ levels of between 61 and 75 points. No results of the kindergarten programme were available. The interested reader will want to consult the more recent report by Hayden and Haring (1976).

What are the problems? Most obvious is the need for comparison group data. It should not be difficult to evaluate across treatment groups (home training, custodial training, special programmes) providing a proper match is made for early neuro-maturational status, extent and specificity of handicap, cytogenetic category, and pre-programme conditions. It is possible, moreover, that experimental studies in university centres attract a different DS child and parent than do institutional or other facilities. Carefully managed early stimulation programmes for DS children which show good short-term results but provide no evidence of durability or spread of gains can be misleading. Down's syndrome has biological boundaries which are not in the educable range for many such that the major contributions of experimental programmes might be to combat maturational erosion and to exploit residual abilities. Otherwise, it is risky to report high expectations, as does Kysela (1973–74) in his visitors report of the Washington programme. He claimed that at the ages of 4–5 years the DS children were 'exhibiting coordinated motor abilities equivalent to their age mates and social and developmental skills equal to those expected of children at their chronological age'. (p. 62). Further 'These children have shown a capacity to acquire and use language in a way that reflects abilities consistent with their chronological growth'. (p. 62). Gains are evident but Hayden and Dmitriev are not so generous in their claims.

Elizabeth Zausmer offers somewhat similar methods of early intervention (1975) with DS children. Developmental modifiers, she says should be applied early and with a healthy regard for the 'critical periods'. To do so requires that we must not be misled by the quiescence of the DS infant or by the hypotonia which leads one to think of them as fragile.

Programming begins during the first few weeks with the encouragement of head movements. Stimulation of the sucking reflexes is undertaken along with regular changes in body position to increase reflexive movements of both head and trunk. The infant can be manipulated and suspended in a variety of positions to engage anti-gravity musculature. 'Such activities elicit labyrinthine and proprioceptive equilibrium reactions and responses and bring into play muscle groups which otherwise are apt to remain inactive if the child is always held in supported positions.' (p. 141.) Touching, tapping and stroking are used to stimulate activity of the head, trunk and extremities. Assisted movements are associated with various pleasant sights, sounds and tactile opportunities so that the infant learns to chain motor and sensory activity and to self-initiate from either end of the sensorimotor sequence. Another Zausmen example is training for sitting. The use of high chairs, or reposing the child on the floor with legs apart, disposes the head to hang forward, rounds the back, inhibits motility of the arms and reduces fields of vision necessary for later visual-tactile experiencing. A better approach is to set the child in a low chair with feet resting on the floor with a small table in front at a convenient level for arm movement. The back will be more erect, weight shifts can be distributed through the legs, field of vision is improved and hand opportunities increased. Parents are instructed in these techniques and in the use of toys to advance sensorimotor status. The central features of the programme are to identify and exploit stages of maturational readiness, to advance training in small enough steps so that success can be felt and enjoyed, and to involve parents fully. With parents as the major dispensors of the programme, reliable emotional support tends to enhance reciprocation of smiling and vocalization in response to motor stimulation. Parents are also able to see and chart gains with a resulting increase in both their morale and acceptance of the child.

Zausmer does not otherwise concede that the developmental sequence for Down's is much different from other infants, although the presence of cardiac problems and of secondary physical defects are mentioned as complicating the maturational schedule. Her belief is that the growth sequence is merely distorted, as a consequence of an especially immature sensory system and hypotonia of the musculature. These are, however, unique and important artifacts of the syndrome which reverberate more widely than has been supposed.

Barnard (1972, 1975) presents a programme of infant stimulation designed initially for the premature infant. Down's syndrome was conceived by Benda as an 'unfinished child' who presumably has many of the features of a premature birth. Barnard builds on the work of Porter (1972) and the traditional infant stimulation literature. Porter instructed mothers to administer exercise to their infants in the form of cycling movements of the arms and legs. Gesell scale measures showed advances in motor and language growth, the latter as a result both of motor system strengthening and the favourable social-emotional context in which the exercise is administered. Kinaesthetic, tactile and auditory stimulation programmes have been shown to be beneficial to premature infants, even while still in incubators. Schedules of rocking and the administration of heart beat sounds were useful for improving sleep and advancing growth (Barnard, 1972). For normal infants, there is sufficient drive level to expect self-initiation of stimulus opportunity with training. Down's syndrome exhibits sensory system immaturity, depressed arousal level and hypotonia-related inertia of the motor systems thereby requiring early and systematic intervention. Future study will determine if the heavy manpower commitment to infant stimulation programmes for DS does in fact slow the characteristic deceleration of growth by one year, and beyond, and if the 'gains' are held and generalized to other areas of development. At this time, there is reason for optimism, even in the face of a significant neurophysiological literature which suggests an inevitable maturational process decline for the syndrome.

Barnard illustrates her principles of early intervention using the Zausmer, Peuschel and Shea (1972) demonstration. For example, the visual stimulation programme demands the manipulation of a variety of objects according to colour, shape and distance along with experience in visual tracking and permanency. Auditory stimulation engages sounds of differing quality, frequency and intensity, manipulating both direction and distance. Kinaesthetic stimulation includes body position change so as to elicit vestibular reaction. Symmetrical, alternate and reciprocal motion patterns are encouraged. Each segment of the regime can be combined with motor-tactile experience, as for example tying sounds to facial expressions and gestures. Sound production is enhanced by oral stimulation related to sucking, licking, chewing, tongue movement and closure of the mouth.

Additional general guidelines are offered: (i) that an intervention programme, involving the parents, be started ideally before 30 months of age, (ii) that baseline assessment data on the DS child and the family situation be assembled, e.g., will the stimulation be maturationally important, is the mother–infant interaction a generally positive one. Over-stimulation is evident when the child shows undue irritability. An individually suited rest–activity balance must, therefore, be determined from the assessment data. The programme should be continually adjusted in the face of any evidence of negative effects on the parents and normal siblings.

The early intervention regimes considered so far, for DS, are comprised essentially of strengthening the sensory system to provide a firmer platform for the later applications of formal motor training. A number of additional programmes, designed primarily for the mentally retarded or brain-injured child, give a nod to the DS child (Stephens, Baumgartner, Smeets & Wolfinger, 1970; Thomas, 1969; Cratty, 1969).

Stephens *et al.* (1970) provide an experimental schedule of motor exercise in the three areas of gross motor control: balance, arm–hand coordination and manual dexterity. The areas correspond to Bruner's (1966) three levels of representation: enactive (physical guidance of child through motor activity), iconic (demonstration of activity) and symbolic (explanation of tasks to student). The stages are tailored for the ages of 7–12 years. Assessment is first undertaken using the Valett (1966) developmental survey. Individual performance was not always uniform across areas of development. An 8-year-old DS boy, for instance, was more proficient in the area of gross motor facility and balance but less so for arm–hand coordination and manual dexterity. The approach used can be illustrated by enumerating the typical items. Training for gross motor control, below the age of 30 months, might involve the instructor demonstrating a roll and then helping the child perform the exercise. Those above the 30-month motor standard go on to practice rolling over and over on a mattress or on the grass. Crawling is similarly handled by demonstration, manipulation and by practice movement through tunnels, around objects, on a 12-inch board, etc. A similarly graded sequence is followed for walking, running, jumping and climbing instruction. Balance training involves standing on a mattress or trampoline, crawling or walking on a slightly elevated balance board, tiptoe and skipping activity, balancing on one foot and walking on toes. Arm–hand coordination training requires rolling and throwing a ball, ring toss games, bean bag in bucket, rolling large objects, drum tapping, bowling and pouring (sand and water). Manual dexterity training uses block building, clay play, sponge play, stringing beads and scissors practice. Motor improvement after 3 months of treatment was evidently superior to gains made by an untreated control group. There is no report of longer term effects or of whether or not the DS group advanced equally well in all areas and across individual subjects.

An attempt has been made to extract the key techniques from a number of DS demonstration programmes so as to identify principles in common. The aspiring specialist should consult original sources for further details of method. Motor-system evaluation and programming for the atypical child, as a class, has been covered by Cratty (1969). His book presents remedial and developmental procedures for the control of large muscle groups, the encouragement of strength, flexibility and endurance, improvement of arousal level, games and body-image promotion, the use of music and rhythm and the encouragement of more refined coordination leading to first stage academic work. Most are relevant to the DS child.

The Doman–Delacato methods (Thomas, 1969) is another packaged programme which can be adapted to the training of the DS child. While the neurophysiological assumptions are not convincingly established, the techniques employed are resourceful. Among the assumptions are (i) that motor and sensory system strengthening, by stimulus manipulation and magnification, somehow 'programme' the brain and (ii) that sensory tract capacity precedes motor output facility, developmentally. The method was designed for the brain-damaged child, the fancied outcome being that damaged cortical areas will regenerate or that undamaged areas will provide compensation. Be that as it may, the DS child does exhibit weak sensory systems reactivity and hypotonic motor output which would justify the adaptation of some of the Doman–Delecato procedures. Sensory strengthening tactics include the use of strong odours (e.g., smelling salts), the manipulation of auditory and tactile situations and the variation of illumination to raise the level of sensory consciousness in the retarded infant. The regime is applied for short periods throughout the day. Motor training employs 'forced' bilateral movements (crawling, head turning, etc.) for perhaps 10 minutes every waking hour and over a period of several years. Lateralization programmes follow, leading eventually to speech training. The motor techniques are not much different from those described earlier. The procedures are labour intensive and of long duration with the danger that limited gains will be at the expense of more effective alternatives.

The experimental approach to behavioural treatment, considered thus far, has engaged environmental releasors timed to exploit maturational events. The other extreme, direct chemical intervention, will be considered shortly. An intermediate approach, though speculative, is taken by Fehr (1976). His hypothesis is that spontaneous fluctuation of peripheral physiological response systems act as 'energizers' of CNS activity, that DS individuals are less labile in this regard and that these spontaneous fluctuations can be experimentally influenced. The effect should be an increased alertness necessary for attending to and processing relevant stimuli. If physiological changes accompany environmental enrichment then two possibilities arise; peripheral physiological measures can be used to monitor the effectiveness of training programmes and peripheral physiological status might be more directly alterable thereby reducing the need for extraceptive programming.

Fehr demonstrates his point of view using ten DS children (mean age 6 years) and ten normal controls matched for age and sex. Mental age and number of intelligent verbalizations were physiologically and behaviourally measured during the life of the study. The enrichment plan monitored by Fehr (over a period of 12 months) included self-help, language, motor and recreational training (see also Chalfant, Silikovitz & Tawney, 1973). Post-enrichment measures indicated reaction time and physiological changes close to those of the normal group. These were taken as an indication that environmental stimulation enhances physiological responsiveness. For example, the greater the MA and verbalization increase, during the period of the study, the greater the decrease in reaction time and the increase in HR and skin response fluctuations. The findings are consistent with the Lacey (1967) formulation that increased heart rate accompanies the performance of internal mental tasks. Other studies, using normal subjects, have shown that gradations of task difficulty are correlated with heart rate level (Kaufman, Gibson and Adamowicz 1967; Adamowicz and Gibson, 1972). Recent attempts to manipulate cardiovascular status directly, so as to influence problem solving efficiency, show some promise (Hershman and Gibson, 1977) and might have relevance for the remediation of learning deficits in mental retardation.

Chemical management

Chemical methods for the control of difficult behaviours or the enhancement of cognitive, psychomotor or sensory facility for Down's syndrome have been consistently popular because such approaches promise cure, are mystical and require little effort. Parents will spend considerable money and time in search of the 'magic bullet' and a few promoters will profit, long after a given method has been explored under controlled conditions and dismissed as valueless. Not all drug treatments for DS are impotent, however. Previous chapters have touched on established regimens for the management of psychoneurotic and psychotic states in Down's syndrome. Pharmacological techniques also exist for the reduction of hypotonia (see Baselon & Paine, 1967), the elevation of arousal and attention thresholds, the abatement of physical stigmata, improvement of circulatory system function, supplementation of nutrition and the treatment of those infections to which DS is especially susceptible. These methods often enhance behavioural status by improving accessibility for training. Our concern here is specifically with chemical methods which claim to alter the fundamental competency ratings of the syndrome.

Physical treatments attract attention proportional to the magnitude of the curative claim. These include the thyroid therapies, the use of pituitary extract, the administration of glutamic acid and its salts, various vitamin therapies, 5-hydroxytryptophan (5-HTP), siccacell therapy, dehydroepiandrosterone for the improvement of neuromuscular control, testis hormone, x-rays in the pituitary region, skull irradiation, ephedrine stimulation, serotonin related therapies, the administration of thymus extracts and combination regimes which include various of these procedures. A body of validation research exists for each.

The claims made for roentgen therapy date from Wieser (1931) who irradiated five different fields of the skull at one-month intervals for up to two years. General development and resistance to infection were said to improve. Later studies found no benefits (Jervis, 1942, Lazar, 1953). Testis hormone and thymus extract therapies have been similarly discredited (Oster, 1953).

Thyroid extract was used first by Smith (1896). Its continuing application was prompted by the clinical similarities between cretinism and Down's and by the ever-changing claims for benefits; ranging across alleged improvements of adiposity, constipation, stature, activity level, stigma count and mental status. Benda (1969) reported some benefits in preventing the raucous voice and thick scrotal tongue. Lethargy is reduced, teething aided and circulation improved, he says. Any enhancement of the development of the vascular system, surgical or chemical, has presumed benefits for the brain. Koch, Share and Graliker (1965) could find no measurable differences among 73 non-institutionalized DS children in a six-year longitudinal double-blind study using cytomel. A few DS patients with intercurrent hypothyroidism have benefited but, on the whole, Down's does not differ from normals for thyroxine values nor do they appear to have a special need for stimulation of thyrotropic hormone (Hillman, 1969).

Benda (1969) continues to be optimistic about pituitary hormone therapy, especially in combination with thyroid and vitamin treatments (Cook, 1950). Pituitary powder alone, however, has no influence on human growth (Keith, 1958). On the other hand, obtaining good quantities of somatotropine from human pituitaries is difficult (Benda, 1969). The effects are said to be improved alertness, mental growth and physical development. In addition, deterioration is expected to slow. These claims were supported in part by Carter and Maley (1958) and Blumberg (1959). Later research by Berg, Kerman, Stern and Mittwoch (1961) and by Diamond and Moon (1961) has produced negative findings.

Siccacell therapy, first promoted by Niehans (1964), assumes that injected embryonic cells migrate to analogous organs to stimulate growth. Haubold, Loew and Haefele-Niemann (1960) reported improvement for DS children under cytotherapy. General developmental, intellectual and social status is claimed to advance. Work by Bardon (1964), using five matched pairs of subjects, failed to confirm these findings. A more extensive study by Black, Kato and Walker (1966) using psychometric, teacher and parent ratings in a double-blind experiment, produced negative results.

Vogel, Broverman, Draguns and Klaiber (1965) and Share (1976) found the status of glutamic acid therapy equivocal although other reviewers have concluded against its usefulness (Penrose and Smith, 1966; Oster, 1953). Zimmerman, Burgemeister and Putnam (1949) first advocated glutamic acid therapy for DS children. Gains in physical growth and IQ were shown after 6 months of treatment but non-DS controls yielded even greater gains. While these findings have not been supported for the mentally retarded in general (Lombard, Gilbert and Donofrio, 1955), there is no adequately controlled test with DS samples. For the mentally retarded, as a group, most positive findings have emerged from studies with only token controls whereas the more tightly designed experiments are substantially negative (Astin and Ross, 1960).

Vitamin treatments have tended to be used with hormonal and other preparations. Benda (1969) recorded weight gains and improved mental growth on a combination of Vitamin B_{12}, pituitary and thyroid therapy. Turkel (1963) described a mixture of vitamins, minerals and enzymes (his U series) which are intended to flush toxic metabolites from the tissues and thus promote normal growth. Bumbalo, Morelewicz and Berens (1964) have been unable to substantiate these claims, although the complexity of formulae and the vagaries of administration have hampered evaluation. White and Kaplitz (1964), White (1969) and Smith (1975) view these findings with skepticism. General improvement from vitamin therapy has been recorded in some cases, presumably where serious nutritional deficiency is present (Houze, Wilson and Goodfellow, 1964). Heaton-Ward (1960, 1961) noted increased appetite and activity using Niamid with 51 hospitalized DS cases but no expected increase in speech quality or intelligence. Indeed, the greatest MA increase occurred in the control group. Griffiths and Behrman (1967) applied dark adaptometry to DS subjects and MR controls finding substantial dark adaptation improvement for the syndrome which led them to suspect disordered metabolism of Vitamin A. The value of the vitamin and combination therapies appears to be in the same order as for the general population, any effects which related directly to mental growth being unproven.

Considerable interest has been expressed recently in the use of 5-hydroxytryptophan to accelerate motor progress by improving muscle tone. It is thought that 5-HTP is a precursor of serotonin in brain metabolism and that 5-HTP levels are reduced in DS infants. Bazelon et al. (1970) detected abatement of hypotonia, reduction of tongue protrusion and acceleration of the motor landmarks. Weise et al. (1974) and Coleman (1973) were unable to establish beneficial effects during the early years of life but did note undesirable side effects (e.g., infant spasms). Studies using epridine to advance age at walking are equally disappointing, the main effects being anorexia, thirst, sweating and frequent micturition (Kucera, 1969).

Granting that the results of chemical therapies have been disappointing to date, it is reasonable to hope for the future. The problem is that preliminary chemical findings are enthusiastically presented as cures even though comparison groups are often not used, samples are small and monitoring is terminated at the point 'something' seems to be happening. Later controlled studies discredit the early findings and the area is abandoned, perhaps prematurely. Smith (1975) has observed that IQ, DQ and SQ scores are too gross to reflect changes which are either subtle or highly particular. Outcome objectives should be refined and measured experimentally. Other problems in chemical research with DS children include the possibilities that effects are limited to critical periods, developmentally, or are gradual and cumulative over a long period; the gains being below the level of detection over months or even several years of treatment. Wolfensberger and Menolascino (1968) have discussed some of these problems as well as the need to test drug effects against environmental conditions which are sufficiently rich and varied to act as releasors to altered metabolic states. In the final analysis, DS children are often affectionate, suggestible and eager to please. Thus, any uncontrolled experiment, using drugs, might produce desirable behavioural changes entirely as placebo effect.

Formal education and work preparation

Some assumptions

The educational and industrial training capacity of the DS child and adult is poorly understood and directed because the various professional, scientific and lay groups in the field have different working assumptions and goals. There are a number of sources of disagreement.

(1) Trainability studies do not agree well for the initial physical and later psychological status of their samples. A disproportionate number of custodial calibre cases find their way to residential settings where simple activity programmes are deemed sufficient. The less impaired (moderate to mild retardation) undertake formal academic and vocational training in community settings. Research studies of the educability or work capacity of DS as a whole will differ according to where the samples are selected – the home, community residence or hospital. As a result, maturational, clinical and case history differences, relevant to educational planning, are likely to be overlooked.

(2) Studies of relatively high educational achievement among certain DS individuals carry the attractive implication that all are capable, with training. Extrapolation from single-case reports does not recognize the maturational lead of the rarer partial, mosaicism and translocation states of DS and thus distorts our understanding of the modal trainability potential of the majority standard trisomy condition.

(3) The assessed learning potential of DS individuals will vary by degree and quality depending on age at examination. Indices of prediction are seldom corrected for regression of maturation or for extent of secondary handicap adjusted between subjects. Optimistic predictions for trainability are often based on test results from early childhood.

(4) Certain less damaged DS children who have received intensive early stimulation appear to retain the lower end of the 'educable' range into later childhood. The costs-over-benefits ratio is high, raising issues of parent and community resource priorities and the extent to which sustained intensive training is effective for all cases.

Uniform educational and vocational expectations for DS are thus un-founded. It would be more useful to build programmes around the special qualities of the syndrome, as a clinical entity, supplemented by the ongoing assessment of individual ability-deficit profiles. A better delineation of post-academic goals for DS adults, in terms of what might be educationally relevant to various life style options, is needed as well.

Academic preparation

The preliminary findings of recent experimental programmes for pre-school DS children and biographical accounts by parents are now taken as models of academic expectation. The orthodox position has been that DS individuals do not profit much from academic study, although a few are observed to develop reading and writing skills. Hultgren (1914), Wallin (1944) and Engler (1949) have recorded these exceptions but add that the level of understanding is notably impoverished, e.g., word calling versus language appreciation. Oster (1953) claimed that 'nobody has found mongols able to add sums' (p. 49). Pearce, Rankine and Ormond (1910) observed some progress in writing skills for the more intelligent but with 'great perseverance on the part of the teacher' (p. 187). An increasing degree of interference from impulsivity and attention disorder, among the more intellectually intact, was noticed in later years.

With respect to reading skills, Seagoe (1964) proposed that the teaching in-vestment be appropriate to age, intellectual potential and life goals. Because the educational commitment is a heavy one, in proportion to gains, the typical DS child would be taught little more than the identification of road and door signs. The plus 50 IQ group can profit from grades I and II reading training by the age of 9 or 10 years but this decision should be governed by anticipated life circumstances or delayed in favour of extended pre-school foundation programmes. Sinson and Wetherick (1973, 1975, 1976) have found that certain educationally relevant skills are late to appear in DS individuals. Using a test of short-term memory for colours, the 8-year-old group failed whereas a 15-year-old group could manage the task. For most, finite teaching resources might better be directed to social, motor and habit training goals. Orthodox academic preparation for the typical DS child has not, in any case, been promising (Cain and Levine, 1963; Dunn and Hottel, 1958; Guskin and Spicker, 1968). The reasons include poor retention and spread of specific academic skills, problems of shallow motivation, the disparity between simple recognition-recall and conceptual ability and the influence of peripheral skeletal and muscular system limitations on finer coordination. Many DS children are exposed to traditional academic training simply because it has parent status value. The outcome is frequently an increase in stress levels for the child and a decline in self regard without any useful educational gain.

Reasons for the failure of standard educational procedures with the DS child include a simple lack of general cognitive capacity, the special problems of arousal and temperament, disadvantage in speech apparatus, skeletal system and musculature and the more subtle limitations of auditory circulating, kinaesthetic feedback and relational capacity. Dedicated parents or teachers have had some success with the brighter DS child, probably because they have made intuitive adjustments in teaching to accommodate the disability profile of the syndrome and of the individual. Dunsdon, Carter and Huntley (1960) demonstrated that while word recognition scores were appropriate to mental age, arithmetic performance, was poorly related to overall mental ability and that social age and social quotient were stronger indicators of educational achievement than was IQ. A similar study of less impaired DS children, undertaken by Pototzky and Grigg (1942) showed a low correspondence between mental age and academic achievement in reading and arithmetic. Several cases achieved a grade six result in the Monroe reading test. Arithmetic skills were especially difficult to acquire, 50% being unable to master simple addition and even fewer to work with single digit division.

Follow-up studies tend to confirm these academic difficulties. Delp and Lorenz (1953) monitored 15 DS children with IQ less than 50 points. Subjects had attended a special class programme for almost 5 years. Median age at re-examination was 22 years. Many of the adults were able to shop, ride public transport, etc. The few who had learned to read, continued to employ the skill for picture captions, television schedules and comics. Longevity of personal habit training was established (eating, grooming) whereas many classroom skills had fallen into disuse (printing, needle-work). Despite concentrated training in time-telling many depended on television programme changes to index their day. Parent opinion was that the major gains of special education were not academic. They mentioned, most often, improvements of pride and posture, growth of motor and emotional control, reduction in fearfulness and an ability to self-direct. Some speech improvement was noted. Again, the social and personal profits overwhelmed the academic gains. The authors concluded that a little reading skill can serve well but requires continuing reinforcement past school leaving age. Arithmetic instruction was least successful judging from the inability of the adult follow-up group to manage money. Since a non-school comparison group was not employed in the study, it is impossible to assign even the secondary gains to the formal academic exposure.

Proven academic programmes specific to the DS child simply do not exist, at least in the open literature. Rosenzweig (1953) offered two reasons: (i) we assume that DS children are like all other retardates and (ii) many professionals reject formal education as relevant. Brousseau (1928) advised against formal education on the grounds that average life expectancy did not justify the effort. Rosenzweig disagreed because DS children who survive to adulthood show a continuing mental plasticity which is of value educationally. Talbot (1937) claimed that when sensory defects, complications of tonsils and adenoids and hypotonia related coordination difficulties are improved later in childhood, scholastic promise increases. The nub of the argument is that scholastic training should build on some years of pre-academic remediation and that once the academic programmes are started they should continue well into adulthood. Against this precept is the gathering evidence for the psychological effects of progressive neuropathology in Down's syndrome, clinically visible even before the onset of adolescence and accompanied by increasing behavioural rigidity and impulsivity. The dilemma, therefore, is that special academic training should capitalize on readiness, which is usually quite late, yet be underway well before secondary deteriorative processes have damaged learning potentials. The equation will differ among DS individuals. The most exciting prospect for solution is found in the early intervention programmes; environmental and medical, where sensorimotor readiness can be advanced and the onset of deterioration delayed.

The proposition that DS children require selective educational handling, appropriate to characteristic patterns of behavioural limitations and assets, has research support. So has the proposition that DS children display qualities of learning handicap similar to other more severely retarded children, in particular the brain-damaged child. Attention deficit, impulsivity, perceptual-learning handicap and motor dysfunction are examples of shared handicaps for which there are an increasing number of remedial 'packages' in the educational marketplace. Innovators of academic regimes for DS children will find something of relevance in most of them. Fuller (1974) described a ball-stick-bird method of teaching reading which exploits association memory and the compulsion to motion. The student manipulates three colour-coded forms comprised of a line (stick), circle (ball) and angle (bird). These three forms can combine to make all letters of the alphabet. Tactile and kinaesthetic feedback is enhanced, an important consideration since efficiency of feedback loops is especially retarded in DS children. Words are formed after two letters are learned and then built to 52 configurations through the use of motivationally compelling action stories. An 18-year-old DS subject with IQ 35 was able to learn to read, print and use spontaneous speech. The Doman (1964) method, explained in *How to teach your baby to read*, is equally straightforward. Children with mental age levels of less than 2 years, it is claimed, can be exposed to simple words printed large on a cue card. The trials are brief and frequent throughout the day. A recognition response (DADDY), through repetition of visual and auditory exposure, is amply rewarded. When recognition of a few dozen words is conditioned, sentences can be undertaken. Doman contends that very young children can recognize large colourful symbols (EXXON) because they are exaggerated and keyed to non-symbolic cues. Moreover, individual letters would be meaningless and would have little stimulus impact. Enhancement of stimulus quality (size, colour, frequency), manipulation of duration of exposure, and the suitable use of reward or praise are claimed to strengthen immature sensory pathways and 'programme' the brain. Whatever the mechanism, any technique which can exploit short attention span, breach the sensory mask, and capitalize on emotional states must be considered suitable for DS children. A similar method for teaching reading to DS children is outlined briefly by Brinkworth and Collins (1969) but is not elaborated. Whether these methods will prove to be of ultimate value for the DS child will depend upon the outcome of experimental study. A step in the right direction is made by Sidman and Cresson (1973) using machine teaching where cross-modal transfer can be exploited in the learning process.

More advanced teaching techniques, appropriate for DS, can be found in the educational literature for minimally brain damaged (MBD) children. (Kephart, 1960; Frostig, 1964). The older DS child has some of the qualities of the MBD child; chiefly his distractability, short attention and impulsivity. These handicaps provide the foundations of perceptual-learning disorder, including the failure to perceive simultaneous stimulus events, to differentiate figure and ground, and to achieve closure. The techniques for stimulus patterning, described by Kephart, are designed for MBD children who are not seriously impaired cognitively and are applied early in life so as to build the abstract attitude, leading to symbol manipulation skills. Especially valuable are the programmes of motor, eye–hand, spatial–temporal, perceptual scanning and ocular control exercises. Prescriptions for laterality and directionality training are included. Stimulus delimitations techniques and perceptual patterning programmes could be modified for use with less handicapped and older DS children, subject to readiness and tailored to more modest goals.

Other aetiologically undifferentiated training programmes in mental retardation are appropriate if the user has in mind the special boundaries and unique developmental patterning of his subjects. Among these publications are Bernard and Powell, *Teaching the mentally retarded child: a family care approach* (1972) and Gibson and Brown, *Managing the severely retarded* (1977), the latter aimed chiefly at group care workers. An integrated programme is offered by Myers, Sinco and Stalma (1973) in their curriculum for the more severely mentally retarded. In recent years, behaviour modification approaches (Gardner, W. I. *Behaviour modification in mental retardation*, 1971) have been used with good results, especially in institutions. Schemes for training in feeding, dressing, toileting and personal grooming are readily available and have been generally successful. Operant and classical conditioning approaches to self-abuse, destructive behaviours, and aggressiveness have been most helpful when combined with sensorimotor upgrading, medical therapies and the appropriate arrangement of the care mileau. Shaping procedures have been least successful in the areas of language development, although training for receptive vocabularies is promising when behaviour modification methods are combined with modelling, environmental manipulation techniques and the remediation of relevant structural and sensorimotor deficiency. Social contact training and techniques of psychological mothering are especially applicable to DS children (Forman, 1967) but have been researched only for the mentally retarded as a class. Systems approaches involve the creation of therapeutic environments such as the experimental 'family' unit in institutions, the arrangement of wards and cottages for optimal stimulation, the training of group management personnel (including the older retarded as surrogate or adjunctive care agents) and the use of total token economies. It is not possible yet to evaluate these approaches for the DS child because follow-up studies are few in number and do not distinguish on a treatments by aetiologies basis. Moreover, the prevailing trend to home care, the increasing fractionation of responsibility among various community supports groups, and the tendency to undervalue professional guidance, inhibits the application of these technologies.

Job preparation

Vocational expectations for DS youth, in contrast to the claims made on behalf of trainability in childhood, have been meagre. Among the reasons are a low survival rate of DS individuals into adulthood, possibly biased in favour of the less competent, and employer discrimination influenced by the superficial stigmata of the condition. Brousseau and Bernard (1928) recommended against work training because of depressed physical stamina related to heart and respiratory difficulties. Benda (1960) added inherent clumsiness as a reason to discount vocational prowess. At best, boys were expected to be garden helpers and girls, house helpers. Engler (1949) simply dismissed skill training because DS individuals cannot retain instruction. Vocational aspirations for DS individuals, when entertained at all, were limited to arts and crafts such as plasticine modelling, bead work and knitting (Brushfield, 1924). Pototzky and Grigg (1942) shared the low vocational expectation because, in their opinion, the DS adult cannot use tools. What is left for them is mother's helper, grounds work, manual labour in a shipping room, laundry work, etc. Thompson (1963) agreed that coordination is poor in DS children but that continuing training can benefit both the motor and visual components of coordination. She has observed DS adults in workshops using soldering irons and proposed that if suitable eye–hand training is given, in the primary stages of schooling, vocational promise will improve. Fitzpatrick (1959) tested the notion that training, through the exploitation of rhythm, might advance vocational productivity. A lever-manipulation task was performed to the beat of a metronome but DS subjects were not superior to other retarded individuals. We need to recognize the motor, sensory and cognitive peculiarities of DS children, applied to work training, and to begin the shaping process as early as individual readiness permits.

Whatever the prejudgements, DS adults are now to be found in sheltered workshops and protected industry doing a wide variety of repair and assembly tasks. A few are employed in unprotected service, manufacturing, and agricultural enterprises. The long-term stability of these placements is not known. The assumption is that since all children engage in academic pursuits, graduating to some identifiable vocation, then so must the DS individual. The result can be inappropriate education followed by a dull job for poor wages. The alternatives are to extend the training process into adulthood, consistent with tested economic outcomes, and to develop satisfying adult activity patterns whether or not they are of commercial importance. Our compulsion that earned income is the measure of life success for mentally handicapped individuals is possibly self-serving. One extreme opinion, offered by Farber (1968), is that the working handicapped among us perpetuate social class by providing evidence that low-level work output attracts meagre rewards. Moreover, the care of the mentally handicapped is itself a major industry which has an extensive budget and personnel network. Maintenance of the care infrastructure depends to some extent on a product which meets the social bias, i.e., ability to adjust to open society and to work for wages. The quality of the community or vocational–economic adjustment has not been a significant concern to date because the preferences of the mentally handicapped adult, in respect to his life goals, are unknown. In any event, these would be difficult to separate from sanctioned beliefs and the emotional investment of parents and pressure groups. The problem is one which deserves dispassionate consideration.

A second problem area is the relation of work success to the social and affective aspects of the syndrome. Swanson (1975) described the success and failure of a number of DS adults employed in a large government agency. One boy delivered mail and did Xerox work. He sang as he worked, was reliable and generally cheerful. On the negative side were the 'mad days' for which staff made allowances. Most evident was a dependency on rigid routine, the breaking of any link in the activity sequence producing immobility. Interruptions of these tasks by friendly staff also tended initially to disturb his concentration and routine. These characteristics are evident in many DS youth and adults. They can be managed by counselling normal employees and managers to make allowances, within practical limits, or by job placement in types of employment where cognitive and personal rigidity are advantages or where the occasional pout does not lower productivity. Much depends on preparing fellow workers and in having some individual in the work setting who will act as 'sponsor' on a continuing basis (Edgerton, 1967). Not every work setting will accommodate a DS individual, objective skill requirements aside. The preparation of Down's individuals for industrial employment continues, nevertheless, as part of general programmes for the mentally retarded. These catch-all schemes have had little demonstrable effectiveness (Windle, 1962; Cobb, 1967). Gibson and Fields (1970) found that hospital trained retardates survived in the community quite independent of duration or type of formal vocational preparation. Job success or failure was a function of general competence (IQ levels), type of handicap and temperament. These essentially biological dimensions of mental retardation might be expected to influence survival on the job and to relate to quality of co-worker or community sponsorship.

Newer methods of vocational education for the moderately to severely retarded, including the DS individual, apply principles of operant discrimination and chaining (Crosson, 1969). Each vocational task is re-defined in terms of operations appropriate to the client. Modelling and assistance procedures are used along with suitable reinforcement (praise, treats, etc.). Assistance is gradually faded. Crosson et al. (1970) have extended these methods to 'transenvironmental' programming. An entire workshop programme is analysed for the functional relationships between environmental event and individual behaviour. The appropriate target behaviours are selected and the critical elements of the 'natural' environment are 'compressed'. Performance repertoires emerge which can be gradually broadened to approach natural conditions. Cue manipulation provides an important component of these schemes. Gold (1975) describes the assembly of a bicycle brake in which form dimension (the shape of each part) is strengthened by a colour dimension (each part colour coded). Pay (reinforcement and incentive) should be meaningful to the trainee and tied to short-term production goals, initially. Units and types of work, schedules of non-monetary reward, feedback procedures and modelling techniques are each designed to be client specific. Later in the programme, instructors are required to determine individual client reaction to bonus pay, the effectiveness of competitive over cooperative work conditions (assembly lines versus solitary work stations) and the client-to-task relevance of quantity over quality output. Some trainees were found to function better in situations where fellow workers rather than managers acted as reinforcers. These more artful approaches to industrial training have not been tested for durability of gains or against older training methods.

Gold (1975) presents three questions for the future: (i) The extent to which pre-vocational training (language acquisition, social skills, self-help behaviours, etc.) can be aligned with vocational training and job targets. (ii) The extent to which principles of industrial engineering are applicable to the mentally handicapped, e.g., the worker controlling his own pace, choosing work methods, monitoring the quality of his product and other aspects of 'job enlargement'. (iii) How to achieve a balance between habilitation preparation for personal growth as against work productivity. Acceptance in modern society is still contingent upon 'real' productivity and deviance is tolerated to that extent. Unfortunately, job failure is often not specific to a particular task, social and general behavioural characteristics being the more frequent determinants of acceptance or rejection by both peers and managers.

A fourth point can be made; that educational and vocational habilitation practices for the mentally handicapped could be made more powerful by tailoring them to the structural and physiological artifacts of individuals and causal groups. Ability profiles for DS as a whole are sufficiently homogeneous to warrant recognition in training procedures. Ability differences within a Down's population are also important to vocational training and are more easily recognized if the performance parameters for the disorder as a class are understood. These similarities and differences have been shown to exist at birth (Carr, 1975) and to survive through adulthood (Menolascino, 1974). Present methods of training demonstrate meagre results and considerable variability of outcome. Schachter (1974) traced the economic and social development for young DS adults over a ten year period. All had been raised under optimal medical, educational and family circumstances. Yet psychological status at adulthood was described as marginal. It will be of interest, in the coming years, to follow the progress to maturity of DS children fostered in specialized community or hospital programmes as compared with those reared under 'optimal' conditions; the usual home, school and sheltered workshop regimes.

Conclusion

The welfare of DS individuals has been advanced by improvements in physical care and by our growing understanding of their special maturational and behavioural qualities. Health gains have been achieved through more effective feeding practices, the control of respiratory and circulatory systems dysfunction and the correction of certain of the structural defects of the syndrome. Psychological gains have been made by adjusting early environment intervention programmes to the sensory, motor and arousal systems properties of the disorder and by building on improved general health. It is too soon yet to pronounce on ultimate results: whether or not behavioural and medical intervention during infancy significantly slows the deterioration curve into adulthood and if the positive effects, overall, will be hidden statistically by the increasing survival of less viable cases of the disorder. We do know that significant remission of the condition is unlikely because most of the damage has occurred *in utero* and is morphologically or physiologically apparent at birth. If, however, certain of these anomalies can be modified then the behavioural phenotypes will be less severe.

There are a number of dangers for the future. The first is to hold out hope for 'magic bullet' (drugs, vitamins, hormones) cures. Parents react with great expectation and are subsequently disenchanted both with the proposed cure and with their DS child. They will continue to be deceived by proposals for chemical reversals of the condition because guilt and frustration are very close to the surface for them and because the purveyors of such methods will continue to hold the public stage to the disadvantage of less glamorous methods of intervention. Two other continuing risks come to mind. These grow out of the belief that DS children are like all others and a conviction that mental handicap is in the eye of the beholder. The first leads to the position that the DS child has few special needs and that undifferentiated family and community care are sufficient. The evidence now favours much more sophisticated remediation which can be undertaken on a group basis but involving skilled parent participation and ongoing professional guidance. The second is a belief that the DS individual will succeed in society or not depending substantially on citizen tolerance. Experience with other handicapping conditions, in adulthood and in unprotected settings, is that community acceptance is given in proportion to the coping skills of the handicapped. These can be improved for most DS individuals but within limits which preclude fully independent functioning or complete community accommodation for the majority. What we need for the immediate future is an integrated DS treatment programme beginning with a full paediatric and psychological assessment soon after birth to be followed by life-span management regimes continually adjusted to within-syndrome variability. The programmes reviewed in the present chapter have demonstrated that the ingredients of a full-scale campaign are available. Orchestration of the parts and validation of outcomes are the next obvious steps.

12

Overview

Laying ghosts

Behavioural research on Down's syndrome is at a stage which only imperfectly sustains the syntheses reached at the end of each chapter and supports, certainly, no further attempt to generalize. This, the final section, speculates instead on the more immediate prospects for DS children and adults and on the place of a bio-behavioural research and service approach to problems of developmental arrest.

But first there are a few ghosts to lay. The DS literature is characteristic of the gap between basic and applied study in MR and between the biological and social sciences at the level of remediation. The separation has encouraged a number of propositions having the regrettable status of working assumptions. Major among them is that patterns of psychological potential are more or less similar across categories of developmental arrest, the only noteworthy distinctions being quantitative. Thus the management burden is more heavy for the severely than for the moderately or mildly retarded but is otherwise similar in kind. The foregoing belief owes something to a second assumption which is curiously discordant with the first, i.e., that adjustment capacity for the mentally retarded is quite plastic so that the clever manoeuvring of environments is both necessary *and* sufficient. There are several corollaries: (i) the elaboration of nosological schema within MR is pointless and possibly dangerous, (ii) bio-behavioural patterns are not sufficiently reliable across the mental retardations to sustain differential management practices, and (iii) psycho-assessment procedures are relatively unimportant in the context of active treatment and training.

These propositions are being confronted by a growing body of evidence which supports distinctive ability–disability profiles for the many causal subgroups within mental retardation. It was suggested in the opening chapter that management programmes, based solely on the foregoing assumptions, have not had impressive results and that alternative positions should be

321

examined for the future. One general impression from the DS literature is that behavioural capacities and incapacities are not substantially random in origin or expression and can be related to the physiological characteristics of the condition. A first priority will be to intervene as close to the basic somatic properties of the disorder as possible. The second priority requires that the external operations, which make up a given management approach, give maximum benefit appropriate to these properties.

Most inhibiting to an eclectic research and remediation approach to Down's syndrome is the fear that physical states are unalterable; that if psychological capacity is governed importantly by physiological and morphological factors, treatment and training opportunities are somehow diminished. There is ample evidence that DS is not defined at birth and that the sensorimotor particulars can be manipulated by maturationally specific programmes of early intervention. There is additional support that affect the socialization potentials are comparatively more intact than cognitive potentials and that the former can provide a platform for directed compensatory growth. In each instance, the requirement is that interstitial activity be attuned to the developmental phasing of the syndrome.

An equally dubious argument is that members of a single aetiological class should exhibit identical physical and psychological consequences. Otherwise, within-syndrome differences must have been acquired through the nurtural process. We now appreciate that common primary causes do not produce identical outcomes. Clinical sequalae are complicated by extent and quality of secondary damage which fluctuates from case to case. Developmental sequencing, while codified within DS to a significant degree, is thus not uniform in expression between and among cases. Data variability, associated with quantitative dissimilarity, can be separated statistically from that related to qualitative similarities across the syndrome. In either event, the sources are mainly syndromic. A practical difficulty with the viewpoint is that parents and professionals read about the exceptional DS child who reaches an educable level and is able to make a place in open society. The observer all too easily assumes that sensitive, loving and educationally intensive environments are the prime prescriptions – and then wonders why all DS children do not reach similar goals based on similar experience. Love, dedication and hard work are essential to rearing the DS child but fall short of maximum remedial impact if not built on the known bio-behavioural features of the condition.

A further impediment to sharpening our working assumptions about the mental retardations is that labelling is viewed as prejudicial to the child and his family. When naming has the single purpose of excluding certain groups

from community services, it is a failure. The present epistemology is substantially a product of nineteenth-century physicians who believed that symptom coalescence is based on shared cause and that prevention and clinical
treatment would be advanced in proportion to the precision of diagnosis.
Little, however, was then known about the substrata of the clinical anomalies
of MR because the biological sciences were in their infancy. Effective
remediation did not automatically follow upon the identification of the
disorders which make up the mental retardations and physicians cooled to
the cause. It was the social worker, psychologist, educator, public health
worker and parent who filled the management void; at least to recent times.

An early phase of the interest of psychology and education in the MR field
was to reject the 'medical' model. These disciplines denied the validity of
even the venerable term 'mental deficiency' because it embodied the notion
of inexplicit biological forces and irreversible deficit. Terms such as mental
retardation, exceptionality and intellectual disadvantage were more readily
acceptable because they implied growth lag or developmental differences
which could somehow be interpreted within the constructs of S–R psychology. The environmentalist view of programme direction within MR
produced a flood of scholarship and services which have, in retrospect,
served control and disposal goals. The upshot was that laymen, mainly the
parents of the retarded, organized to declare a plague on both the medically
originated structuralists and the social sciences based functionalists. The new
parent pressure groups were politically potent and preached that the mentally
handicapped are rejected in the community because stereotypes, medical or
social, generate prejudice and prejudice sustains stereotypes. Segregation,
justified by labels, was viewed as diagnostically self-fulfilling because deficit
is a function of its naming. Diagnosogenesis is a genuine phenomenon in some
areas of behavioural handicap but has little force in relation to the severe
forms of mental arrest. The next logical step, following denial of the problem,
was the movement to full integration of the MR into regular classes and
regular jobs. It was imagined that the generosity of the community, at large,
would guarantee acceptance of the new citizens and treat non-acceptance
as a product of willful discrimination.

That has not happened and clearly the emperor has no clothes. Public
attitudes toward the de-institutionalized and community 'integrated' mentally retarded are still uncertain. Attempts to buttress integration with hard-sell
programmes of sponsorship, citizen advocacy, legislated rights and job
creation incentives are equally unreliable for tactical and practical reasons.
There is evidently a need for both the general public and the mentally
retarded in the community to protect their respective life space and integrity.

It is conceivable, indeed, that the social integration of the MR will prove workable only to the extent that support and re-training services are continually available over the life span of the client and if the MR adult has the right to 'opt out' in favour of periods of cloistering. Parents, employers, sponsors, etc., also require the right of disassociation when and if the need arises. As things stand now, we expect too much from the MR as potential citizens and from ourselves as resource providers. To invite the DS adult to survive in the community without specialized early management or a significant following infrastructure of services is not consistent with the evidence of de-institutionalization research and we are in danger of coming full tilt from an unthinking abandonment of the MR, in decades past, to a planned abandonment now. These are hard words only if we fail to acknowledge that much of our management research is of poor quality and that programme accountability studies have not, thus far, supported idealized goals.

Options and assumptions

What are the possibilities? Scientists from all participating disciplines are again interested in the effective treatment of disorders of developmental origin. They accept subgroups of MR as having discrete causes and identifiable consequences which can be modified in part. They acknowledge the ethics and economics of prevention and of direct biological intervention, where possible. Large-scale preventative methods are now available for Down's syndrome but political systems, legal codes and social values inhibit implementation. The future for habilitation services includes semi-independent community placement, community residential-work units, industrial and agricultural communes, and worker colonies sponsored by institutions and community agencies. Whatever plan is deemed suitable for a given DS individual, at a given time in his development, a continuing network of support and re-programming services will be essential.

The most contentious of the foregoing options is likely to be the institutional route. The old establishments were unnecessarily large, remote from parents and from centres of post-secondary education, had few research facilities and were poorly funded. The result was a progressively degraded form of custodial care. The newer and smaller residential centres are offered here as a preferred model because community access can be assured on a balanced basis. The drive for community integration, failing the design of long-term support services, will lead to little more than ghetto status for the mentally handicapped. Moreover, small community residences are too frequently unstable in staffing, have few in-house or other training services and provide limited access to specialized professional counsel. They became orphanages for the adult MR; unspecialized institutions without walls which serve to remind the public of the failure of their programmes and of their clients. A management alternative, intermediate between the old and the new, is the smaller community-related institution. The advantages are many. Assessment, training, treatment and outreach supervision can be coordinated from a single point regionally. Parents can be involved in professional treatment programmes and family-based clients can be monitored as out-patients or have access to intensive services as in-patients for limited periods. Parent relief services are easily arranged and can help insure that the DS child will remain in a family setting even if that setting is unstable from time to time. Within the community institution, professional services can be grouped economically according to client problems held in common. The training of care technologists and the undertaking of applied and bridging research is enhanced insofar as centres of advanced study are close at hand. Present pressures to integrate services for the mentally handicapped, even if approached piecemeal, will achieve many of the same ends because the centralized coordination of proliferating community services is inevitable. Cost control and ease of administration are two-reasons. The process, though, will be a painful one because social agencies have a reputation for resisting intrusions, are often insular, avoid external evaluation and compete among themselves for the tax dollar.

A number of general impressions emerge from the review of many hundreds of behavioural studies of Down's syndrome. The first is of the relatively poor quality of research design and data management represented by these investigations. It has been possible to reach conclusions, on a tentative basis, by assuming that consensus has power and that methodological error is randomly distributed. Both arguments are subject to dispute. A second impression is that research specialists from education, the social sciences and medicine have a tendency to interpret their findings without regard to related data from outside their fields. The inferences made by each are thereby weakened. A final observation is that fundamental and programme scientists, in our domain, do not communicate very well. There are problems in the way we bridge research to practice and how we train MR researchers, professionals and technologists. The search for solutions will continue to be impeded by our traditional beliefs and habits. A number of these warrant closer inspection.

(1) The term 'mental retardation', or any of its euphemisms, has ongoing value if we expect no more than administrative or legal convenience and if

we accept that severity of disorder, exclusive of the nature of the disorder, has meaning for management purposes. Both rationales are under pressure. Parents fret about the stigmatizing influence of broad descriptive labels and functionalists *cum* radical behaviouralists continue to defend the questionable position that antecedent biological conditions cannot or need not be recognized in the search for remedial tools. Thus our management and research enterprises can be fruitful only to the extent that the mentally retarded are similarly dissonant with the child care practices of family and society. We overlook the possibility that distinct causal groups within MR present distinctive problems with respect to learning and mentation. Further refinements in classification will be justified where the labelling function represents special disorders, implies special needs and dictates special services. Down's syndrome meets these criteria.

(2) The proposal for a stronger bio-behavioural approach to managing disorders of maturational origin suggests a syndromic model and that, in turn, a medical model. The medical model has been in disrepute for reasons suggested earlier. In addition, there are the several misunderstandings that remediation, to be successful, must be totally curative and that only one group among the helping professions possesses the necessary skills. The medical model addresses similarities within conditions. The bio-behavioural model is less specific; it also deals with similarities across conditions and differences within conditions. It presupposes that bio-behavioural variability can be apportioned according to source; between causal categories, within causal categories, and on the basis of interacting nurtural or situational events across maturational periods. There need be, therefore, no exclusive explanatory or remedial model if all available data is incorporated into programming.

(3) Just as the integration of the major theoretical and serving modes in MR is urgent, so is the need to train applied scientists and professionals more flexibly. It is possible, even commonplace, to be a 'specialist' in MR while knowing little about human genetics, or learning theory, or neuropsychology, or social process or educational technology. It is also evident from the literature that applied research into mental retardation has not exploited advances in data management of the kind which permit the processing of complex simultaneous events. We have had an over-sufficiency of research comparing two forms of a test for undifferentiated MR, contrasting unspecified MR samples with normal children, drawing conclusions from single case data, and demonstrating programmes without the adequate use of control or follow-up procedures. Service workers suffer because multidiscipline leadership is rare and faddish treatments soon peak and retreat,

leaving behind an irrelevant or redundant technology. Operant procedures, chemical and surgical intervention, sensorimotor training, attention to health and diet problems, perceptual-learning and other stimulus patterning procedures, modelling approaches, and milieu management are helpful when used in concert and balanced to fit the needs of individuals and classes of individuals.

(4) A final area of concern is that we should validate our methods and programmes. Most have suitable short term results, if only for placebo reasons. Each engages resources and absorbs client time but none prove equally effective under all circumstances. Excuses are made that controlled study is unethical, that outcomes are uncertain over time because community criteria of success are unstable and that human achievement cannot be weighed and sized as if a commodity. There are, admittedly, problems with cost-benefit and social outcome studies, but none which can escape innovative research strategies. What is increasingly appreciated for Down's syndrome is that remediation must be specific to the given individual, intensive and early off the mark. Improved assessment methods should facilitate the selection of programme streams to match projected ability–disability configurations and to help avoid stressing the DS child by inappropriate expectation.

In the end, the outcome options for the DS adult will be dictated by the community at large. The protectors of public funds work invariably to priorities which favour demonstrated capacity and select against services which do not meet social needs at fair cost. We counter with statements about the rights of the disadvantaged when the fundamental issues are those of responsibility; of concerned parents, professionals and other staff. The call then is two-fold: (i) to reduce the observable gap in performance between the DS individual and the average citizen by hard-nosed remediation tailored to all dimensions of the disorder and (ii) to understand that community tolerance is founded on the self-interest of the majority of its members.

References

Abraham, W. (1958). *Barbara: a prologue*. New York: Rinehart.

Adamowicz, J. K. and Gibson, D. (1970). Cue screening, cognitive elaboration and heart-rate change. *Canadian Journal of Psychology*, **24**, 240–8.

Adamowicz, J. K. and Gibson, D. (1972). Verbalization, cognitive effort and heart rate alteration. *Canadian Journal of Psychology*, **26**, 1–10.

Akesson, H. O. and Forssman, H. (1966). A study of maternal age in Down's syndrome. *Annals of Human Genetics*, **29**, 271–6.

Aldrich, C. A. (1947). Preventative medicine and mongolism. *American Journal of Mental Deficiency*, **52**, 127–9.

Alley, G. R. (1968). Perceptual-motor performance of mentally retarded children after systemic visual–perceptual training. *American Journal of Mental Deficiency*, **73**, 247–50.

American Association on Mental Deficiency (1973). Rights of mentally retarded persons. *Mental Retardation*, **11** (5), 56–8.

Antley, M. A., Ray, M. and Hartlage, L. C. (1973). Effects of genetic counselling on parental self concept. *Journal of Psychology*, **83**, 335–8.

Apert, E. (1914). *Le Mongolisme*. English edn. Paris: Mode Medicale.

Ardran, G. M., Harker, P. and Kemp, F. H. (1972). Tongue size in Down's syndrome. *Journal of Mental Deficiency Research*, **16**, 160–6.

Arey, L. B. (1954). *Developmental anatomy*. 6th edn. Philadelphia: W. B. Saunders Co.

Armstrong, R. G. (1959). Review of the current theories and findings concerning mongolism. *Psychology Newsletter, NYU*, **10**, 151–8.

Astin, A. W. and Ross, S. (1960). Glutamic acid and human intelligence. *Psychological Bulletin*, **57**, 429–34.

Astrup, C., Sersen, E. A. and Wortis, J. (1967). Further psychophysiological studies of retarded, neurotic, psychotic and normal children. In *Recent advances in biological psychiatry*, ed. J. Wortis, vol. 9. New York: Plenum Press.

Bae, A. Y. (1968). Factors influencing vocational efficiency of institutionalized retardates in different training programs. *American Journal of Mental Deficiency*, **72**, 871–4.

Bardon, L. M. (1964). Siccacell treatment in mongolism. *Lancet*, **2**, 234.

Barkla, D. H. (1963). Congenital absence and fusion in the deciduous dentition in mongols. *Journal of Mental Deficiency Research*, **7**, 102–6.

Barkla, D. H. (1966). Ages of eruption of permanent teeth in mongols. *Journal of Mental Deficiency Research*, **10**, 190–7.

Barnard, K. E. and Powell, M. L. (1972). *Teaching the mentally retarded child: a family care approach*. Saint Louis: Mosby.

Barnard, K. E. (1975). Infant stimulation. In *Down's syndrome (mongolism): research, prevention and management*, ed. R. Koch and F. F. de la Cruz. New York: Brunner/Mazel.

Barnet, A. B. and Lodge, A. (1967). Click evoked EEG responses in normal and developmentally retarded infants. *Nature*, **214**, 252–5.

Barnet, A. B., Ohlrich, E. S. and Shanks, B. L. (1971). EEG evoked responses to repetitive auditory stimulation in normal and Down's syndrome infants. *Developmental Medicine and Child Neurology*, **13**, 321–9.

Barr, M. W. (1904). *Mental defectives: their history, treatment and training.* Philadelphia: Philip Blakiston's Son.

Barthel, E. (1952). Diagnosis and therapeutic successes in mongolian idiocy. *Psychiatry, Neurology and Medical Psychology* (Leipzig), **4**, 152–9.

Baumeister, A. A. and Williams, J. (1967). Relationship of physical stigmata to intellectual functioning of mongolism. *American Journal of Mental Deficiency*, **71**, 586–92.

Bavin, J. T. R., Marshall, R. and Delhanty, J. D. A. (1963). A mongol with a 21:22 type chromosomal translocation. *Journal of Mental Deficiency Research*, **7**, 84–9.

Bayley, N. (1955). On the growth of intelligence. *American Psychologist*, **10**, 805–18.

Bayley, N., Rhodes, L. and Gooch, B. (1966). A comparison of the development of institutionalized and home reared mongoloids. A follow-up study. *California Mental Health Research Digest*, **4**, 104–5.

Bayley, N., Rhodes, L., Gooch, B. and Marcus, M. (1971). Environmental factors in the development of institutionalized children. In *Exceptional Infant*, ed. J. Hellmuth, vol. 2, studies in abnormalities. New York: Brunner/Mazel.

Bazelon, M. and Paine, R. (1967). Reversal of hypotonia in infants with Down's syndrome by administration of 5-hydroxytryptophan. *Lancet*, **1**, 1130.

Bazelon, M., Paine, R. S., Cowie, V., Hunt, P., Houck, J. C. and Mahanand, D. (1970). Reversal of hypotonia in infants with Down's syndrome by administration of 5-hydroxytryptophan. *Lancet*, **2**, 365.

Beach, F. (25 March 1882). On types of imbecility. *Medical Times and Gazette*, 300–2.

Beal, G. and Stanton, R. G. (1945). Reduction in the number of mongolian defectives – a result of family limitations. *Canadian Journal of Public Health*, **36**, 33–7.

Becker, K. L. and Albert, A. (1963). Familial translocation mongolism: a carrier exhibiting non acrocentric translocation. *Proceedings Staff Meetings Mayo Clinic*, **38**, 216–67.

Becker, K. L. (1966). Translocation mongolism. *Postgraduate Medicine*, **40**, 459–64.

Beddie, A. and Osmund, H. (1955). Mothers, mongols and mores. *Canadian Medical Association Journal*, **73**, 167–170.

Beidleman, B. (1945). Mongolism: a selective review. *American Journal of Mental Deficiency*, **50**, 35–53.

Beley, A. P. L. and Lecuyer, R. (1960). Les enfants arrieres mongoliens. *Revue de Neuropsychiatrie Infantile et d'Hygiène Mentale de l'Enfance*, **8**, 37–51.

Belmont, J. M. (1971). Medical–Behavioural Research in Retardation. In *International Review of Research in Mental Retardation*, ed. N. R. Ellis, vol. 5. New York: Academic Press.

Benda, C. E. (1946). *Mongolism and cretinism*, 1st edn. New York: Grune & Stratton.

Benda, C. E. (1949). *Mongolism and cretinism*, 2nd edn. New York: Grune & Stratton.

Benda, C. E. (1953). Research in congenital acromicria (mongolism) and its treatment. *Quarterly Review Pediatrics*, **8**, 79–96.

Benda, C. E. (1956). Mongolism: A comprehensive review. *Archives of Pediatrics*, **73**, 391–407.

Benda, C. E. (1957). Discussion of the paper of Grace M. Sawyer MD and Albert J. Shatter PhD on reproduction in a mongoloid. A follow-up. *American Journal of Mental Deficiency*, **61**, 796–7.

Benda, C. E. (1960*a*). *The child with mongolism.* New York: Grune & Stratton.

Benda, C. E. (1960*b*). Mongolism: Clinical manifestations, pathology and etiology. In *Mental Retardation*, ed. P. W. Bowman, First International Medical Conference. New York: Grune & Stratton.

Benda, C. E. (1969). *Down's syndrome: mongolism and its management.* New York: Grune & Stratton.

Berg, J. M., Kerman, B. H., Stern J. and Mittwoch, U. (1961). Treatment of mongolism with pituitary extract. *Journal of Mental Science,* **107**, 475–80.

Berg, J. M. and Stern, J. (1963). Observations on children with mongolism. *Proceedings, 2nd International Congress Mental Retardation, Vienna, 1963,* **1**, 367–72.

Berg, J. M., Gilderdale, S. and Way, J. (1969). On telling parents of a diagnosis of mongolism. *British Journal of Psychiatry,* **115**, 1195.

Berkson, G. (1960). An analysis of reaction time in normal and mentally deficient young mongoloids. III: variation of stimulus and response complexity. *Journal of Mental Deficiency Research,* **4**, 69–77.

Berkson, G. (1963). Psychophysiological studies in mental deficiency. In *Handbook of Mental Deficiency,* ed. N. R. Ellis. New York: McGraw-Hill.

Berkson, G., Hermelin, B. and O'Connor, N. (1961). Physiological responses of normals and institutionalized mental defectives to repeated stimuli. *Journal of Mental Deficiency Research,* **5**, 30–9.

Berry, D. M. (1924). An investigation of fifty cases of mongolian imbecility. *British Journal of Childrens Diseases,* **21**, 259.

Berry, M. F. and Eisenson, J. (1956). *Speech Disorders; principles and practices of therapy.* New York: Appleton-Century-Crofts.

Bertrand, I. and Koffas, D. (1946). Cas d'idiotie mongolienne adulte avec nombreuses plaques seniles et concretions calcaires pallidales. *Revue Neurologique,* **78**, 338.

Biesele, J. J., Schmid, W. and Lawlis, M. G. (1962). Mentally retarded schizoid twin girls with 47 chromosomes. *Lancet,* **1**, 403.

Bigum, H. B., Beck E. C. and Dustman, R. E. (1966–67). Visual and somatosensory evoked responses of mongoloid and normal children. *Research Relating to Children,* **21**, 16.

Bigum, H. B., Dustman, R. E. and Beck, E. C. (1970). Visual and somato-sensory evoked responses from mongoloid and normal children. *Electroencepholography and Clinical Neurophysiology Journal,* **28**, 576–85.

Bilovsky, D. and Share, J. (1965). The ITPA and Down's syndrome: an exploratory study. *American Journal of Mental Deficiency,* **70**, 78–82.

Birch, H. E. and Belmont, L. (1961). The problems of comparing home rearing versus foster-home rearing in defective children. *Pediatrics,* **28**, 956–61.

Birch, H. G. and Demb, H. (1959). The formation and extinction of conditioned reflexes in 'brain-damaged' and mongoloid children. *Journal of Nervous and Mental Diseases,* **129**, 162–70.

Black, A. H. and Thomas, L. D. (1966). Differential effectiveness of primary, secondary, and social reinforcement in discrimination learning of mongoloids: preliminary note. *Perceptual and Motor Skills,* **23**, 585–6.

Black, D. B., Kato, J. G. and Walker, G. W. R. (1966). A study of improvement in mentally retarded children accruing from Siccacell therapy. *American Journal of Mental Deficiency,* **70**, 499–508.

Blacketer-Simmonds, D. A. (1953). An investigation into the supposed differences existing between mongols and other mentally defective subjects with regard to certain psychological traits. *Journal of Mental Science,* **99**, 702–19.

Blackwood, W., McMenemy, W. H., Meyer, A., Norman, R. M. and Russell, D. S. (1963). *Greenfield's Neuropathology.* Baltimore: Williams & Wilkins.

Blanchard, I. (1964). Speech pattern and etiology in mental retardation. *American Journal of Mental Deficiency,* **68**, 612–17.

Blank, C. E. (1962). Mosaicism in a mother with a mongol child. *British Medical Journal,* **2**, 378.

Blessing, K. R. (1959). The middle range mongoloid in trainable classes. *American Journal of Mental Deficiency,* **63**, 812–21.

Block, J. D., Sersen, E. A. and Wortis, J. (1970). Cardiac classical conditioning and reversal in the mongoloid, encephalopathic, and normal child. *Child Development*, **41**, 771–85.

Blount, W. R. (1968). Language and the more severely retarded: a review. *American Journal of Mental Deficiency*, **73**, 21–9.

Blumberg, E. (1959). Two years of pituitary treatment on mongoloids. *Journal of the Maine Medical Association*, **50**, 120.

Borselli, L. and Sferlazzo, R. (1963). Considerazioni sul problema dell'epilessia nei mongoli. *Rivista di Clinica Pediatria*, **62**, 45.

Bourne, H. (1955). Protophrenia: a study of perverted rearing and mental dwarfism. *Lancet*, **2**, 1156.

Bowlby, J. (1952). *Maternal care and mental health*. Geneva: WHO monograph, series no. 2.

Brauner, A. and Brauner, F. (1964). *Raising the mentally defective child*. Seine, France: Groupement de Recherches Practiques.

Brink, M. and Grundlingh, E. M. (1976). Performance of persons with Down's syndrome on two projective techniques. *American Journal of Mental Deficiency*, **81**, 265–70.

Brinkworth, R. (1967). The effects of early training on the mongoloid infant, doctoral dissertation (unpublished), University of Birmingham.

Brinkworth, R. and Collins, J. (1969). *Improving mongol babies*. Belfast: National Society for Mentally Handicapped Children.

Brogger, A. (1967). *Translocation in human chromosomes*. Oslo, Norway: Scandinavian University Books.

Brooks, D. N. and Woolley, H. (1972). Hearing loss and middle ear disorders in patients with Down's syndrome. *Journal of Mental Deficiency Research*, **16**, 21–9.

Brousseau, K. and Brainerd, M. G. (1928). *Mongolism: a study of the psychical and mental characteristics of mongoloid imbeciles*. Baltimore: Williams & Wilkins.

Brown, R. I. and Clarke, A. D. B. (1963). The effects of auditory distraction on institutionalized subnormal and severely subnormal persons. *Journal of Mental Deficiency Research*, **7**, 1–8.

Bruner, J. S. (1966). *Toward a theory of instruction*. Cambridge: Harvard University Press.

Brushfield, T. (1924). Mongolism. *British Journal of Children's Diseases*, **21**, 240.

Buck, C., Valentine, G. H. and Hamilton, K. A. (1966). Reproductive performance of mothers of mongols. *American Journal of Mental Deficiency*, **70**, 886–93.

Buck, C., Valentine, G. H. and Hamilton, K. A. (1969). A study of microsymptoms in the parents and sibs of patients with Down's syndrome. *American Journal of Mental Deficiency*, **73**, 683–92.

Buck, J. N. (1955). The sage: an unusual mongoloid. In *Clinical studies of personality*, ed. A. Burton and R. E. Harris, pp. 455–81. New York: Harper & Row.

Buddenhagen, R. G. (1967–68). Operant conditioning as a technique for establishing vocal verbal behavior in non-talking institutionalized mongoloid children. *Dissertation Abstracts*, **1804A** (University of Rochester, 1967).

Buddenhagen, R. G. (1971). *Establishing vocal verbalizations in mute mongoloid children*. Champaign, Illinois: Research Press.

Buddenhagen, R. G. and Sickler, P. (1969). Hyperactivity: a forty-eight hour sample plus a note on etiology. *American Journal of Mental Deficiency*, **73**, 580–9.

Buium, N., Rynders, J. and Turnure, J. (1974). Early maternal linguistic environment of normal and Down's syndrome language-learning children. *American Journal of Mental Deficiency*, **79**, 52–8.

Bullard, W. N. (1911). Mongolian idiocy. *Boston Medical Surgical Journal*, **164**, 56.

Bumbalo, T. S., Morelewicz, H. V. and Berens, D. E. (1964). Treatment of Down's syndrome with the 'U' series of drugs. *Journal American Medical Association*, **178**, 361.

Buresch, M. A. (1975). *Mongoloid psychology: questions and principles concerning the Down's syndrome child*. Detroit, Michigan: Mongoloid Achievements Foundation, Troy, Michigan, Harlo Press.

Butler, A. J. (1960). Investigation of homogeneity of mongoloid traits. *Research Relating to Children*, US Department of Health and Welfare **1**, 21.

Buttlerfield, E. C. (1961). A provocative case of overachievement by a mongoloid. *American Journal of Mental Deficiency*, **66**, 444–8.

Byck, M. (1968). Cognitive differences among diagnostic groups of retardates. *American Journal of Mental Deficiency*, **73**, 97–101.

Caccamo, J. M. and Yater, A. C. (1972). The ITPA and Negro children with Down's syndrome. *Exceptional Children*, **38**, 642–3.

Cain, L. F. and Levine, S. (1963). Effects of community and institutional school programs on trainable mentally retarded. *CEC Research Monographs* (series E).

Caldwell, B. M. and Guze, S. B. (1960). A study of the adjustment of parents and siblings of institutional and non-institutional retarded children. *American Journal of Mental Deficiency*, **64**, 845–8.

Canbanas, R. (1954). Some findings in speech and voice therapy among mentally deficient children. *Folia Phoniatrica*, **6**, 34–7.

Cant, N. H. P., Gerrard, J. W. and Richards, B. W. (1953). A girl of mongolian appearance and normal intelligence. *Journal of Mental Science*, **99**, 560–3.

Cantor, G. N. and Girardeau, F. L. (1959). Rhythmic discrimination ability in mongoloid and normal children. *American Journal of Mental Deficiency*, **63**, 621–5.

Carr, J. (1970). Mental and motor development in young mongol children. *Journal of Mental Deficiency Research*, **14**, 205–20.

Carr, J. (1975). *Young children with Down's syndrome*. London: Butterworths.

Carson, J. C. (1907–8). The mongolian type. *Journal of Psychoasthenics*, **12**, 44–8.

Carter, C. H. (1967). Unpredictability of mental development in Down's syndrome. *Southern Medical Journal*, **60**, 834.

Carter, C. and Maley, M. (1958). Preliminary report on treatment of mongoloids. *Journal Florida Medical Association*, **44**, 709–13.

Carter, C. O. (1958). A life table for mongols with the causes of death. *Journal of Mental Deficiency Research*, **2**, 64–74.

Carter, C. O., Hamerton, J. L., Polani, P. E., Dunlap, A. and Weller, S. D. (1960). Chromosome translocation as a cause of familial mongolism. *Lancet*, **2**, 678–80.

Carter, D. and Clark, L. (1973). MA intellectual assessment by operant conditioning of Down's syndrome children. *Mental Retardation*, **11** (3), 39–41.

Cassel, M. E. (1953). A note on exogenous factors on the case histories of mongoloid individuals. *Training School Bulletin*, **50**, 65–70.

Cassel, R. H. (1949). Design reproduction in mental deficiency. *Journal Consulting Psychology*, **13**, 425–8.

Castellan-Paour, M. T. and Paour, J. L. (1971). (Attempt at re-education of syntactic structuration in the adolescent mongol.) *Revue de Neuropsychiatrie Infantile et d'Hygiene Mentale de l'Enfance*, **19**, 449–61.

Centerwall, S. W. and Centerwall, W. R. (1958). *An introduction to your child who has mongolism*. Los Angeles: College of Medical Evangelists.

Centerwall, S. W. and Centerwall, W. R. (1960). A study of children with mongolism reared in the home compared to those reared away from the home. *Pediatrics*, **25**, 678–85.

Chalfant, J., Silikovitz, R. and Tawney, J. (1973). *Systematic instruction for retarded children: the Illinois program*. Danville: Interstate.

Chaudhuri, A. and Chaudhuri, K. C. (1965). Chromosome mosaicism in an Indian child with Down's syndrome. *Journal of Medical Genetics*, **2**, 131.

Chigier, E. (1972). *Down's syndrome: a cross-cultural study of child and family*. Lexington, Massachusetts: Heath.

Chitham, R. G. and MacIver, E. (1965). A cytogenetic and statistical survey of 105 cases of mongolism. *Annals of Human Genetics*, **28**, 309.

Clark, R. M. (1933). The mongol: a new explanation. *Journal of Mental Science*, **79**, 328–36.

Clarke, C. M., Edwards, J. H. and Smallpeice, V. (1961). Trisomy/normal mosaicism in an intelligent child with some mongoloid characters. *Lancet*, 1028–30.

Clarke, C. M., Ford, C. E., Edwards, J. H. and Smallpeice, V. (1963). 21-trisomy/normal mosaicism in an intelligent child with some mongoloid characteristics. *Lancet*, **2**, 1229.

Clausen, J. (1966). *Ability structure and subgroups in mental retardation.* Washington: Sparton.

Clausen, J. (1968). Behavioral characteristics of Down's syndrome subjects. *American Journal of Mental Deficiency*, **73**, 118–26.

Clausen, J., Lidsky, A. and Sersen, E. A. (1975). Measurement of autonomic functions in mental deficiency. In *Developmental psychophysiology of mental retardation and learning disability*, ed. R. Karrer. Springfield, Illinois: C. C. Thomas.

Clements, P. R., Bates, M. V. and Hafer, M. (1976). Variability within Down's syndrome (trisomy-21): empirically observed sex differences in IQs. *Mental Retardation*, **14** (1), 30–1.

Clift, M. W. (1922). Roentgenological findings in mongolism. *American Journal Roentgenology*, **9**, 420.

Cobb, H. V. (1967). The prediction of adult adjustment of the retarded. *Proceedings of the first congress of the international association for the scientific study of mental deficiency*, pp. 314–22. Surrey, England: Michael Jackson.

Coleman, M. (ed.) (1973). *Serotonin in Down's syndrome.* New York: American Elsevier Publishing Co.

Coleman, T. W. (1960). A comparison of young brain-injured and mongolian mentally defective children on perception, thinking and behavior, doctoral dissertation (unpublished), University of Michigan.

Collman, R. D. and Stoller, A. (1962). A survey of mongoloid births in Victoria, Australia, 1942–57. *American Journal of Public Health*, **52**, 813.

Collman, R. D. and Stoller, A. (1963 a). A life table for mongols in Victoria, Australia. *Journal of Mental Deficiency Research*, **7**, 53–9.

Collman, R. D. and Stoller, A. (1963 b). Data on mongolism in Victoria, Australia: Prevalence and life expectation. *Journal of Mental Deficiency Research*, **7**, 60–8.

Collman, R. D. and Stoller, A. (1963 c). Comparison of age distributions for mothers of mongols born in high and in low birth incidence areas and years in Victoria, 1942–57. *Journal of Mental Deficiency Research*, **7**, 79.

Colton, R. E. (1973). A study of pure tone thresholds and intelligence in institutionalized and non-institutionalized Down's syndrome. *Dissertation Abstracts International*, **34** (5-A), 2420.

Conel, J. L. (1939). *The postnatal development of the human cerebral cortex.* Cambridge, Massachusetts: Harvard University Press.

Connor, F. P. and Goldberg, I. I. (1960). Opinions of some teachers regarding their work with trainable children: Implications for teacher education. *American Journal of Mental Deficiency*, **64**, 658–70.

Cook, B. A. (1950). Mongolism in one of twins. *Medical Journal of Australia*, **2**, 445–6.

Cooke, R. E. (1970). Seen in a report on 'Premature senility found in brains of mongoloids'. *Pediatric News* (January), **4**, 1.

Coppen, A. and Cowie, V. (1960). Maternal health and mongolism. *British Medical Journal*, **1**, 1843.

Coriat, L. F. de (1965). Evolucion de las Actitudes Posturales del Lactante. *Archivos Argentinos de Pediatria*, Buenos Aires.

Coriat, L. F. de, Theslenco, L. and Waksman, J. (1967). The effects of psychomotor stimulation on the IQ of young children with trisomy-21. *Proceedings of the first congress of the international association for the scientific study of mental deficiency*, 377–85.

Cornwell, A. C. (1974). Development of language, abstraction and numerical concept formation in Down's syndrome children. *American Journal of Mental Deficiency*, **79**, 179–90.

Cornwell, A. C. and Birch, H. G. (1969). Psychological and social development in home-reared children with Down's syndrome (Mongolism). *American Journal of Mental Deficiency*, **74**, 341–50.

Cowie, V. A. (1970). *A study of the early development of mongols*. Oxford: Pergamon Press.

Cratty, B. J. (1969). *Motor activity and the education of retardates*. Philadelphia: Lea & Febiger.

Crissey, S. (1975). Mental retardation: past, present and future. *American Psychologist*, **30**, 800–8.

Crome, L., Cowie, V. and Slater, E. (1966). A statistical note on the cerebellar and brain stem weight in mongolism. *Journal of Mental Deficiency Research*, **10**, 69–72.

Crookshank, F. G. (1924). *The mongol in our midst*. London: Kegan Paul.

Crookshank, F. G. (1925). *The mongol in our midst: a study of man and his three faces*, 2nd edn. New York: E. P. Dutton & Co.

Crosson, J. E. (1969). A technique for programming sheltered workshop environments for training severely retarded workers. *American Journal of Mental Deficiency*, **73**, 814–18.

Crosson, J. E., Youngberg, C. D. and White, O. R. (1970). Transenvironmental programming: an experimental approach to the rehabilitation of the retarded. In *Rehabilitation research and training center in mental retardation*, ed. H. J. Prehm, pp. 19–34. University of Oregon.

Cummins, H. and Midlo, C. (1943). *Finger-prints, palms and soles*. Philadelphia: Blakiston.

Cytryn, L. and Lourie, R. S. (1972). Prevention of mental illness in the mentally retarded. In *Mental Health Services for the mentally retarded*, ed. E. Katz. Springfield: C. C. Thomas.

Dalton, A. J., Crapper, D. R. and Schlotterer, G. R. (1974). Alzhemer's disease in Down's syndrome: visual retention deficits. *Cortex*, **10**, 366–77.

Dameron, L. E. (1963). Development of intelligence of infants with mongolism. *Child Development*, **34**, 733–8.

Davidenkova, E. F. (1966). *Down's disease: clinical and genetical investigations*. Leningrad: 'Medicine' Publishing House.

Davis, R. C. (1940). *Set and muscular tension*, vol. 10. Indiana: Indiana University.

Day, R. W. (1966). Genetic counselling and eugenics. In *Prevention and treatment of mental retardation*, ed. I. Philips. New York: Basic Books.

Decker, H., Herberg, E., Haythornthwaite, M., Rupke, L. and Smith, D. (1968). Provision of health care for institutionalized retarded children. *American Journal of Mental Deficiency*, **73**, 283–93.

Degenkolb, J. (1906). Friederichs Ataxie und Mongoloide Idiotie. *Referate Neurologie Zentralblatter*, 693.

Deisher, R. W. (1957). Role of physician in counselling. *Journal of Pediatrics*, **50**, 231–5.

Delp, H. A. and Lorenz, M. (1953). Follow-up of 84 public school special class pupils with IQ's below 50. *American Journal of Mental Deficiency*, **58**, 175–82.

Demidov, A. U. (1972). (The influence of sex on the phenotypic characteristics of Down's syndrome.) *Defektologia*, **4** (1), 33–7.

De Vries-Krutt (1971). *Small ship, great sea*. New York: Collins.

Diamond, E. F. and Moon, M. S. (1961). Neuromuscular development in mongoloid children. *American Journal of Mental Deficiency*, **66**, 218–21.

Dicks-Mireaux, M. J. (1966). Development of intelligence of children with Down's syndrome. Preliminary report. *Journal of Mental Deficiency Research*, **10**, 89–93.

Dicks-Mireaux, M. J. (1972). Mental development of infants with Down's syndrome. *American Journal of Mental Deficiency*, **77**, 26–32.

Dittmann, L. L. (4 May 1957). Home training for retarded children. *Children*.

Dobzhansky, T. (1955). *Evolution, genetics and man*. New York: Wiley.

Dodd, B. (1976). A comparison of the phonological systems of mental age matched, normal, severely subnormal and Down's syndrome children. *British Journal of Disorders of Communication*, **11**, 27–42.

Dodd, B. J. (1972). Comparison of babbling patterns in normal and Down's syndrome infants. *Journal of Mental Deficiency Research*, **16**, 35–40.

Dodd, B. J. (1975). Recognition and reproduction of words by Down's syndrome and non-Down's syndrome retarded children. *American Journal of Mental Deficiency*, **80**, 306–11.

Doll, E. A. (1935). The measurement of social competence. *Proceedings American Association Mental Deficiency*, **40**, 103–26.

Doll, E. A. (1953). *Measurement of social competence: a manual for the Vineland social maturity scale*, Educational Test Bureau. New Jersey, USA: Educational Publishers Inc.

Doman, G. (1964). *How to teach your baby to read*. New York: Random House.

Domey, R. G. (1969). Taxonomies and correlates of physique. *Psychological Bulletin*, **62**, 411–26.

Domino, G. (1965). Personality traits in institutionalized mongoloids. *American Journal of Mental Deficiency*, **69**, 568–70.

Domino, G., Goldschmid, M. and Kaplan, M. (1964). Personality traits of institutionalized mongoloid girls. *American Journal of Mental Deficiency*, **68**, 498–502.

Domino, G. and Newman, D. (1965). Relationship of physical stigmata to intellectual subnormality in mongoloids. *American Journal of Mental Deficiency*, **69**, 541–7.

Donaldson, D. D. (1961). The significance of spotting of the iris in mongoloids: Brushfield's spots. *AMA Archives Ophthalmology*, **65**, 26–31.

Down, J. L. N. (1866). Observations on an ethnic classification of idiots. *Clinical Lectures and Reports, London Hospital*, **3**, 259.

Down, J. L. H. (1867). Observations on ethnic classification of idiots. *Mental Science*, **13**, 121–8.

Down, R. L. (1909). Discussion following Shuttleworth's paper. *British Medical Journal*, **2**, 665.

Drillien, C. M. and Wilkinson, E. M. (1964). Emotional stress and mongoloid births. *Developmental Medicine and Child Neurology*, **6**, 140–3.

Duché, D. J. and Lecuyer, R. (1966). Psychoneurotic states in mongoloids. *Annales Medico Psychologiques*, **2**, 107.

Dunn, L. M. and Hottel, J. V. (1958). The effectiveness of special day classes for trainable children. US Office of Education, Department of Health, Education and Welfare Report.

Dunsdon, M. I., Carter, C. O. and Huntley, R. (1960). Upper end of range of intelligence in Mongolism. *Lancet*, **1**, 565–8.

Durling, D. and Benda, C. E. (1952). Mental growth curves in untreated institutionalized mongoloid patients. *American Journal of Mental Deficiency*, **56**, 578.

Dutton, G. (1959). The physical development of mongols. *Archives Diseases of Children*, **34**, 46.

Dutton, G. (1961). The fasting blood sugar of mongols. *Journal of Mental Deficiency Research*, **5**, 10–16.

Earl, C. J. C. (1934). The primitive catatonic psychoses of idiocy. *British Journal of Medical Psychology*, **14**, 3–11.

Eck, M. (1966). Psychological problems posed by trisomy-21. *Medicine Infantile*, **73**, 479–81.

Edgerton, R. B. (1967). *Cloak of competence*. Berkeley: University of California Press.

Edgerton, R. B. (1975). Community attitudes and Down's syndrome. In *Down's syndrome (mongolism): research prevention and management*, ed. R. Koch and F. F. de la Cruz. New York: Brunner/Mazel.

Editorial (1953). Early home care or institution for the retarded child. *Journal of Pediatrics*, **42**, 396.

Ellingson, R. J., Eisen, J. D. and Ottersberg, G. (1973). Clinical electroencephalographic observations on institutionalized mongoloids confirmed by karyotype. *Electroencephalography and Clinical Neurophysiology*, **34**, 193–6.

Ellingson, R. J. and Lathrop, G. H. (1973). Intelligence and frequency of the alpha rhythm. *American Journal of Mental Deficiency*, **78**, 334–8.

Ellingson, R. J., Menolascino, F. J. and Eisen, J. D. (1970). Clinical–EEG relationships in mongoloids confirmed by karyotype. *American Journal of Mental Deficiency*, **74**, 645–50.

Ellis, A. and Beechley, R. M. (1950). A comparison of matched groups of mongoloid and non-mongoloid feebleminded children. *American Journal of Mental Deficiency*, **54**, 464–8.

Ellis, N. R. and Anders, T. R. (1968). Short-term memory in the mental retardate. *American Journal of Mental Deficiency*, **72**, 931–6.

Engler, M. (1949). *Mongolism*. Bristol: John Wright & Sons.

Ertl, J. P. and Schafer, E. W. (1969). Brain response correlates of psychometric intelligence. *Nature*, **223**, 421–2.

Esley, G. W. (1957). Emotional problems presented by handicapped children and their families. *Pennsylvania Medical Journal*, **60**, 721.

Evans, D. and Hampson, M. (1969). The language of mongols. *British Journal of Disorders of Communication*, **3**, 171–81.

Evans, K. and Carter, C. O. (1954). Care and disposal of mongolian defectives. *Lancet*, **1**, 960–3.

Faber, B. (1960). Family organization and crisis: maintenance of integration in families with a severely mentally retarded child. *Monograph of the Society for Research in Child Development*, **25**, 75.

Fabia, J. and Drolette, M. (1970). Malformations and leukemia in children with Down's syndrome. *Pediatrics*, **45**, 60.

Fallstrom, K. and Aronson, M. (1972). (The effect of early psychological training of mentally retarded children.) *Nordisk Psykaitrisk Tidsskrift*, **26** (8), 467–73.

Fanconi, G. (1939). Die mutationstheorie des mongolismus. *Schweizerische Medizinische Wochenschrift*, **69**, 82.

Farber, B. (1959). Effects of a severely mentally retarded child on family integration. *Social Research Child Development Monographs*, **24** (2), 1–112.

Farber, B. (1968). *Mental retardation: its social concept and social consequences*. New York: Houghton.

Farber, B. and Ryckman, D. B. (1965). Effects of severely mentally retarded children on family relationships. *Mental Retardation Abstracts*, **11**, 1–17.

Farrell, M. J. (1956). The adverse effects of early institutionalization of mentally subnormal children. *American Journal of Diseases of Children*, **91**, 278–81.

Fehr, F. S. (1976). Psychophysiological studies of Down's syndrome children and the effects of environmental enrichment. In *Developmental psychophysiology of mental retardation*, ed. R. Karrer. Springfield, Illinois: C. C. Thomas.

Fennell, C. H. (1904). Mongolian imbecility. *Journal of Mental Science*, **50**, 32.

Fields, D. L. and Gibson, D. (1969). Validities of regression based IQ forecasts from developmental landmarks in mental retardation. *Proceedings of the Canadian Psychological Association*, Toronto, **10** (2), 202.

Fields, D. L. and Gibson, D. (1971). Forecasting mental growth for at-home mongols (Down's syndrome). *Journal of Mental Deficiency Research*, **15**, 163–8.

Finley, S. C., Finley, W. H., Rosecrans, C. J. and Phillips, C. (1965). Exceptional intelligence in a mongoloid child of a family with a 13–15/partial 21 (D/partial G) translocation. *New England Journal of Medicine*, **272**, 1089–92.

Finley, W. H., Finley, S. C., Rosecrans, C. J. and Tucker, C. (1966). Normal/21-trisomy mosaicism. *American Journal of Diseases of Children*, **112**, 444–7.

Fish, C. H. (1957). Causes of death of mongoloids in an institution for the mentally retarded. *Proceedings American Association on Mental Deficiency*, Hartford, Connecticut.

Fisher, L. (1970). Attention deficit in brain damaged children. *American Journal of Mental Deficiency*, **74**, 502–8.

Fishler, K. (1975). Mental development in mosaic Down's syndrome as compared with trisomy-21. In *Down's syndrome (mongolism): Research, prevention and management*, ed. R. Koch and F. F. de la Cruz. New York: Bruner/Mazel.

Fishler, K., Graliker, B. V. and Koch, R. (1965). The predictability of intelligence with Gesell developmental scales in mentally retarded infants and young children. *American Journal of Mental Deficiency*, **69**, 515–25.

Fishler, K., Koch, R. and Filipelli, J. (1962). Adaptation of Gesell developmental scales for evaluation of development in children with Down's syndrome (mongolism). *Proceedings American Psychological Association Annual Meeting*, St Louis.

Fishler, K., Share, J. and Koch, R. (1964). Adaptation of Gesell developmental scales for evaluation of development in children with Down's syndrome. *American Journal of Mental Deficiency*, **68**, 642–6.

Fisichelli, V. R., Haber, A., David, J. and Karelitz, S. (1966). Audible characteristics of the cries of normal infants and those with Down's syndrome. *Perceptual and Motor Skills*, **23**, 744–6.

Fisichelli, V. R. and Karelitz, S. (1963). The cry latencies of normal infants and those with brain damage. *Journal of Pediatrics*, **62**, 724.

Fisichelli, V. R. and Karelitz, S. (1966). Frequency spectra of the cries of normal infants and those with Down's syndrome. *Psychonomic Science*, **6**, 195–6.

Fitzpatrick, F. K. (1959). The use of rhythm in training severely subnormal patients. *American Journal of Mental Deficiency*, **63**, 981–7.

Flavell, J. H. (1963). *The developmental psychology of Jean Piaget*. Princeton, New Jersey: Van Nostrand.

Flesch, R. (1949). *The art of readable writing*. New York: Harper & Bros.

Fletcher-Beach, T. (1882). Types of imbecility. *Medical Times and Gazette*, London.

Ford, C. E., Jones, K. W., Miller, O. J., Mittwoch, V., Penrose, L. S., Ridler, M. and Shapiro, A. (1959). The chromosomes in a patient showing both mongolism and Klinefelter syndrome. *Lancet*, 709.

Forman, T. M. (1967). The mongoloid child – behavioural description. *Special Education in Canada*, **41**, 9–11.

Forssman, H. (1960). Mongolism among inmates of Swedish institutions for mentally deficient: rate and age distribution. *American Journal of Mental Deficiency*, **65**, 32–6.

Forssman, H. and Thysell, T. (1957). A woman with mongolism and her child. *American Journal of Mental Deficiency*, **62**, 500–3.

Fotheringham, J. B., Skelton, M. and Hoddinott, B. A. (1971). *The retarded child and his family*, monograph series/11. Toronto: Ontario Institute for Studies in Education.

Francis, S. H. (1970). Behavior of low-grade institutionalized mongoloids: changes with age. *American Journal of Mental Deficiency*, **75**, 92–101.

Franklin, A. W. (1958). Care of the mongol baby – the first phase. *Lancet*, 256–8.

Fraser, J. and Mitchell, A. (1876–7). Kalmuc idiocy: report of a case with autopsy with notes on 62 cases. *Journal of Mental Science*, **22**, 161.

Freeman, J. C. and Simpson, R. M. (1938). Skin resistancer and muscular tension. *Journal of General Psychology*, **19**, 319–25.

French, E. L. and Scott, J. C. (1960). *Child in the shadows*. Philadelphia: J. B. Lippincott.

Friedlander, B. Z., McCarthy, J. J. and Soforenko, A. Z. (1967). Automated evaluation with severely retarded institutionalized infants. *American Journal of Mental Deficiency*, **71**, 909–19.

Friedman, A. (1955). Mongolism in twins. *American Journal of Diseases of Children*, **90**, 43–50.

Frith, U. and Frith, C. D. (1974). Specific motor disabilities in Down's syndrome. *Journal of Child Psychology and Psychiatry and Allied Disciplines*, **15**, 293–301.

Frostig, M. and Horne, D. (1964). *The Frostig program for the development of visual perception: teacher's guide*. Chicago: Follett.

Fuller, R. (1974). *Severely retarded people can learn to read*. Ziff-Davis.

Fulton, R. T. and Loyd, L. L. (1968). Hearing impairment in a population of children with Down's syndrome. *American Journal of Mental Deficiency*, **73**, 298–302.

Gant, S. (1957). *One of those: the progress of a mongoloid child*. New York: Pageant.

Gardner, W. I. (1971). *Behavior modification in mental retardation*. Chicago: Aldine Atherton.

Gath, A. (1974). Sibling reactions to mental handicap: a comparison of the brothers and sisters of mongol children. *Journal of Child Psychology and Psychiatry and Allied Disciplines*, **15** (3), 187–98.

Gesell, A. and Amatruda, C. S. (1964). *Developmental diagnosis: normal and abnormal child development*, 2nd edn. (See also 1941 and 1949 edns.) New York: Harper & Row.

Giannini, M. J. and Goodman, L. (1963). Counselling families during the crisis reaction to mongolism. *American Journal of Mental Deficiency*, **67**, 740–7.

Gibbs, E. L., Gibbs, F. A. and Hirsch, W. (1964). Rarity of 14- and 6- per second positive spiking among mongoloids. *Neurology*, **14**, 581–7.

Gibson, D. (1960). Intellectual status and the cardinal stigmata of mongolism; a study in the dimensions of mongolism. Unpublished manuscript.

Gibson, D. (1962). The disputed bond between stigma frequency and amentia in mongolism. *American Journal of Mental Deficiency*, **67**, 90–2.

Gibson, D. (1965). Dermatoglyphic characteristics in trisomy and translocation mongolism: a reply. *American Journal of Mental Deficiency*, **70**, 490.

Gibson, D. (1966a). Early developmental staging as a prophecy index in Down's syndrome. *American Journal of Mental Deficiency*, **70**, 825–8.

Gibson, D. (1966b). Amentia level and physical concomitants of Down's syndrome: a curvilinear resolution. *American Journal of Mental Deficiency*, **71**, 433–6.

Gibson, D. (1967). Intelligence in the mongoloid and his parent. *American Journal of Mental Deficiency*, **71**, 1014–16.

Gibson, D. (1973). Karyotype variation and behavior in Down's syndrome: methodological review. *American Journal of Mental Deficiency*, **78**, 128–33.

Gibson, D. (1974). Involuntary sterilization of the mentally retarded: a western Canadian phenomenon. *Canadian Psychiatric Association Journal*, **19**, 59–63.

Gibson, D. (1975). Chromosomal psychology and Down's syndrome (Mongolism). *Canadian Journal of Behavioural Science*, **7**, 167–91.

Gibson, D. and Brown, R. I. (eds.) (1977). *Managing the severely retarded*. Springfield, Illinois: C. C. Thomas.

Gibson, D. and Butler, A. J. (1954). Culture as a possible contributor to feeble-mindedness. *American Journal of Mental Deficiency*, **58**, 490–5.

Gibson, D. and Fields, D. L. (1970). Habilitation forecast in mental retardation; the configural search strategy. *American Journal of Mental Deficiency*, **74**, 558–62.

Gibson, D. and Frank, H. F. (1959). Dual occurrences of mongolism in two sibships. *American Journal of Mental Deficiency*, **63**, 618–20.

Gibson, D. and Frank, H. F. (1961). Dimensions of mongolism. I. Age limits for cardinal mongol stigmata. *American Journal of Mental Deficiency*, **66**, 30–4.

Gibson, D. and Gibbins, R. J. (1958). The relation of mongolian stigmata to intellectual status. *American Journal of Mental Deficiency*, **63**, 345–8.

Gibson, D., Jephcott, A. E. and Wilkins, R. (1959). Academic success among high grade hospitalized mentally retarded children as a function of intelligence and etiological classification. *American Journal of Mental Deficiency*, **63**, 852–9.

Gibson, D. and Pozsonyi, J. (1965). Morphological and behavioural consequences of chromosome subtype in mongolism. *American Journal of Mental Deficiency*, **69**, 801–4.

Gibson, D., Pozsonyi, J. and Zarfas, D. (1964). Dimensions of mongolism: II. The interaction of clinical indices. *American Journal of Mental Deficiency*, **68**, 503–10.

Gilliland, A. R. (1948). The measurement of the mentality of infants. *Child Development*, **19**, 155–8.

Girardeau, F. L. (1959). The formation of discrimination learning sets in mongoloid and normal children. *Journal of Comparative and Physiological Psychology*, **52**, 566–70.

Giraud, P., Bernard, R., Stahl, A., Giraud, F., Hartung, N. and Lebeuf, M. (1963). Mosaique chromosomique chez une mongolienne avec un IQ 85. *Pediatrie*, **18**, 753.

Gliddon, J. B., Busk, J. and Galbraith, G. C. (1975). Visual evoked responses as a function of light intensity in Down's syndrome and non-retarded subjects. *Psychophysiology*, **12**, 416–22.

Gliddon, J. B., Galbraith, G. C. and Busk, J. (1975). Effects of preconditioning visual stimulus duration on visual-evoked responses to a subsequent test flash in Down's syndrome and nonretarded individuals. *American Journal of Mental Deficiency*, **80**, 186–90.

Glovsky, L. (1966). Audiological assessment of a mongoloid population. *Training School Bulletin*, **63**, 27–36.

Glovsky, L. (1972). A communication program for children with Down's syndrome. *Training School Bulletin*, **69**, 5–9.

Goddard, H. H. (1912). *The Kallikak family*. New York: Macmillan.

Goddard, H. H. (1916). *Feeblemindedness; its causes and consequences*. New York: Macmillan.

Godinova, A. M. (1963). (Electroencephalographic changes in Down's syndrome.) *Zhurnal Nevropatologii i Psikhiatrii imeni S. S. Korsakova*, **63**, 1058–64.

Gold, M. C. (1973). Research on the vocational habilitation of the retarded: The present, the future. In *International review of research in mental retardation*, ed. N. R. Ellis, vol. 6. New York: Academic Press.

Gold, M. C. (1975). Vocational training. In *Mental Retardation and Developmental Disabilities*, ed. S. Wortis. New York: Brunner/Mazel.

Goldberg, I. I. (1957). Current status of education and training in the US for trainable mentally retarded children. *Exceptional Children*, **24**, 146–54.

Goldie, L., Curtis, J. A. H., Svendsen, U. and Robertson, N. R. C. (1968). Abnormal sleep rhythms in mongol babies. *Lancet*, **1**, 229–30.

Goldstein, H. (1954 a). A study of mongolism and non-mongoloid mental retardation in children. *Archives of Pediatrics*, **71**, 11–20.

Goldstein, H. (1954 b). Treatment of mongolism and non-mongoloid mental retardation in children. *Archives of Pediatrics*, **71**, 77–98.

Goldstein, H. (1956 a). Congenital acromicria syndrome. *Archives of Pediatrics*, **73**, 115–24.

Goldstein, H. (1956 b). Treatment of congenital acromicria syndrome in children. *Archives of Pediatrics*, **73**, 153–67.

Gordon, A. M. (1944). Some aspects of sensory discrimination in mongolism. *American Journal of Mental Deficiency*, **49**, 55.

Gordon, A. M. (1946). Some aspects of idiocy mongolism. *American Journal of Mental Deficiency*, **50**, 402–10.

Gotkin, L. (1967). *Manual for matrix games*. New York: Appleton-Century-Crofts.

Gottsleben, R. H. (1955). The incidence of stuttering in a group of mongoloids. *Training School Bulletin*, **51**, 209–18.

Goueffic, S., Vallancien, B. and Leroy-Boisivon, A. (1967). *La Voix des mongoliens*. *Journal Français d'Oto-Rhino-Laryngologie et Chirurgie Maxillo-Faciale*, **16**, 139.

Graliker, B. V., Parmelee, A. H. Sr. and Koch, R. (1959). Attitude study of parents of mentally retarded children. II. Initial reaction and concerns of parents to a diagnosis of mental retardation. *Pediatrics*, **24**, 819.

Graliker, B. V., Fishler, K. and Koch, R. (1962). Teenage reactions to a mentally retarded sibling. *American Journal of Mental Deficiency*, **66**, 838–43.

Gramza, A. F. and Witt, P. A. (1969). Choices of colored blocks in the play of pre-school children. *Perceptual and Motor Skills*, **29**, 783–7.

Gramza, A. F., Witt, P. A., Linford, A. G. and Jeanrenaud, C. (1969). Responses of mongoloid children to colored block presentation. *Perceptual and Motor Skills*, **29**, 1008.

Gratz, R. T., Henderson, N. D. and Katz, S. (1972). A comparison of the functional and intellectual performance of phenylketonuric, anoxic and Down's syndrome individuals. *American Journal of Mental Deficiency*, **76**, 710–17.

Green, M. (1966). *Elizabeth*. Stoughton.

Griffiths, A. W. and Behrman, J. (1967). Dark adaptation in mongols. *Journal of Mental Deficiency Research*, **11**, 23–36.

Gunnarson, S. (1945). Electroencephalographic examination of imbeciles. *Acta Paediatrica* (Stockholm), **32**, 426–34.

Gunzburg, H. C. and Sinson, J. (1973). *Progress assessment chart of the social development of 'mongol' children*. Birmingham: SEFA Publications.

Guskin, S. (1963). Social psychologies of mental deficiencies. In *Handbook of mental deficiency*, ed. N. R. Ellis. New York: McGraw-Hill.

Guskin, S. and Spicker, H. (1968). Educational research in mental retardation. In *International review of research in mental retardation*, ed. N. R. Ellis, vol. 3. New York: Academic Press.

Gustafson, J. M. (1973). Mongolism, parental desires and the right to life. *Perspectives in Biology and Medicine*, **16** (4), 529–57.

Gustavson, K. H. (1964). *Down's syndrome: a clinical and cytogenetical investigation*. Uppsala (Sweden): Almquist & Wilksells.

Haggerty, H. E. and Nash, H. B. (1924). IQ of children in relation to father's occupational level. *Journal of Educational Psychology*, **15**, 569.

Hall, B. (1964). Mongolism in new borns. *Acta Pediatrics*, supp. 154.

Hall, B. and Dohlgvist, D. (1969). Galactose-1-phosphate-urid-1 transferase activity in blood in translocation Down's syndrome. *Lancet*, 907–8.

Hallenbeck, P. N. (1960). A survey of recent research in mongolism. *American Journal of Mental Deficiency*, **64**, 827–34.

Hamerton, J. L., Gianelli, F. and Polani, P. E. (1965). Cytogenetics of Down's syndrome (mongolism). I. Data on a consecutive series of patients referred for genetics counselling and diagnosis. *Cytogenetics*, **4**, 171.

Harrell, T. W. and Harrell, M. S. (1945). Army classification test scores for civilian occupations. *Educational and Psychological Measurement*, **5**, 229–39.

Harrison, S. (1958). A review of research in speech and language development of the mentally retarded child. *American Journal of Mental Deficiency*, **62**, 236–40.

Harvey, A., Yept, B. and Sellin, D. (1966). Developmental achievement of trainable mentally retarded children. *Training School Bulletin*, **63**, 100–8.

Haubold, H., Loew, W. and Haefele-Niemann, R. (1960). Possibilities and limitations of a post-maturation treatment of retarded and especially of mongoloid children. *Landarzt*, **36**, 378–83.

Hayashi, T. (1963). Karyotypic analysis of 83 cases of Down's syndrome in Harris County, Texas. *Texas Reports on Biology and Medicine*, **21**, 28.

Hayashi, T., Hsu, T. C. and Chao, D. (1962). A case of mosaicism in mongolism. *Lancet*, **1**, 218–19.

Hayden, A. H. and Dmitriev, V. (1975). The multidisciplinary preschool program for Down's syndrome children at the University of Washington model pre-school center. In *Exceptional infant*, ed. B. Z. Friedlander, G. M. Sterritt and G. E. Kirk, vol. 3, Assessment and intervention. New York: Brunner/Mazel.

Hayden, A. H. and Haring, N. G. (1976). Early intervention for high risk infants and young children: programs for Down's syndrome children. In *Intervention strategies for high risk infants and young children*, ed. T. D. Tjossem. Baltimore: University Park Press.

Heaton-Ward, W. A. (1960). The effects of NIAMID, a mono-amine oxidase inhibitor on the IQ and behaviour of mongols. In *Proceedings of the London Conference on the Scientific Study of Mental Deficiency*, 1960, p. 42. London: The Shenval Press.

Heaton-Ward, W. A. (1961). An interim report on a controlled trial of the effects of NIAMID on the mental age and behavior of mongols. In *Stoke Park studies; mental subnormality*, ed. J. Jancar. Bristol: John Wright & Sons.

Hellmann, P. (1908–9). Anatomische studien uber den mongolismus. *Archiv fur Kinderheilkunde* (Stuttgart), **49**, 329–41.

Hermelin, B. (1964). Effects of variation in the warning signal on reaction time of severe subnormals. *Quarterly Journal Experimental Psychology*, **16**, 241–9.

Hermelin, B. (1969). Some behavioral studies of mongolism. In *Proceedings, American Academy on mental retardation*, San Francisco.

Hermelin, B. and O'Connor, N. (1961). Shape perception and reproduction in normal children and mongol and non-mongol imbeciles. *Journal of Mental Deficiency Research*, **5**, 67–71.

Hermelin, B. and Venables, P. (1964). Reaction time and alpha blocking in normal and subnormal subjects. *Journal of Experimental Psychology*, **67**, 365–72.

Hersher, L. (1962). Letter to the Editor. *Pediatrics*, **30**, 1007–8.

Hershman, A. I. and Gibson, D. (1977). Heart rate alteration and cognitive efficiency. In *Proceedings, Canadian Psychological Association Annual Meeting*, Vancouver.

Hillman, J. C. (1969). Thyroid-stimulating hormone and thyroxine levels in the plasma of patients with Down's syndrome. *Journal of Mental Deficiency Research*, **13**, 191–6.

Hilliard, L. T. and Kirman, B. H. (1957). *Mental deficiency*. London: Tindall & Cox.

Himwich, H. E. and Fazakas, J. E. (1940). Cerebral metabolism in mongolian idiocy and phenylpyruvic oligophrenia. *Archives of Neurology and Psychiatry*, **44**, 1213–18.

Hirai, T. and Izawa, S. (1964). An electroencephalographic study of mongolism. *Psychiatria et Neurologia Japonica*, **66**, 166–77.

Hoak, E. (1973). Behavioural implications of the human XYY genotype. *Science*, **179**, 139–50.

Hobbs, N. (ed.) (1975). *Issues in the classification of children*. (Vols I and II). San Francisco: Jossey-Bass.

Hollien, H. and Hopeland, R. H. (1965). Speaking fundamental frequency (SFF) characteristics of mongoloid girls. *Journal of Speech and Hearing Disorders*, **30**, 344–9.

Holroyd, J. and McArthur, D. (1976). Mental retardation and stress on the parents: a contrast between Down's syndrome and childhood autism. *American Journal of Mental Deficiency*, **80**, 431–6.

Holt, K. S. (1958). The influence of a retarded child upon family limitation. *Journal of Mental Deficiency Research*, **2**, 28–36.

Holt, S. B. (1959). The correlations between ridge counts on different fingers estimated from a population sample. *Annals of Human Genetics*, **23**, 459.

Holt, S. B. (1964). Finger print patterns in mongolism. *Annals of Human Genetics*, **27**, 279.

Horackova, M. and Hrubcova, M. (1959). (The problem of education mongoloid children.) *Československa Pediatrica*, **14**, 1023–30.

Hormuth, R. P. (1953). Home problems and family care of the mongoloid child. *Quarterly Review Pediatrics*, Nov., 275–80.

Houze, M., Wilson, H. D. and Goodfellow, H. D. (1964). Treatment of mental deficiency with Alpha Tocopherol. *American Journal of Mental Deficiency*, **69**, 328–9.

Hultgren, E. O. (1914). Om den mongoloida idiotien. *Nyt Tidsskrift f. Abnormvaesenet*, **16**, 177 and 209.

Hunt, J. V. (1966). A comparison of normal infants and children with Down's syndrome (mongolism) on free play behaviour and galvanic skin response. *Dissertation Abstract*, **26** (7), 4090.

Hunt, N. (1967). *The world of Nigel Hunt: the diary of a mongoloid youth*. New York: Garrett/Helix.

Iida, M. (1973). A clinical statistical, biochemical and developmental psychological research on children with Down's syndrome. *Journal of Mental Health* (in Japanese), **21**, 211–48.

Illingsworth, R. S. (1961). The predictive value of developmental tests in the first year with special reference to the diagnosis of mental subnormality. *Journal of Child Psychology and Psychiatry*, **2**, 210–15.

Illingsworth, R. S. (1962). *An introduction to developmental assessment in the first year*. London: National Spastics Society.

Ingalls, T. H. (1953). Possibilities of prevention of mongolism. *Quarterly Review of Pediatrics*, August, 135–8.

Itard, J-M-G. (1894). *The wild boy of Aveyron* (translated in 1964 from the reprinted Paris edition of 1894). New York: Appleton-Century-Crofts.

Jackson, M. (1974). Visual feedback in word acquisition behaviour in moderately retarded subjects. *Slow Learning Child: The Australian Journal on the Education of Backward Children*, **21** (3), 155–63.

Jackson, R. N. (1968). Employment adjustment of educable mentally handicapped ex-pupils in Scotland. *American Journal of Mental Deficiency*, **72**, 924–30.

Jarvik, L. F., Falek, A. and Pierson, W. (1964). Down's syndrome (mongolism): The heritable aspects. *Psychological Bulletin*, **61**, 388–98.

Jebsen, R. H., Johnson, E. W., Knobloch, H. and Grant, D. K. (1961). Differential diagnosis of infantile hypotonia. *American Journal Diseases of Children*, **101**, 34–43.

Jeffree, D., Wheldall, K. and Mittler, P. (1973). Facilitating two-word utterances in two Down's syndrome boys. *American Journal of Mental Deficiency*, **78**, 117–22.

Jelliffe, S. E. and White, W. A. (1923). *Diseases of the nervous system*. New York: Lea & Febiger.

Jensen, A. R. (1969). How much can we boost IQ and scholastic achievement? In *Environment, heredity and intelligence, Harvard Educational Review*, preprint series, no. 2.

Jensen, R. A. (1950). The clinical management of the mentally retarded child and the parents. *American Journal of Psychiatry*, **106**, 831.

Jervis, G. A. (1942). Recent progress in the study of mental deficiency. Mongolism, a review of the literature of the last decade. *American Journal of Mental Deficiency*, **47**, 467.

Jervis, G. A. (1948). Early senile dementia in mongoloid idiocy. *American Journal of Psychiatry*, **105**, 102–6.

Jervis, G. A. (1953). A note on the etiology of mongolism. *Quarterly Review of Pediatrics*, **8**, 126.

Jervis, G. A. (1970a). Report on 'Premature senility found in brains of mongoloids'. *Pediatric News*, 1970, **4**, 1 and 46.

Jervis, G. A. (1970b). Premature senility in Down's syndrome. *Annals of the New York Academy of Sciences*, **171**, 559–61.

Johnson, C. D. and Barnett, D. C. (1961). Relationship of physical stigmata to intellectual status in mongoloids. *American Journal of Mental Deficiency*, **66**, 435–7.

Johnson, J. T. and Olley, J. G. (1971). Behavioral comparisons of mongoloid and nonmongoloid retarded persons: a review. *American Journal of Mental Deficiency*, **75**, 546–59.

Johnson, R. C. (1970). Prediction of independent functioning and of problem behavior from measures of IQ and SQ. *American Journal of Mental Deficiency*, **74**, 591–3.

Johnson, R. C. and Abelson, R. B. (1969a). Intellectual, behavioral and physical characteristics associated with trisomy, translocation and mosaic types of Down's syndrome. *American Journal of Mental Deficiency*, **73**, 852–5.

Johnson, R. C. and Abelson, R. B. (1969b). The behavioral competence of mongoloid and non-mongoloid retardates. *American Journal of Mental Deficiency*, **73**, 856–7.

Jolly, D. H. (1953). When should the seriously retarded child be institutionalized? *American Journal of Mental Deficiency*, **57**, 632–6.

Jones, B. E., Croley, H. T. and Levy, J. M. (1960). The relation between physical and mental retardation in mongolism. *Research Relating to Mentally Retarded Children*. U.S. Department Health, Education and Welfare, **1**, 22.

Jones, H. B. (1963). An investigation to determine the validity of voice quality as a criterion of mongolism, Master's Thesis, Hunter College.

Joruik, L. F., Falek, A. and Pierson, W. P. (1964). Down's syndrome (mongolism): The hereditable aspects. *Psychological Bulletin*, **61**, 388–98.

Junkala, J. B. (1966). Changes in PMA relationships in noninstitutionalized mongoloids. *American Journal of Mental Deficiency*, **71**, 460–4.

Kaariainen, R. and Dingman, H. F. (1961). The relation of the degree of mongolism to the degree of subnormality. *American Journal of Mental Deficiency*, **66**, 438–43.

Kaback, M. M. (1970). Seen in 'Premature senility found in Brains of mongoloids'. *Pediatric News*, **4**, 1 and 46.

Kanner, L. (1957). *Child psychiatry*. Springfield, Illinois: C. C. Thomas.

Kanner, L. (1964). *A history of the care and study of the mentally retarded*. Springfield, Illinois: C. C. Thomas.

Kaplan, A. R. and Zsako, S. (1966). Down's syndrome associated with family history of malignancy in mothers of affected children. *American Journal of Mental Deficiency*, **70**, 866–72.

Kaplan, B. J. (1955). Mongolism in the Bantu, including a case report. *South African Medical Journal*, **29**, 1041–3.

Karelitz, S. and Fishichelli, V. R. (1962). The cry thresholds of normal infants and those with brain damage. *Journal Pediatrics*, **61**, 679.

Karelitz, S., Karelitz, R. and Rosenfelt, L. (1959). Infants vocalizations and their significance. In *Mental retardation: proceedings of the first internation conference on mental retardation*, ed. P. Bowman and H. Mautner. New York: Grune & Stratton.

Karlin, I. W. and Strazzulla, M. (1952). Speech and language problems of mentally deficient children. *Journal of Speech and Hearing Disorders*, **17**, 286–94.

Karrer, R. (1966). Autonomic nervous system functions and behavior: a review of experimental studies with mental defectives. In *International review of research on mental retardation*, ed. N. R. Ellis, vol. II. New York: Academic Press.

Karrer, R. (ed.) (1975). *Developmental psychophysiology of mental retardation*. Springfield, Illinois: C. C. Thomas.

Karrer, R. and Clausen, J. (1964). A comparison of mental deficient and normal individuals upon four dimensions of autonomic activity. *Journal Mental Deficiency Research*, **8**, 149–63.

Katz, E. (1972). *Mental Health Services for the Mentally Retarded*. Springfield, Illinois: C. C. Thomas.

Kaufman, D., Gibson, D. and Adamowicz, J. K. (1967). Heart rate change under variable auditory and mental task conditions. *Psychonomic Science*, **9** (8), 471–2.

Kaufman, M. E. and Alberto, P. A. (1976). Research on efficacy of special education for the mentally retarded. In *International review of research in mental retardation*, ed. N. R. Ellis. New York: Academic Press.

Keegan, D. L., Pettigrew, A. and Parker, Z. (1974). Amitriptyline in the psychotic states of Down's syndrome: the comparison of two cases. *Diseases of the Nervous System*, **35** (8), 381–3.

Keith, H. (1958). Mongolism. *Postgraduate Medicine*, **23**, 629–35.

Kellner, H. (1906). (A case study.) *Munchener Medizinische Wochenschrift*, 6 March, 497.

Kelman, H. R. (1959). The effects of a group of noninstitutionalized mongoloid children upon their families as perceived by their mothers. *Dissertation Abstracts* (Microfilm. HQ 754. M7 K4).

Kennedy, M. and Sheridan, C. (1973). Tactile-visual equivalence of shape and slant in brain-damaged and mongoloid children. *Perceptual and Motor Skills*, **36** (2), 632.

Kephart, N. C. (1960). *The slow learner in the classroom*. Columbus, Ohio: Charles E. Merrill.

Kirk, S. (1957). Public school provisions for severely retarded children. *Special Report to the Interdepartmental Health Resources Board*, Albany, N.Y., July.

Kirk, S., Karnes, M. B. and Kirk, W. D. (1955). *You and your retarded child*. New York: MacMillan.

Kirk, S. and Kirk, W. D. (1971). *Psycholinguistic learning disabilities*. Urbana, Illinois: University of Illinois Press.

Kirman, B. H. (1951). Epilepsy in mongolism. *Archives Diseases of Childhood*, **26**, 501.

Kirman, B. H. (1953). Mongolism: diagnosis and management at home. *Medical World*, **78**, 258.

Klebba, J. T. (1973). Psychological and bio-clinical studies of Down's syndrome. *Dissertation Abstracts International*, May, **33** (11-B), 5496.

Knights, R. M., Atkinson, B. R. and Hyman, J. A. (1967). Tactual discrimination and motor-skills in mongoloid and non-mongoloid retardates and normal children. *American Journal of Mental Deficiency*, **71**, 894–900.

Knights, R. M., Hyman, J. A. and Wozny, M. A. (1965). Psychomotor abilities of familial, brain-injured and mongoloid retarded children. *American Journal of Mental Deficiency*, **70**, 454–7.

Knobloch, H. and Pasamanick, B. (1963). Predicting intellectual potential in infancy. *American Journal of Diseases of Children*, **106**, 43–51.

Koch, R., Graliker, B. V. and Parmelee, A. H. Sr. (1959). Attitude studies of parents with mentally retarded children. *Pediatrics*, **23**, 582–4.

Koch, R., Share, J. B. and Graliker, B. V. (1965). The effects of Cytomel on children with Down's syndrome – A double-blind longitudinal study. *Pediatrics*, **66**, 776–8.

Koch, R., Share, J., Webb, A. and Graliker, B. V. (1963). The predictability of Gesell developmental scales in mongolism. *Journal of Pediatrics*, **62**, 93–7.

Kohn, G., Taysi, K., Atkins, T. E. and Mellman, W. J. (1970). Mosaic mongolism. I. Clinical correlations. *Journal of Pediatrics*, **76**, 874–9.

Kolstoe, O. P. (1958). Language training of low-grade mongoloid children. *American Journal of Mental Deficiency*, **63**, 17–30.

Komiya, M. (1973). (Comparative studies of Down's syndrome and physiologically mentally retarded children on figure-copying ability.) *Japanese Journal of Special Education*, **11**, 31–8.

Kostrzewski, J. (1963 a). The level and dynamics of mental development in Down's syndrome. Doctoral Dissertation, Lubin, Poland.

Kostrzewski, J. (1963 b). Investigations on the level of mental development in Down's syndrome. *Pediatria Polska*, **38**, 781–9.

Kostrzewski, J. (1965). The dynamics of intellectual and social development in Down's syndrome: Results of experimental investigation. *Roczniki: Filozoficzne*, **13** (4), 5–32.

Kraepelin, E. (1919). *Dementia Praecox*. Edinburgh: E. & S. Livingston.

Kralovich, A. M. (1959). A study of performance differences on the Cattell infant intelligence scale between matched groups of organic and mongoloid subjects. *Journal of Clinical Psychology*, **15**, 198–9.

Kramer, B. (1953). The problems of mongolism. In *Mongolism, a symposium*, p. 77. New York: New York Association for the Help of Retarded Children.

Kramm, E. R. (1963). *Families of mongoloid children*. U.S. Department of Health, Education and Welfare, Welfare Administration, Children's Bureau.

Kraus, B., Clark, A. and Oka, S. (1968). Mental retardation and abnormalities of the dentition. *American Journal of Mental Deficiency*, **72**, 905–17.

Kreezer, G. (1939). Intelligence level and occipital alpha rhythm in the mongolian type of mental deficiency. *American Journal of Psychology*, **52**, 503–32.

Krogman, W. M. (1941). Growth of man. *Tabulae Biologicae*, **20**, 652.

Kucera, J. (1969). Age at walking, age at eruption of decidious teeth and response to Ephedrine in children with Down's syndrome. *Journal of Mental Deficiency Research*, **2**, 143–8.

Kuenzel, M. W. (1929). A survey of mongolian traits. *Training School Bulletin*, **26**, 49–59.

Kugel, R. B. (1970). Combatting retardation in infants with Down's Syndrome. *Children*, **17**, 188–92.

Kugel, R. B. and Mohr, J. (1963). Mental retardation and physical growth. *American Journal of Mental Deficiency*, **68**, 41–8.

Kugel, R. B. and Reque, D. (1961). A comparison of mongoloid children. *Journal of the American Medical Association*, **175**, 959–61.

Kuhlmann, F. (1904). Experimental studies in mental deficiency: three cases of imbecility (mongolian) and six cases of feeblemindedness. *American Journal of Psychology*, **15**, 391–446.

Kysela, G. M. (1973–4). Early childhood education for children with Down's syndrome. *Mental Retardation Bulletin*, **2** (2), 58–63.

Lacey, J. I. (1967). Somatic response patterning and stress: some revisions of activation theory. In *Psychological stress: issues in research*, ed. M. A. Appley and R. Turnbull. New York: Appleton-Century-Crofts.

Lacey, J. I., Kagan, J., Lacey, B. C. and Moss, H. A. (1962). The visceral level: situational determinants and behavioral correlates of autonomic response patterns. In *Expressions of the emotions in man*, ed. P. Knapp. International Universities Press.

Lacey, J. I. and Lacey, B. C. (1958). The relationship of resting autonomic activity to motor impulsivity. *Proceedings of the Association for Research in Nervous and Mental Disease*, **36**, 144–209.

Lang, J. L. (1974). Psychology and psychopathology of the child with Down's syndrome: structural features. *Revue de Neuropsychiatrie Infantile et d'Hygiène Mentale de l'Enfance*, **22**, 19–39.

Lapage, C. P. (1911). *Feeblemindedness in children of school age*, pp. 109–10 (1920 edn. p. 75). Manchester: University Press.

Launay, C. and Bayen, M. (1964). Mental development in mongoloids, *Revue du Practicien*, **14**, 21–31.

Laurie, L. A. (1935). Conduct disorders of intellectually subnormal children. *American Journal of Psychiatry*, **91**, 1025–38.

LaVeck, G. D. and de la Cruz, F. F. (1963). Electroencephalographic and etiological findings in mental retardation. *Pediatrics*, **31**, 478–85.

Lazar, M. (1953). Etiology of mongolism. *Psychiatric Quarterly Supplement*, **27**, 197–206.

Leberman, P. (1968). Primate vocalizations and human linguistic ability. *Journal of Acoustic Society of America*, **44**, 1574–84.

Lenneberg, E. H. (1967). *Biological foundation of languages*. New York: Wiley.

Lenneberg, E. H., Nichols, I. A. and Rosenberger, E. F. (1962). Primitive stages of language development in mongolism. *Proceedings, Association Research in Nervous and Mental Disease*, **42**, 119–37.

Lerman, J. W., Powers, G. R. and Rigrodsky, S. (1965). Stuttering patterns observed in a sample of mentally retarded children. *Training School Bulletin*, May, **62**.

Lesser, A. J. (1958). New program for mentally retarded children. *American Journal of Public Health*, **48**, 9.

Levinson, A. and Bigler, J. A. (1960). *Mental retardation in infants and children*. Chicago: The Year Book Publishers, Inc.

Levinson, A., Friedman, A. and Stamps, F. (1955). Variability of mongolism. *Pediatrics*, **16**, 43.

Lieberman, P. (1968). Primate vocalizations and human linguistic ability. *Journal of Acoustic Society of America*, **44**, 1574–84.

Lilienfeld, A. M. and Benesch, A. (1969). *Epidemiology of mongolism*. Baltimore: Johns Hopkins Press.

Lind, J., Vuorenkoski, V., Rosberg, G., Partanen, T. J. and Wasz-Hockert, O. (1970). Spetographic analysis of vocal response to pain stimuli in infants with Down's syndrome. *Developmental Medicine and Child Neurology*, **12**, 478–86.

Lindstein, J., Alvin, A., Gustavson, K. H. and Fraccaro, M. (1962). Chromosomal mosaicism in a girl with some features of mongolism. *Cytogenetics*, **1**, 20–31.

Little, T. M. and Masotti, R. E. (1974). The palmo-mental reflex in normal and mentally retarded subjects. *Developmental Medicine and Child Neurology*, **16**, 59–63.

Littman, R. W. and Rosen, E. (1950). Molar and molecular. *Psychological Review*, **57**, 58–65.

Liu, M. C. and Corlett, K. (1959). A study of congenital heart defects in mongolism. *Archives Disorders of Childhood*, **34**, 410–19.

Liverant, S. (1960). Intelligence: A concept in need of re-examination. *Journal of Consulting Psychology*, **24**, 101–10.

Lobo, E. de H. and Webb, A. (1970). Parental reactions to their mongol baby. *The Practitioner*, **204**, 412–15.

Loeffler, F. and Smith, G. F. Unpublished observations, 1964. Seen in Penrose, L. S. and Smith G. F., *Down's Anomaly*. Boston: Little, Brown & Co., 1966.

Loesch-Mdzewska, D. (1968). Some aspects of the neurology of Down's syndrome. *Journal of Mental Deficiency Research*, **12**, 237–46.

Lombard, J. P., Gilbert, J. G. and Donofrio, A. F. (1955). The effects of glutamic acid upon the intelligence, social maturity and adjustment of a group of mentally retarded children. *American Journal of Mental Deficiency*, **60**, 122–32.

Lubman, C. G. (1955). Speech program for severely retarded children. *American Journal of Mental Deficiency*, **60**, 297–300.

Luria, A. R. (1963). *The mentally retarded child*. London: Pergamon.

Lurie, L. A. (1935). Conduct disorders of intellectually subnormal children. *American Journal of Psychiatry*, **91**, 1379.

Lyle, J. G. (1959). The effect of an institution environment upon the verbal development of imbecile children. I. Verbal intelligence. *Journal of Mental Deficiency Research*, **3**, 122–8.

Lyle, J. G. (1960a). The effect of an institution environment upon the verbal development of imbecile children. II. Speech and language. *Journal of Mental Deficiency Research*, **4**, 1–13.

Lyle, J. G. (1960b). The effect of an institution environment upon the verbal development of imbecile children. III. The Brookland Residential Family Unit. *Journal of Mental Deficiency Research*, **4**, 14–23.

Lyle, J. G. (1960c). Some factors affecting the speech development of imbecile children in an institution. *Journal of Child Psychology and Psychiatry*, **1**, 121–9.

Lyle, J. G. (1961). Some personality characteristics of trainable children in relation to verbal ability. *American Journal of Mental Deficiency*, **66**, 69–75.

MacDonald, J. D. (1974). An experimental parent-associated treatment program for preschool language-delayed children. *Journal of Speech and Hearing Disorders*, **39** (4), 395–415.

MacGillivray, R. C. (1967). Epilepsy in Down's anomaly. *Journal of Mental Deficiency Research*, **11**, 43–8.

MacGillivray, R. (1968). Congenital cataract and mongolism. *American Journal of Mental Deficiency*, **72**, 631–3.

Malzberg, B. (1950). Some statistical aspects of mongolism. *American Journal of Mental Deficiency*, **54**, 266.

Malzberg, B. (1953). Sex differences in the prevalence of mental deficiency. *American Journal of Mental Deficiency*, **58**, 301–5.

Mansfield, J. T. (1972). The operant conditioning of abstract motor responses to prepositional speech in mongoloids. Doctoral Dissertation, University of California, Los Angeles.

Martin, W. E. and Blum, A. (1961). Interest generalization and learning in mentally normal and subnormal children. *Journal of Comparative and Physiological Psychology*, **54**, 28–32.

Masland, R. L., Sarason, S. B. and Gladwin, T. (1958). *Mental subnormality*. New York: Basic Books.

Mauer, I. and Noe, O. (1964). Triple stem-line chromosomal mosaicism in Down's syndrome. *Lancet*, **1**, 666.

Mautner, H. (1959). *Mental retardation*. New York: Pergamon.

Mayer-Gross, W., Slater, E. and Roth, M. (1960). *Clinical Psychiatry*, 2nd edn. Baltimore: Williams & Wilkins.

McCarthy, J. J. (1964). The importance of linguistic ability in the mentally retarded. *Mental Retardation*, **2**, 90–6.

McCarthy, J. M. (1965). Patterns of psycholinguistic development of mongoloid and non-mongoloid severely retarded children. Doctoral Dissertation. University of Illinois.

McCarver, R. B. and Craig, E. M. (1974). Placement of the retarded in the community: prognosis and outcome. In *International Review of Research in Mental Retardation*, ed. N. R. Ellis. New York: Academic Press.

McCaw, W. R. (1958). A curriculum for the severely mentally retarded. *American Journal of Mental Deficiency*, **62**, 616–21.

McCord, H. (1956). The hypno-ability of the mongoloid-type child. *Journal of Clinical and Experimental Hypnosis*, **4**, 19–20.

McDonald, G. and MacKay, D. N. (1974). The effects of proximal and distal proactive interference on recall by subnormals. *Journal of Mental Deficiency Research*, **18**, 377–91.

McIntire, M. S. and Dutch, S. J. (1964). Mongolism and generalized hypotonia. *American Journal of Mental Deficiency*, **68**, 669–70.

McIntire, M. S., Menolascino, F. J. and Wiley, J. H. (1965). Mongolism – some clinical aspects. *American Journal of Mental Deficiency*, **69**, 794–9.

McLean, J. E., Yoder, D. E. and Schiefelbusch, R. L. (eds.) (1972). *Language Intervention with the Retarded*. Baltimore: University Park Press.

McNeill, Wm D. D. (1955). Developmental patterns of mongoloid children: a study of certain aspects of their growth and development. *Dissertation Abstracts*, **15**, 86–7.

Mein, R. (1961). A study of the oral vocabularies of severely subnormal patients. II. Grammatical analyses of speech samples. *Journal of Mental Deficiency Research*, **5**, 52–9.

Mein, R. and O'Connor, N. (1960). A study of the oral vocabularies of severely subnormal patients. *Journal of Mental Deficiency Research*, **4**, 130.

Meindl, J. L., Barclay, A. G., Lamp, R. E. and Yater, A. C. (1971). Mental growth in non-institutionalized mongoloid children. *Proceedings APA annual meeting*, vol. 6, part 2, 621–2.

Mellon, J. P., Pay, B. Y. and Green, D. M. (1963). Mongolism and thyroid autoantibodies. *Journal of Mental Deficiency Research*, **7**, 31–7.

Melyn, M. A. and White, D. T. (1973). Mental and developmental milestones of non-institutionalized Down's syndrome children. *Pediatrics*, **52**, 542.

Menolascino, F. J. (1965). Psychiatric aspects of mongolism. *American Journal of Mental Deficiency*, **69**, 653–60.

Menolascino, F. J. (1967). Psychiatric findings in a sample of institutionalized mongoloids. *Journal of Mental Subnormality*, **13**, 67–74.

Menolascino, F. J. (1974). Developmental attributes in Down's syndrome. *Mental Retardation*, **12** (3), 13–17.

Michejda, M. and Menolascino, F. J. (1975). Skull base abnormalities in Down's syndrome. *Mental Retardation*, **13** (1), 24–6.

Michel, J. F. and Carney, R. J. (1964). Pitch characteristics of mongoloid boys. *Journal of Speech and Hearing Disorders*, **29**, 121–5.

Mickelthwart, G. W. (1910). Mongolian Imbeciles. *British Medical Journal*, **2**, 659.

Midgeon, B. N., Kaufman, B. N. and Young, W. J. (1962). A chromosome abnormality with fragment in a para-mongol child. *Bulletin of Johns Hopkins Hospital*, **111**, 221.

Miezejeski, C. M. (1974). Effect of white noise on reaction time of mentally retarded subjects. *American Journal of Mental Deficiency*, **79**, 39–43.

Miranda, S. B. and Frantz, R. L. (1973). Visual preferences of Down's syndrome and normal infants. *Child Development*, **44**, 555–61.

Mittler, P., Gillies, S. and Jukes, E. (1966). Prognosis in psychotic children: Report of a follow up study. *Journal of Mental Deficiency Research*, **10**, 73–83.

Mongolism – A symposium (1953). Reprinted from the *Quarterly Review of Pediatrics*, 1953. New York: Association for the Help of Retarded Children.

Mongoloid Conference Proceedings (1969). Wisconsin: Wisconsin Association for Retarded Children, Madison.

Montague, J. C., Brown, W. S. and Hollien, H. (1974). Vocal fundamental frequency characteristics of institutionalized Down's syndrome children. *American Journal of Mental Deficiency*, **78**, 414–18.

Montague, J. C. and Hollien, H. (1973). Perceived voice quality disorders in Down's syndrome children. *Journal of Communication Disorders*, **6**, 76–87.

Montague, J. C. and Hollien, H. (1974). Perceived voice quality disorders in Down's syndrome Children. *Training School Bulletin*, **71**, 80–9.

Moore, B. C. (1973). Some characteristics of institutionalized mongols. *Journal Mental Deficiency Research*, **17**, 46–51.

Moore, B. C., Thuline, H. C. and Capes, La V. (1968). Mongoloid and non-mongoloid retardates: a behavioral comparison. *American Journal of Mental Deficiency*, **73**, 433–6.

Mordock, J. B. (1968). Paired associate learning in mental retardation: a review. *American Journal of Mental Deficiency*, **72**, 857–65.

Morris, J. V. (1957). Mongolism in a twin. *British Medical Journal*, 1038.

Morris, J. V. and MacGillivray, R. C. (1953). Mongolism in one of twins. *Journal of Mental Science*, **99**, 557–9.

Mosier, D. H. (1962). Mechanisms of regulation of growth. In *40th Ross Conference on Pediatric Research, Monograph of the Ross Laboratories*, Columbus, Ohio.

Moskowitz, H. and Lohmann, W. (1970). Auditory threshold for evoking an orienting reflex in mongoloid patients. *Perceptual and Motor Skills*, **31**, 879–82.

Muir, J. (1903). An analysis of twenty-six cases of mongolism. *Archives of Pediatrics*, **20**, 161.

Myers, C. R. (1938). An application of the control group method to the problem of the etiology of mongolism. *Proceedings American Association on Mental Deficiency*, **62**, 42.

Myers, D. G., Sinco, M. E. and Stalma, E. S. (1973). *The right-to-education child: a curriculum for the severely and profoundly mentally retarded*. Springfield, Illinois: C. C. Thomas.

Murphy, A., Pueschel, S. M. and Schneider, J. (1973). Group work with parents of children with Down's syndrome. *Social Casework*, **54** (2), 114–19.

Murphy, M. M. (1956). Comparison of developmental patterns of three diagnostic groups of middle grade and low grade mental defectives. *American Journal of Mental Deficiency*, **61**, 164–9.

Nadler, H. L., Inouyo, T. and Hasia, E. Y. (1967). Enzymes in cultivated human fibroblasts derived from patients with autosomal trisomy syndrome. *American Journal of Human Genetics*, **19**, 94–9.

Nakamura, H. (1961). Nature of institutionalized adult mongoloid intelligence. *American Journal of Mental Deficiency*, **66**, 456–8.

Nakamura, H. (1965). An inquiry into systematic differences in the abilities of institutionalized adult mongoloids. *American Journal of Mental Deficiency*, **69**, 661–5.

Nassau, A. and Kornik, R. (1957). Educable mongoloids. *Dapim Refuiyim*, **16**, 1943–5.

Neeman, R. L. (1971). Preceptual-motor attributes of mental retardates: a factor analytic study. *Perceptual and Motor Skills*, **33**, 927–34.

Neville, J. (1959). Paranoid schizophrenia in a mongoloid defective: some theoretical considerations derived from an unusual case. *Journal of Mental Science*, **105**, 444–7.

Newman, A. F. (1960). An investigation of the relation between physical stigmata frequency and intellectual status in mongolism. MA Thesis, University of Toronto, Canada.

Niehans, P. (1964). *Cellular therapy from the viewpoint of doctor and patient*. Switzerland: Ott Verlang Thun.

Norris, D. (1971). Crying and laughing in imbeciles. *Developmental Medicine and Child Neurology*, **13**, 756–61.

O'Connor, N. and Berkson, G. (1963). Eye movement in normals and defectives. *American Journal of Mental Deficiency*, **68**, 85–90.

O'Connor, N. and Hermelin, B. (1961). Visual and stereognostic shape recognition in normal children and mongol and non-mongol imbeciles. *Journal of Mental Deficiency Research*, **5**, 63–6.

O'Connor, N. and Hermelin, B. (1963). *Speech and thought in severe subnormality*. New York: Pergamon/MacMillan.

O'Connor, N. and Tizard, J. (1956). *The social problem of mental deficiency*. London: Pergamon.

O'Hara, P. T. (1972). Electron microscopic study of the brain in Down's syndrome. *Brain*, **95** (4), 681–4.

O'Hare, M. G. (1966). Concept formation in children with Down's syndrome (mongolism). *Dissertation Abstracts*, **27** (6B), 2143.

Ong, B. H., Rosner, E., Mahanand, D., Houck, J. C. and Paine, R. S. (1967). Clinical, psychological and radiological comparisons of trisomic and translocation Down's syndrome. *Developmental Medicine and Child Neurology*, **9** (3), 307–12.

Orel, H. (1926). Zur Atiologie des mongolismus. *Zeitschrift fur Kinderpsychiatrie*, **42**, 440.

Oster, J. (1953). *Mongolism*. Copenhagen: Danish Science Press.

Oster, J. (1960). Etiologic aspects of mongolism. In *Proceedings 1st International Medical Conference*. New York: Grune & Stratton.

Owens, D., Dawson, J. C. and Losin, S. (1971). Alzheimer's disease in Down's syndrome. *American Journal of Mental Deficiency*, **75**, 606–12.

Paluck, R. J. and Esser, A. H. (1971). Controlled experimental modification of aggressive behavior in territories of severely retarded boys. *American Journal of Mental Deficiency*, **76**, 23–9.

Parmelee, A. H. (1956). Management of mongolism in childhood. *International Record of Medicine*, **69**, 358–61.

Parsloe, P. and Rose, J. (1972). The mother of a mongol girl talks about her experience. *British Journal Social Work*, **2** (i), 5–19.

Pavlov, I. P. (1932). 'The Function of the Brain'. A film presented at the International Congress of Physiology, Rome.

Pearce, F. H., Rankine, R. and Ormond, A. W. (1910). Notes on 28 cases of mongoloid imbeciles. *British Medical Journal*, **2**, 185–90.

Penrose, L. S. (1933). *Mental defect*. London: Sidgwick & Jackson.

Penrose, L. S. (1949 a). *The biology of mental defect*. London: Sidgwick & Jackson.

Penrose, L. S. (1949 b). The incidence of mongolism in the general population. *Journal of Mental Science*, **95**, 685.

Penrose, L. S. (1951). Maternal age in familial mongolism. *Journal of Mental Science*, **97**, 738.

Penrose, L. S. (1963 a). Finger-prints, palms and chromosomes. *Nature*, **197**, 933–8.

Penrose, L. S. (1963 b). *The biology of mental defect*, revised edn. New York: Grune & Stratton, Inc.

Penrose, L. S. (1963 c). Measurements of likeness in relatives of trisomics. *Annals of Human Genetics*, **27**, 183–7.

Penrose, L. S. (1967). The effects of chance in maternal age distribution upon the incidence of mongolism. *Journal of Mental Deficiency Research*, **11**, 54–7.

Penrose, L. S. and Delhanty, J. D. A. (1961). Familial Langdon Down anomaly with chromosome fusion. *Annals of Human Genetics*, **25**, 243–52.

Penrose, L. S., Ellis, J. N. and Delhanty, J. D. A. (1960). Chromosomal translocations in mongolism and in normal relatives. *Lancet*, **2**, 409–10.

Penrose, L. S. and Loesch, D. (1967). A study of dermal ridge width in the second (palmar) interdigital area with special reference to aneuploid states. *Journal of Mental Deficiency Research*, **2**, 36–42.

Penrose, L. S. and Smith, G. F. (1966). *Down's anomaly*. London: J. & A. Churchill, 1966.

Perry, T. L., Tischler, B. and Chapple, J. A. (1966). The incidence of mental illness in the relatives of individuals suffering from phenylketonuria or mongolism. *Journal of Psychiatric Research*, **4**, 51–7.

Pertego, J. (1950). La Escala metrica de Oseretzky para el examen de la motorica. *Revista de Psicologia General y Aplicada*, **15**, 539–53.

Peterson, D. L. (1960). The age generality of personality factors derived from ratings. *Educational and Psychological Measurement*, **20**, 461–74.

Pitt, D. (1960). Mongolism: the modern management. *Medical Journal of Australia*, **2**, 971.

Pitt, D. (undated). *Your Down's syndrome child*. Arlington, Texas: National Association for Retarded Citizens.

Polani, P. E. (1963). Cytogenetics of Down's syndrome. In *Symposium on Genetics*, ed. L. I. Gardner, **10**, pp. 423–48. Pediatric Clinics of North America.

Porter, L. S. (1972). The impact of physical-physiological activity on infants' growth and development. *Nursing Research*, May–June, 210–19.

Pototzky, C. and Grigg, A. E. (1942). A reversion of the prognosis in mongolism. *American Journal of Orthopsychiatry*, **12**, 503.

Pozsonyi, J. and Gibson, D. (1965). Biochemical consequences of supernumerary chromosome subtype in mongolism. *American Journal of Mental Deficiency*, **70**, 213–17.

Pozsonyi, J., Gibson, D. and Zarfas, D. E. (1964). Skeletal maturation in mongolism (Down's syndrome). *Journal of Pediatrics*, **64**, 75–8.

Preus, A. (1972). Stuttering in Down's syndrome. *Scandinavian Journal of Educational Research*, **16**, 89–104.

Prysiazniuk, A. W. and Wicijowski, P. J. (1964). Learning sets in mongoloid and non-mongoloid children: a replication. *American Journal of Mental Deficiency*, **69**, 76–8.

Pueschel, S. M. Early intervention in children with Down's syndrome. Unpublished report, Child Development Center, Rhode Island Hospital, Providence.

Pueschel, S. M., Rothman, K. J. and Ogilby, J. D. (1967). Birth weights of children with Down's syndrome. *American Journal of Mental Deficiency*, **80**, 442–5.

Quaytman, W. (1953). The psychological capacities of mongoloid children in a community clinic. *Quarterly Review of Pediatrics*, **8**, 255–67.

Rarick, G. L. and Seefeldt, V. (1974). Observations from longitudinal data on growth of stature and sitting height of children with Down's syndrome. *Journal of Mental deficiency Research*, **18**, 63–78.

Razran, G. (1961). The observable unconscious and the inferable conscious in current Soviet psychophysiology: introceptive conditioning. Semantic conditioning and the orienting reflex. *Psychological Review*, **68**, 81–147.

Reed, S. C. (1963). Genetic counselling for Down's syndrome (mongolism). *Eugenics Quarterly*, **10**, 139–42.

Rehn, A. T. and Thomas, E. Jr. (1957). Family history of a mongoloid girl who bore a mongoloid child. *American Journal of Mental Deficiency*, **62**, 496–9.

Reinecke, M. E. (1973). An analysis of the intellectual characteristics of Down's syndrome and non-Down's syndrome retarded children. *Dissertation Abstracts International* (Ap.), **33** (10-A), 5588.

Reisman, L. E. (1966). Relationship between cytogenic constitution, physical stigmata and intelligence in Down's syndrome. In *Proceedings American Association Mental Deficiency Meeting*, Chicago.

Reisman, L. E., Shipe, D. and Williams, R. D. B. (1966). Mosaicism in Down's syndrome: studies in a child with an unusual chromosome constitution. *American Journal of Mental Deficiency*, **70**, 855–9.

Rempel, E. D. (1974). Psycholinguistic abilities of Down's syndrome children. In *Proceedings of the annual meeting of the American Association on Mental Deficiency*, Toronto.

Rhodes, L., Gooch, B., Siegelman, E. Y., Behrns, C. and Metzger, R. (1969). *A language stimulation and reading program for severely retarded mongoloid children.* California Mental Health Research Monograph No. 11, State of California, Department of Mental Hygiene.

Ribble, M. (1943). *The rights of infants.* New York: Columbia University Press.

Richards, B. W. (1965). The diagnosis of Down's syndrome. *Developmental Medicine and Child Neurology*, **7**, 285–8.

Richards, B. W. (1969). Mosaic mongolism. *Journal of Mental Deficiency Research*, **13**, 66–83.

Richards, B. W. and Stewart, A. (1962). Mosaicism in a mongol. *Lancet*, **2**, 275.

Richards, B. W., Stewart, A., Sylvester, P. E. and Jasiewicz, V. (1965). Cytogenetic survey of 225 patients diagnosed clinically as mongols. *Journal of Mental Deficiency Research*, **9**, 245–59.

Richards, B. W. and Sylvester, P. E. (1969). Mortality trends in mental deficiency institutions. *Journal of Mental Deficiency Research*, **13**, 276–92.

Richmond, J. B. (1954). Self-understanding for the parents of handicapped children. *Public Health Reports*, **69**, 702.

Ridler, M. A. C. (1965). A mosaic mongol with normal leucocyte chromosomes. *British Journal of Psychiatry*, **111**, 183.

Rigrodsky, S., Prunty, F. and Glovsky, G. (1961). A study of the incidence, types and associated etiologies of hearing loss in an institutionalized mentally retarded population. *Training School Bulletin*, **58**, 30–44.

Rimland, B., Stone, I. and Dameron, L. (1969). The relationship between the IQ's of institutionalized mongoloids and their normal siblings. (Unpublished manuscript.)

Rinaldi, F. (1972). The spontaneous cerebral electro-activity faster than 14 c/s: EEG findings among mongoloids. *Acta Neurologica*, **27** (3), 291–304.

Roberts, N. and Roberts, B. (1968). *David.* Richmond, Virginia: John Knox Press.

Robinson, H. B. and Robinson, N. M. (1965). *The mentally retarded child.* New York: McGraw-Hill.

Robinson, N. M. and Robinson, H. B. (1976). *The mentally retarded child*, 2nd edn. New York: McGraw-Hill.

Roche, A. F. (1964). Skeletal maturation rates in mongolism. *American Journal Roentgenology*, **91**, 979.

Roche, A. F. (1965). The stature of mongols. *Journal of Mental Deficiency Research*, **9**, 131–45.

Roche, A. F. and Barkla, D. H. (1964). The eruption of deciduous teeth in mongols. *Journal of Mental Deficiency Research*, **8**, 54–64.

Roche, A. F., Roche, P. J. and Lewis, A. B. (1972). The cranial base in trisomy-21. *Journal of Mental Deficiency Research*, **16**, 7–20.

Roith, A. I. (1961). Psychotic depression in a mongol. *Journal of Mental Subnormality*, **7**, 45–7.

Rollin, H. R. (1946). Personality in mongolism with special reference to the incidence of catatonic psychosis. *American Journal of Mental Deficiency*, **51**, 219–37.

Rosecrans, C. J. (1968). The relationship of normal/21-trisomy mosaicism and intellectual development. *American Journal of Mental Deficiency*, **72**, 562–5.

Rosecrans, C. J. (1971). A longitudinal study of exceptional cognitive development in a partial translocation Down's syndrome child. *American Journal of Mental Deficiency*, **76**, 291–4.

Rosenfeld, M. J., Peterson, R. M. and Koch, R. (1969). Down's syndrome: intelligence and chromosome findings. *Proceedings American Academy on Mental Retardation*, San Francisco, 1969.

Rosenzweig, L. E. (1953). School training of the mongoloid child. *Quarterly Review of Pediatrics*, Nov., 281–9.

Rosner, F., Ong, B., Paine, R. and Mahanand, D. (1965). Biochemical differentiation of trisomic Down's syndrome (mongolism) from that due to translocation. *New England Journal of Medicine*, December, 1356–61.

Rosner, F., Paine, R. and Mahanand, D. (1965). Blood serotonin activity in trisomic and translocation Down's syndrome. *Lancet*, 1191–3.

Ross, L. E., Headrick, M. W. and Mackay, P. B. (1967). Classical eyelid conditioning of young mongoloid children. *American Journal of Mental Deficiency*, **72**, 21–9.

Ross, R. T. (1962). The mental growth of mongoloid defectives. *American Journal of Mental Deficiency*, **66**, 736–8.

Ross, R. T. (1971). A preliminary study of self-help skills and age in hospitalized Down's syndrome patients. *American Journal of Mental Deficiency*, **76**, 373–7.

Rotter, J. B. (1960). Some implications of a social learning theory for the production of goal directed behavior from testing procedures. *Psychological Review*, **67**, 301–16.

Rowe, R. D. and Uchida, I. A. (1961). Cardiac malformation in mongolism. *American Journal of Medicine*, **31**, 726–35.

Rudel, R. G. (1959). The absolute response in tests of generalization in normal and retarded children. *American Journal of Psychology*, **72**, 401–8.

Rudel, R. G. (1960). The transposition of intermediate size by brain-damaged and mongoloid children. *Journal of Comparative and Physiological Psychology*, **53**, 89–94.

Rundle, A. T., Donoghue, E., Abbas, K. A. and Krstic, A. (1972). A catch-up phenomenon in skeletal development of children with Down's syndrome. *Journal of Mental Deficiency Research*, **16**, 41–7.

Runge, G. H. (1959). Glucose tolerance in mongolism. *American Journal of Mental Deficiency*, **63**, 822–8.

Sackett, G. P. (1967). Response to differentiated visual complexity in four groups of retarded children. *Journal of Comparative and Physiological Psychology*, **64**, 200–5.

Saenger, G. (1960). Factors influencing the institutionalization of mentally retarded individuals in New York City. A report to the New York State Interdepartmental Health Resources Board, January, 1960.

Sapon, S. M. (1968). *Verbal behavior management series*. Kit I, tacting. Rochester, New York: Mono Press.

Sapon, S. M. and Reeback, R. (1966). Shaping vocal behavior in a nine-year-old mongoloid boy. University of Rochester, Verbal Behavior Laboratory Report No. 1.

Sawyer, G. M. and Shafter, A. J. (1957). Reproduction in a mongoloid: a follow up. *American Journal of Mental Deficiency*, **61**, 793–5.

Scano, V. (1958). A study of body build in children with mongolism during the first two years of life. *Annali Italiani di Pediatria*, **11**, 3, 242–5.

Schachter, M. (1960). Psychological problems with parents of mongol children. In *Proceedings, London Conference on the Scientific Study of Mental Deficiency*, p. 65.

Schachter, M. (1974). (Long-term psychological and social prognosis in cases of mongolian retardation followed for more than 10 years.) *Annales Médico-Psychologiques*, **1** (2), 195–224.

Scheffelin, M. (1968 a). Comparison of four stimulus response modalities in paired-associate learning with Down's syndrome children. *Dissertation Abstract* (University of Illinois), **28** (12-B), 5220–1.

Scheffelin, M. (1968 b). A comparison of four stimulus-response channels in paired-associate learning. *American Journal of Mental Deficiency*, **73**, 303–7.

Schiefelbusch, R. L., Copeland, R. H. and Smith, J. O. (1967). *Language and Mental Retardation*, New York: Holt, Rinehart & Winston.

Schlanger, B. and Christensen, N. J. (1964). Effects of training upon audiometry with the mentally retarded. *American Journal of Mental Deficiency*, **68**, 469–75.

Schlanger, B. and Gottsleben, R. H. (1957). Analysis of speech defects amongst the institutionalized mentally retarded. *Journal of Speech and Hearing Disorders*, **22**, 98–103.

Schipper, M. T. (1959). The child with mongolism in the home. *Pediatrics*, **24**, 132–44.

Schlottmann, R. S. and Anderson, V. H. (1973). Social and play behavior of children with Down's syndrome in sexually homogeneous and heterogeneous dyads. *Psychological Reports*, **33**, 595–600.

Schlottmann, R. S. and Anderson, V. H. (1975). Social and play behaviors of institutionalized mongoloid and non-mongoloid retarded children. *Journal of Psychology*, **91**, 201–6.

Schmid, W., Lee Chi Hao and Smith, P. M. (1961). At the borderline of mongolism: Report of a case with chromosome analysis. *American Journal of Mental Deficiency*, **66**, 449–55.

Schonell, F. J. and Watts, B. H. (1956). A first survey of the effects of a subnormal child on the family unit. *American Journal of Mental Deficiency*, **61**, 210–19.

Schroth, M. L. (1975). The use of IQ as a measure of problem solving ability with mongoloid and non-mongoloid retarded children. *Journal of Psychology*, **91**, 49–56.

Schuller, A. (1907). Infailismus. *Wiener Medizinische Wochenschrift*, **57**, 629.

Seagoe, M. V. (1964). *Yesterday was Tuesday, all day and all night: the story of a unique education.* Toronto: Little, Brown & Co.

Seagoe, M. V. (1965). Verbal development in a mongoloid. *Exceptional Children*, **31**, 269–73.

Seitz, S. (1975). Language intervention – changing the language environment of the retarded child. In *Down's syndrome (mongolism): research, prevention and management*, ed. R. Koch and F. F. de la Cruz. New York: Brunner/Mazel.

Semmel, L. I. and Dolley, D. G. (1971). Comprehension and imitation of sentences by Down's syndrome children as a function of transformational complexity. *American Journal of Mental Deficiency*, **75**, 739–45.

Semmel, M. J. (1960). Comparison of teacher ratings of brain-injured and mongoloid severely retarded (trainable) children attending community day-school classes. *American Journal of Mental Deficiency*, **64**, 963–71.

Seppalainen, A. M. and Kivalo, E. (1967). EEG findings and epilepsy in Down's syndrome. *Journal of Mental Deficiency Research*, **11**, 116–25.

Seguin, E. (1846). *Traitement moral, hygiène et education des idiots et des autres enfants arrières.* Paris: J. B. Baillière.

Sersen, E. A., Astrup, C., Foistad, I. and Wortis, J. (1970). Motor conditional reflexes and word associations in retarded children. *American Journal Mental Deficiency*, **74**, 495–501.

Share, J. B. (1975). Developmental progress in Down's syndrome. In *Down's syndrome (mongolism): research, prevention and management*, ed. R. Koch and F. F. de la Cruz. New York: Brunner/Mazel.

Share, J. B. (1976). Review of drug treatment for Down's syndrome persons. *American Journal of Mental Deficiency*, **80**, 388–93.

Share, J. B. and French, R. W. (1974). Early motor development in Down's syndrome children. *Mental Retardation*, **12** (6), 23.

Share, J., Gralicker, B. and Koch, R. (1964). The predictability of Gesell development scales in Down's syndrome. In US Department of Health, Education and Welfare, Children's Bureau: *The case of the retarded child. Therapy and Prognosis*, pp. 39–43. Washington, DC: Superintendent of Documents, US Government Printing Office.

Share, J., Koch, R., Webb, A. and Graliker, B. (1964). The longitudinal development of infants and young children with Down's syndrome (mongolism). *American Journal of Mental Deficiency*, **68**, 685–92.

Share, J. B. and Veale, A. M. (1962). *Developmental landmarks for children with Down's syndrome (mongolism).* University of Otago Press.

Share, J., Webb, A. and Koch, R. (1961). A preliminary investigation of the early developmental status of mongoloid infants. *American Journal of Mental Deficiency*, **66**, 238–41.

Shaw, M. W. (1962). Familial mongolism. *Cytogenetics*, **1**, 141–79.

Sheehan, J., Martyn, M. M. and Kilburn, K. L. (1968). Speech disorders in retardation. *American Journal of Mental Deficiency*, **73**, 251–6.

Shepard, T. H., McGreal, R. and Hammer, S. (1957). Mongolism: grading and intercorrelation of certain measurements. *Journal of Diseases of Children*, **94**, 563.

Sherlock, E. B. and Donkin, H. B. (1911). *The feeble minded. A guide to study and practice.* London: Macmillan & Co.

Shipe, D., Reisman, L. E., Chung, Chin-Young, Darnell, A. and Kelly, S. (1968). The relationship between cytogenetic constitution, physical stigmata, and intelligence in Down's syndrome. *American Journal of Mental Deficiency*, **72**, 789–97.

Shipe, D. and Shotwell, A. M. (1965). The effect of out-of-home care on mongoloid children: A continuation study. *American Journal of Mental Deficiency*, **69**, 649–52.

Shotwell, A. M. (1964). Suitability of the Kuhlmann–Binet infant scale for assessing intelligence of mental retardates. *American Journal of Mental Deficiency*, **68**, 757–65.

Shotwell, A. M. and Shipe, D. (1964). The effect of out-of-home care on the intellectual and social development of mongoloid children. *American Journal of Mental Deficiency*, **68**, 693–9.

Shukowsky, W. and Aisenberg, R. (1912). Uber Mongolismus bei Kindern. *Jahrbucher für Kinderheilkunde*, Berlin, **76**, 317–27.

Shuttleworth, G. E. (1895). *Mentally deficient children*. London: H. Lewis.

Shuttleworth, G. E. (1900). *Mentally deficient children*, 2nd edn. London: P. Blakiston's Sons.

Shuttleworth, G. E. (1906). Comments on R. Langdon Down's Paper. *Journal of Mental Science*, **52**, 189.

Shuttleworth, G. E. (1909). Mongolian imbecility. *British Medical Journal*, **2**, 661–5.

Shuttleworth, G. E. and Potts, W. (1916). *Mentally deficient children*, 4th edn. Philadelphia: Blakiston's Son.

Sidman, M. and Cresson, O. (1973). Reading and cross modal transfer of stimulus equivalences in severe retardation. *American Journal of Mental Deficiency*, **77**, 515–23.

Sidman, M., Cresson, O. and Willson-Morris, M. (1974). Acquisition of matching to sample via mediated transfer. *Journal of the Experimental Analysis of Behavior*, **22**, 261–73.

Siegel, F., Balow, B., Fisch, O. and Anderson, V. E. (1968). School behavior profile ratings of phenylketonuric children. *American Journal of Mental Deficiency*, **72**, 937–43.

Silverstein, A. B. (1964). An empirical test of the mongoloid stereotype. *American Journal of Mental Deficiency*, **68**, 493–7.

Silverstein, A. B. (1966). Mental growth in mongolism. *Child Development*, **37**, 725–9.

Silverstein, A. B. and Owens, E. P. (1968). Factor structure of the social deprivation scale for mongoloid retardates. *American Journal of Mental Deficiency*, **73**, 315–17.

Simon, A., Ludwig, C., Gofman, J. W. and Cook, G. H. (1954). Metabolic studies in mongolism: serum protein-bound iodine, cholestral, and lipo-protein. *American Journal of Psychiatry*, **111**, 138–45.

Sinson, J. and Wetherick, N. E. (1972). Cue salience and learning in severely subnormal children. *Journal of Mental Deficiency Research*, **16**, 112.

Sinson, J. and Wetherlick, N. E. (1973). Short-term retention of colour and shape information in mongol and other severely subnormal children. *Journal of Mental Deficiency Research*, **17**, 177–82.

Sinson, J. C. and Wetherlick, N. E. (1975). The nature of the colour retention deficit in Down's syndrome. *Journal of Mental Deficiency Research*, **19**, 97–100.

Sinson, J. C. and Wetherlick, N. E. (1976). Evidence for increased mental capacity with age in Down's syndrome. *Journal of Mental Deficiency Research*, **20**, 31–4.

Slater, E. and Cowie, V. (1971). *The genetics of mental disorders*. London: Oxford University Press.

Slaughter, S. S. (1960). *The mentally retarded child and his parent*. New York: Harper & Row.

Smith, A. and McKeown, T. (1955). Prenatal growth of mongoloid defectives. *Archives Disease of Childhood*, **30**, 257–9.

Smith, D. W. and Wilson, A. A. (1973). *The child with Down's syndrome (mongolism): causes, characteristics and acceptance*. Toronto: W. B. Saunders.

Smith, G. F., Bat-Miriam, M. and Ridler, M. A. C. (1966). Dermal patterns on the fingers and toes in mongolism. *Journal of Mental Deficiency Research*, **10**, 105–15.

Smith, N. V. (1975). Universal tendencies in the child's acquisition of phonology. In *Language, cognitive deficits and retardation*, ed. N. O. O'Connor. London: Butterworths.

Smith, T. T. (1896). A peculiarity in the shape of the hand in idiots of the mongol type. *Pediatrics*, **2**, 315–20.

Solitaire, G. B. and Lamarche, J. B. (1966). Alzheimer's disease and senile dementia as seen in mongoloids: neuropathological observations. *American Journal of Mental Deficiency*, **70**, 840–8.

Solitaire, G. B. and Lamarche, J. B. (1967). Brain weight in the adult mongol. *Journal of Mental Deficiency Research*, **11**, 79–84.

Soltan, H. C. (1965). Letter to the editor. *American Journal of Mental Deficiency*, **70**, 489–90.

Spicer, T. (1903). Mongolian imbecility with a review of 23 cases; discussion. *Archives of Pediatrics*, **15**, 393–6.

Spitzer, R., Rabinowitch, J. and Wybar, K. (1961). A study of the abnormalities of the skull, teeth and lenses in mongolism. *Canadian Medical Association Journal*, **84**, 567–72.

Spreen, O. (1965 a). Language functions in mental retardation: a review. I. Language development, types of retardation and intellectual level. *American Journal of Mental Deficiency*, **69**, 482–94.

Spreen, O. (1965 b). Language functions in mental retardation: a review. II. Language in higher level performance. *American Journal of Mental Deficiency*, **70**, 351–2.

Spuehler, N. (1929). Contribution à l'étude de l'avenir des enfants atteints de mongolisme. Doctoral Dissertation, Zurich.

Stafferi, J. R. (1968). Body image stereotypes of mentally retarded. *American Journal of Mental Deficiency*, **72**, 841–3.

Stedman, D. J. and Eichorn, D. H. (1964). A comparison of the growth and development of institutionalized and home-reared mongoloids during infancy and early childhood. *American Journal of Mental Deficiency*, **69**, 391–401.

Stein, Z., Susser, M. and Guterman, A. V. (1973). Screening programme for prevention of Down's syndrome. *Lancet*, 305–10.

Stein, Z. A. (1975). Family planning as a method of prevention. In *Down's syndrome (mongolism): research, prevention and management*, ed. R. Koch and F. F. de la Cruz. New York: Brunner/Mazel.

Stephens, W. B. and Peck, J. R. (1968). *Success of young adult male retardates*. CEC Research monograph. Washington DC: Council for Exceptional Children.

Stephens, B., Baumgartner, B. B., Smeets, P. M. and Wolfinger, W. (1970). Promoting motor development in young retarded children. *Education and Training of the Mentally Retarded*, **5**, 119–24.

Sternlicht, M. (1966). *A talk to parents of the mongoloid child*. Published by Staten Island Aid for Retarded Children.

Sternlicht, M. and Wanderer, Z. W. (1962). Nature of institutionalized adult mongoloid intelligence. *American Journal of Mental Deficiency*, **67**, 301–2.

Stickland, C. A. (1954). Two mongols of unusually high mental status. *British Journal of Medical Psychology*, **27**, 80–3.

Stoller, A. and Collman, N. R. D. (1965 a). Virus aetiology for Down's syndrome (mongolism). *Nature*, **208**, 903.

Stoller, A. and Collmann, R. D. (1965 b). Incidence of infective hepatitis followed by Down's syndrome nine months later. *Lancet*, **2**, 1221.

Stoller, A. and Collmann, R. D. (1965 c). Patterns of occurrence of births in Victoria, Australia, producing Down's syndrome (mongolism) and congenital anomalies of the central nervous system: a 21-year prospective and retrospective survey. *Medical Journal of Australia*, **1**, 1.

Stoller, A. and Collmann, R. D. (1966). Area relationship between incidences of infectious hepatitis and of the births of children with Down's syndrome nine months later. *Journal of Mental Deficiency Research*, **10**, 84–7.

Stone, N. D. (1967). Family factors in willingness to place the mongoloid child. *American Journal of Mental Deficiency*, **72**, 16–20.

Stone, N. D. and Parnicky, J. J. (1965). Factors associated with parental decision to institutionalize mongoloid children. *Training School Bulletin*, **61**, 163–72.

Stone, N. D. and Parnicky, J. J. (1966). Factors in child placement: parental response to congenital defect. *Social Work*, **11**, 35–43.

Stott, D. H. (1960). Analysis of parental case histories of mongol children. In *Abstracts, Conference on the Scientific Study of Mental Deficiency*, London, 1960, p. 26.

Straumanis, J. J., Shagass, C. and Overton, D. A. (1973 a). Somatosensory evoked responses in Down's syndrome. *Archives of General Psychiatry*, **29** (4), 544–9.

Straumanis, J. J., Shagass, C. and Overton, D. A. (1973 b). Auditory evoked responses in young adults with Down's syndrome and idiopathic mental retardation. *Biological Psychiatry*, **6**, 75–9.

Strauss, A. A. and Kephart, N. C. (1955). *Psychopathology and education of the brain-injured child*. New York: Grune & Stratton.

Strazzulla, M. (1953). Speech problems of the mongoloid child. *Quarterly Review of Pediatrics*, **8**, 268–72.

Strazzulla, M. (1956). Nursery school training for retarded children. *American Journal of Mental Deficiency*, **61**, 141–51.

Strunk, D. F. (1964). An analysis of the psycholinguistic abilities of a select group of mongoloids. Doctoral dissertation. University of Virginia.

Struwe, F. (1929). Histopathologische Untersuchungen ueber Entstehung und Wesen der senilen plaques. *Zeitschrift ges Neurologie und Psychiatrie*, **122**, 291 (seen in Oster, 1953).

Sutherland, G. A. (1953). A 1907 report seen in Cant *et al.*, 1953.

Sutherland, J. S., Graham, D. M., Gibson, D. and Butler, A. J. (1954). A sociometric study of institutionalized mental defectives. *American Journal of Mental Deficiency*, **59**, 266–71.

Swanson, F. R. (1975). Preparation for employment. In *Down's syndrome (mongolism): research, prevention and management*, ed. R. Koch and F. F. de la Cruz. New York: Brunner/Mazel.

Szurek, S. A. and Philips, I. (1966). Mental retardation and psychotherapy. In *Prevention and treatment of mental retardation*, ed. I. Philips. New York: Basic Books.

Talbot, F. B. (1937). The present status of mongolism. In *Proceedings, 4th Institute Exceptional Children*, vol. 20 (Oct.). Child Research Clinic.

Talbot, M. E. (1964). *Edouard Seguin: a study of an educational approach to the treatment of mentally defective children*. New York: Columbia University.

Talkington, L. W. and Hall, S. M. (1970). Matrix language program with mongoloids. *American Journal of Mental Deficiency*, **75**, 88–91.

Talkington, L. W., Altman, R. and Grinnell, T. K. (1971). Effects of positive and negative feedback on the motor performance of mongoloids. *Perceptual and Motor Skills*, **33**, 1075–8.

Tang, F. C. and Chagnon, M. (1967). Body build and intelligence in Down's syndrome. *American Journal of Mental Deficiency*, **72**, 381–3.

Tarjan, G., Dingman, H., Eyman, R. and Brown, S. (1960). Effectiveness of hospital release programs. *American Journal of Mental Deficiency*, **64**, 609–17.

Tawney, J. W. (1974). Acceleration of vocal behavior in developmentally retarded children. *Education and Training of the Mentally Retarded*, **9**, 22–7.

Taylor, A. I. (1968). Cell selection *in vivo* in normal G trisomic mosaics. *Nature*, **219**, 1028.

Tennies, L. G. (1943). Some comments on the mongoloids. *American Journal of Mental Deficiency*, **48**, 46–8.

Thelander, H. E. and Pryor, H. B. (1966). Abnormal patterns of growth and development in mongolism. *Clinical Pediatrics*, **5**, 493–501.

Thomas, E. W. (1969). *Brain-injured children*. Springfield, Illinois: C. C. Thomas.

Thompson, M. M. (1963). Psychological characteristics relevant to the education of the pre-school mongoloid child. *Mental Retardation*, **1**, 148–51.

Thompson, W. H. (1938). A mongolian with superior attainment in the language arts. *Psychological Bulletin*, **35**, 633.

Thorum, A. R. (1974). A comparative study of certain audio-linguistic skills of children with two selected types of deficits. *Dissertation Abstracts International*, Jan., **34** (7-B), 3555.

Timbury, G. C., McGuire, R. J. and MacGillivray, R. C. (1963). The effect of anti-thyroid treatment on the functioning of a thyrotoxic mongol. *American Journal of Mental Deficiency*, **67**, 822–6.

Timme, W. (1921). The mongolian idiot. *Archives of Neurology and Psychiatry*, **5**, 568.

Tips, R. I., Smith, G. S., Perkins, A. L., Bergman, E. and Myer, D. L. (1963). Genetic counselling problems associated with trisomy-21 Down's disorder. *American Journal of Mental Deficiency*, **68**, 334–9.

Tizard, J. (1960). Residential care of mentally handicapped children. *British Medical Journal*, **1**, 1041–6.

Tizard, J. (1966). Some problems of management of young mentally handicapped children. In *The Application of research to the education and training of the severely subnormal child*, ed. H. C. Gunzburg, monograph supplement to the *Journal of Mental Subnormality*, April 1966, 11–13.

Tizard, J. and Grad, J. C. (1961). *The mentally handicapped and their families*. London: Oxford University Press.

Tredgold, A. F. (1914). *Mental Deficiency*, 2nd edn, New York: William Wood.

Tredgold, A. F. (1937). *Mental Deficiency*, 6th edn, reprinted 1944. Baltimore: Williams & Wilkins.

Tredgold, A. F. (1947). *A textbook of mental deficiency*. London: Bailliere, Tindall & Cox.

Tredgold, R. F. and Soddy, K. (1956). *Tredgold's textbook of mental deficiency*, 9th edn. London: Bailliere, Tindall & Cox.

Tsuang Ming-Tso and Lin Tsung-Yi (1964). A clinical and family study of Chinese mongol children. *Journal of Mental Deficiency Research*, **8**, 84–91.

Turkel, H. (1963). Medical treatment of mongolism. *Proceedings 2nd International Congress Mental Retardation*, Vienna, 1963, **1**, 409.

Uchida, J. A. (1970). Epidemiology of mongolism: the Manitoba study. *Annals of the New York Academy of Sciences*, **171**, 361–9.

Valencia, J. I., de Lozzio, C. B. and de Coriat, L. F. (1963). Heterosomic mosaicism in a mongoloid child. *Lancet*, **2**, 488.

Valett, R. E. (1966). *Valett developmental survey*. Palo Alto: Consulting Psychologists Press.

Van der Hoeven, J. (1968). *Slant-eyed angel*. Gerrards Cross: Colin Smythe.

Van der Scheer, W. M. (1926). On the etiology of mongolism. *Nederlandsch Maadschrift voor Geneeskunde*, Leiden, **13**, 407–44.

Van Riper, C. (1954). *Speech correlation, principles and methods*, 3rd edn. Englewood Cliffs, New Jersey: Prentice-Hall.

Veall, R. M. (1974). The prevalence of epilepsy among mongols related to age. *Journal of Mental Deficiency Research*, **18**, 99–106.

Verghese, A. and Murti, R. D. (1961). Mongolism: a review of some aspects. *Transactions All India Institute Mental Health*, **2**, 20–36.

Verlinskaya, D. K. and Shtil'bans, I. I. (1966). Features of dematoglyphics in chromosomal pathology. *Zhurnal Nevropatologii i Psikhiatrii*, **66**, 1608–13.

Vernon, McCay (1972). Language development's relationship to cognition, affectivity and intelligence. *Canadian Psychologist*, **13**, 360–74.

Verresen, H., van den Berghe, H. and Creemers, J. (1964). Mosaic trisomy in phenotypically normal mother of mongol. *Lancet*, **1**, 526.

Villiger, U. and Mathis, A. (1972). The language of mongoloids. (In German.) *Heilpadogogik*, **41**, 131–8.

Voelker, C. H. (1936–7). Amelioration of dyslogia mongolia. *Journal of Abnormal Social Psychology*, **31**, 266–77.

Vogel, W. (1961). The relationship of age and intelligence to autonomic functioning. *Journal Comparative and Physiological Psychology*, **54**, 133–8.

Vogel, W. and Broverman, D. M. (1964). Relationship between EEG and test intelligence: a critical review. *Psychological Bulletin*, **62**, 132–44.

Vogel, W., Broverman, D. M., Draguns, J. G. and Klaiber, E. L. (1965). The role of glutamic acid in cognitive behaviors. *Psychological Bulletin*, **65**, 367–82.

Wagner, H. R. (1962). Mongolism in orientals. *American Journal Diseases of Children*, **103**, 706–14.

Wagner, T. (1960). The mongoloid child of school age. *Heilpadagogische Werkblatter*, **29**, 59–64.

Walker, G. H. (1950). Social and emotional problems of the mentally retarded child. *American Journal of Mental Deficiency*, **55**, 132.

Walker, N. F. (1956). A suggested association of mongolism and schizophrenia. *Acta Genetica et Statistica Medica*, **6**, 132–42.

Walker, N. F. (1957). The use of dermal configurations in the diagnosis of mongolism. *Journal of Pediatrics*, **50**, 19.

Walker, N. F., Carr, D. H., Sergovich, F. R., Barr, M. L. and Soltan, H. C. (1963). Trisomy-21 and 13–15/21 mongol defectives. *Journal of Mental Deficiency Research*, **7**, 150–63.

Wallace, R. M. and Fehr, F. S. (1970). Heart rate, skin resistance and reaction time of mongoloid and normal children under baseline and distraction conditions. *Psychophysiology*, **6**, 722–31.

Wallin, J. E. W. (1909). Medical and psychological inspection of school children. *Western Journal of Education*, **2**, 434–6.

Wallin, J. E. W. (1944). Mongolism among school children. *American Journal of Orthopsychiatry*, **14**, 104.

Wallin, J. E. W. (1949). *Children with mental and physical handicaps.* New York: Prentice Hall.

Walter, R. D., Yeager, C. L. and Rubin, H. K. (1955). Mongolism and convulsive seizures. *A.M.A. Archives of Neurology and Psychiatry*, **74**, 557–63.

Walthi, U., Salvisber, H. and Auf der Maur, P. (1973). Schweizesische zeitschrift für psychologie und ihre anwendungen. *Separatakzug aus*, **32**, 132–58.

Warburg, M. (1968). Norrie's disease. *Journal of Mental Deficiency Research*, **12**, 247–51.

Ward, E. G. (1941). Mongolism. *Proceedings of the Texas Neurological Society*, 1941.

Warner, E. N. (1935). A survey of mongolism with a review of 100 cases. *Canadian Medical Association Journal*, **33**, 495–500.

Warner, R. (1949). Mongolism in one of twins and in another sibling. *American Journal Diseases of Children*, **78**, 573–88.

Watson, E. H. (1958). Counselling parents of mentally retarded children. Report of a round table discussion. *Pediatrics*, **22**, 401.

Weber, F. P. A 1917 report seen in Cant *et al.*, 1953. ·

Webster, T. E. (1963). Problems of emotional development in young retarded children. *American Journal of Psychiatry*, **120**, 34–41.

Weinberg, B. and Zlatin, M. (1970). Speaking fundamental frequency characteristics of five- and six-year-old children with mongolism. *Journal of Speech and Hearing Research*, **13**, 418–25.

Weinstein, E. D. and Warkany, J. (1963). Maternal mosaicism and Down's syndrome (mongolism). *Journal of Pediatrics*, **63**, 599.

Weise, P., Koch, R., Shaw, K. F. and Rosenfeld, M. J. (1974). The use of 5-HTP in the treatment of Down's syndrome. *Pediatrics*, **54**, 165–8.

Wesner, C. E. (1972). Induced arousal and word recognition learning by mongoloids and normals. *Perceptual and Motor Skills*, **35** (2), 586.

West, R. and Ansberry, M. (1968). *The rehabilitation of speech.* 4th edn. New York: Harper & Row.

West, R., Ansberry, M. and Carr, A. (1957). *The rehabilitation of speech*. 3rd edn. New York: Harper & Bros.

West, R., Kenny, L. and Carr, A. (1947). *The rehabilitation of speech*. New York: Harper.

White, D. (1969). IQ changes in mongoloid children during post-maturation treatment. *American Journal of Mental Deficiency*, **73**, 809–13.

White, D. and Kaplitz, S. E. (1964). Treatment of Down's syndrome with a vitamin-mineral-hormonal preparation. In *Proceedings of the International Congress for the Scientific Study of Mental Retardation*. Copenhagen, pp. 224–30.

Wieser, W. (1931). *Münchener Medizinische Wochenschrift*.

Wilcock, J. C. and Venables, P. H. (1968). Dimensional dominance in discrimination learning: a study of severely subnormal and normal subjects. *British Journal of Psychology*, **59**, 285.

Wile, I. S. and Orgel, S. T. (1928). A study of physical and mental characteristics of mongols. *International Clinics*, Sept. **3**, 38th Series, 1945–147.

Wilks, J. and Wilks, E. (1974). *Bernard: bringing up our mongol son*. London: Routledge & Kegan Paul.

Windle, C. (1962). Prognosis of mental subnormals. *American Journal of Mental Deficiency*, 1962, 66 (Monograph Supplement No. 5).

Wing, L. (1975). A study of language impairment in severely retarded children. In *Language, cognitive deficits and retardation*, ed. N. O. O'Connor. London: Butterworth.

Winschel, L. (1962). A review of the etiology of mongolism. *Exceptional children*, **28**, 279–86.

Wirtz, M. A. (1954). Day classes for severely retarded children. *American Journal of Mental Deficiency*, **58**, 357–70.

Witmer, L. (1896). Practical work in psychology. *Pediatrics*, **1**, 462–71.

Wolf, E. G., Wenar, C. and Ruttenberg, B. A. (1972). A comparison of personality variables in autistic and mentally retarded children. *Journal of Autism and Childhood Schizophrenia*, **2**, 92–108.

Wolf, S. and Lourie, R. S. (1953). Impact of the mentally defective child on the family unit. *Clinical Proceedings of the Children's Hospital*, Washington, **9**, 25.

Wolfensberger, W. (1971). Vocational preparation and occupation. In *Mental retardation: appraisal, education and rehabilitation*, ed. A. A. Baumeister. Chicago: Aldine.

Wolfensberger, W. and Halliday, R. A. (1970). Socio-ecological variables associated with institutionalization of retardates. *Journal of Mental Deficiency Research*, **14**, 1–15.

Wolfensberger, W. and Menolascino, F. (1968). Basic considerations in evaluating ability of drugs to stimulate cognitive development in retardates. *American Journal of Mental Deficiency*, **73**, 414–23.

Wolfensberger, W. and Zauha, H. (1973). *Citizen advocacy and protective services for the impaired and handicapped*. Toronto: N.I.M.R.

Wolinsky, G. F. (1965). Piaget's theory of perception: insights for educational practices with children who have perceptual difficulties. *Training School Bulletin*, **62**, 12–26.

Wolk, S. M. (1958). A survey of the literature on curriculum practices for the mentally retarded. *American Journal of Mental Deficiency*, **62**, 826–39.

Wood, J. (1909). Mongolian imbecility. *Australian Medical Congress*, 1909, Melbourne.

Woodward, M. and Stein, D. J. (1963). Developmental patterns of severely subnormal children. *British Journal of Educational Psychology*, **33** (I).

Wunsch, Wm. L. (1957). Some characteristics of mongoloids evaluated in a clinic for children with retarded mental development. *American Journal of Mental Deficiency*, **62**, 122–30.

Yannet, H. (1953). Pediatric management of the mongolian child. *Quarterly Review of Pediatrics*, Aug., 131–4.

Yates, M. L. and Lederer, R. (1961). Small, short-term group meetings with parents of children with mongolism. *American Journal of Mental Deficiency*, **65**, 467–72.

Zapella, M. and Cowie, V. (1962). A note on time of diagnosis in mongolism. *Journal of Mental Deficiency Research*, **6**, 82–6.

Zausmer, E. (1975). Principles and methods of early intervention. In *Down's syndrome (mongolism): research, prevention and management*, ed. R. Koch and F. F. de la Cruz. New York: Brunner/Mazel.

Zausmer, E., Pueschel, S. M. and Shea, A. (1972). A sensori-motor stimulation program for the young child with Down's syndrome. *MCH Exchange*, **2** (1).

Zeaman, D. and House, B. J. (1962). Mongoloid MA is proportional to log CA. *Child Development*, **33**, 481–8.

Zekulin, X. Y., Gibson, D., Mosley, J. L. and Brown, R. I. (1974). Auditory-motor chanelling in Down's syndrome subjects. *American Journal of Mental Deficiency*, **78**, 571–7.

Zellweger, H. and Abbo, G. (1963). Chromosomal mosaicism and mongolism. *Lancet*, **1**, 827.

Zigler, E. (1966). Research on personality structure in the retardate. In *International review of research on mental retardation*, ed. N. R. Ellis, vol. 1. New York: Academic Press.

Zigler, E., Butterfield, E. C. and Goff, G. (1966). A measure of pre-institutional social deprivation for institutionalized retardates. *American Journal of Mental Deficiency*, **70**, 873–85.

Zimmerman, F. T., Burgemeister, B. B. and Putman, T. J. (1949a). Effects of glutamic acid on intelligence of patients with mongolism. *Archives of Neurology and Psychiatry*, **61**, 275–87.

Zimmerman, F. T., Burgemeister, B. B. and Putman, T. J. (1949b). The effect of glutamic acid upon the mental and physical growth of mongols. *American Journal of Psychiatry*, **105**, 661–8.

Zipperlen, H. R. (1975). Normalization. In *Mental retardation and developmental disabilities*, ed. J. Wortis. Vol. VII. New York: Brunner/Mazel.

Zisk, P. K. and Bialer, I. (1967). Speech and language problems in mongolism: a review of the literature. *Journal of Speech and Hearing Disorders*, **32** (3), 228–41.

Index

DATE DUE